SECTION 21:
Radiology of the Colon

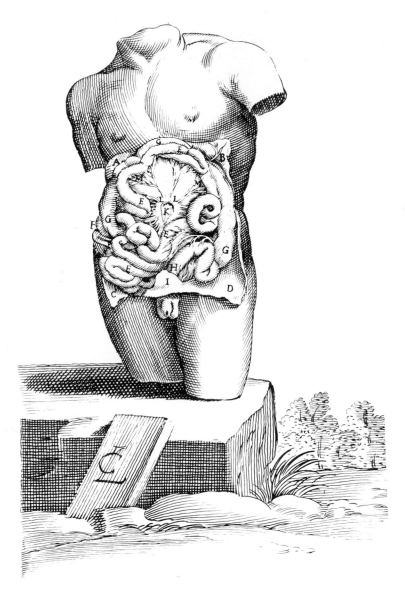

Plate from: *Tabulae Anatomicae* by Pietro Berettini, Rome, 1741.
Courtesy of The Francis A. Countway Library of Medicine, Boston, Mass.

Radiology of the Colon

edited by

JACK R. DREYFUSS, M.D.

Associate Clinical Professor of Radiology, Harvard Medical School; Radiologist,
Massachusetts General Hospital, Boston, Massachusetts

MURRAY L. JANOWER, M.D.

Physician-in-Chief, Department of Radiology, St. Vincent Hospital; Professor of Radiology,
University of Massachusetts Medical School, Worcester, Massachusetts; Lecturer on
Radiology, Harvard Medical School; Clinical Associate in Radiology, Massachusetts
General Hospital, Boston, Massachusetts

SECTION 21
GOLDEN'S DIAGNOSTIC RADIOLOGY
Laurence L. Robbins, M.D., Series Editor

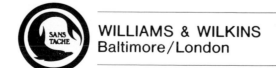

WILLIAMS & WILKINS
Baltimore/London

Successor volume to:
Dreyfuss & Janower: Radiologic Examination of the Colon
Copyright ©, 1969, The Williams & Wilkins Company
Library of Congress Catalog Card Number 72-97176

Copyright ©, 1980
The Williams & Wilkins Company
428 E. Preston Street
Baltimore, Md. 21202, U.S.A.

Made in the United States of America

Library of Congress Cataloging in Publication Data

Main entry under title:

Radiology of the colon.

 (Golden's diagnostic radiology; section 21)
 Includes bibliographical references and index.
 1. Colon (Anatomy—Diseases—Diagnosis. 2. Colon (Anatomy—Radiography. I.
Dreyfuss, Jack R. II. Janower, Murray L. III. Series. [DNLM: 1. Colon—Radiogra-
phy. WN1200 G6182 sect. 21]
RC78.G6 sect. 21 [RC804.R6] 616.07'572'08s
ISBN 0-683-02652-6   [616.3'4] 79-12260

Composed and printed at the
Waverly Press, Inc.
Mt. Royal and Guilford Aves.
Baltimore, Md. 21202, U.S.A.

Volumes of
Golden's Diagnostic Radiology Series

DEDICATION

This book is dedicated
with great affection
to

LAURENCE L. ROBBINS, M.D.

Professor of Radiology at the
Massachusetts General Hospital, Emeritus,
Harvard Medical School;
Senior Radiologist,
Massachusetts General Hospital,
Boston, Massachusetts
Radiologist-in-Chief
Massachusetts General Hospital
from 1946 to 1971

He has been the teacher, colleague,
and friend of each contributor
to this volume.

Foreword

Today, medical textbooks must be very broad in scope and can no longer be readily written by a single author, since expertise in all subjects can rarely be mastered by one mind. *Radiology of the Colon* is therefore appropriately a multi-authored book.

It was a fortunate decision of Dr. Dreyfuss and Dr. Janower to choose their collaborators from among past and present colleagues in their own institution, The Massachusetts General Hospital. Having worked together for many years, the authors have an integrated approach to their subject matter. Obvious care in editing has also avoided the fragmentation of information and style which so frequently characterizes multi-authored books.

One expects an up-to-date text to highlight current knowledge of disease entities and to present controversies where they exist, offering lucid interpretation of available data and clear guidelines based on the best available scientific publications and on the authors' own extensive personal experience. These expectations are met by the text before us.

The chapter on polyps of the colon is a superb example of clear and useful writing. The analysis of controversial statistical data is convincing and the summaries are helpful.

It is apparent that the authors are also teachers. The various chapters are organized along a similar pattern and the presentation is concise but not superficial. The emphasis throughout is on essentials. Thus, the reader emerges with a clear understanding of the material and with sound practical information.

This book will be of prime interest to radiologists in clinical practice or teaching and to those in residency training. It should also have great appeal to internists, surgeons, and pathologists who deal with diseases of the colon in their daily practice as well as to medical students. In view of the rapid progress in all branches of radiology and the use of newer technology, the updating of information on radiology of the colon offered in a single volume is a much needed and invaluable contribution.

ALICE ETTINGER, M.D.

Preface

Publication of *Radiologic Examination of the Colon* by The Williams & Wilkins Company in 1969 marked the first monograph on that subject in a quarter of a century. While this volume is the lineal descendant of our earlier work, it is *not* a second edition. Rather, it is a new book with a new title and 10 additional authors.

In the decade just past, there have been significant advances in technique, particularly in the refinement of air-contrast studies, as well as further elaboration of our understanding of polyps, colitis, diverticular disease, and vascular disorders of the colon which necessitate an up-to-date coverage of these subjects.

The following chapters have been completely rewritten: History; Anatomy and Physiology; Techniques; Congenital Diseases; Diverticular Disease; Colitis; Unusual Inflammatory Lesions; Polyps and Tumors; the Appendix; Obstruction, Trauma and Surgery; and Other Colonic Disorders. In addition, new chapters have been added on: Acquired Diseases of the Pediatric Colon; Ischemic Colitis; Angiography; The Polyposis Disorders; as well as three chapters on the Pathology of Diverticular Disease, Ulcerative and Crohn's Colitis, and Polypoid and Nonpolypoid Tumors of the Colon.

Whereas the 1969 volume was intended to be sparing of both words and illustrations, in fact a monograph, this volume is designed to be broader in scope and more fully illustrated, yet still retain the directness and narrative style of its predecessor. It has also been our goal to achieve a practical, updated approach to diseases of the colon, emphasizing clinical-pathologic correlation. Once again we have deliberately avoided interrupting the text with internal references. Instead, pertinent sources together with classic articles are listed in the bibliography at the end of each chapter.

We are indebted to our 10 co-authors for the expertise they contributed to their individual chapters. We are particularly proud that *Radiology of the Colon* could be written entirely by Massachusetts General Hospital radiologists, although some now practice far from Boston and the Department that nurtured them.

JACK R. DREYFUSS, M.D.
MURRAY L. JANOWER, M.D.

1979

Acknowledgments

This book could not have been produced by the labor of editors and authors alone. We are most grateful to our Massachusetts General Hospital colleagues who have read parts or all of the manuscript, or contributed material for our use: Drs. Laurence L. Robbins, Stanley M. Wyman, Beryl Benacerraf and Rodney J. Butch, Radiologists; Dr. Richard W. Erbe, Geneticist; Dr. Leslie W. Ottinger, Surgeon; Dr. Robert H. Schapiro, Gastroenterologist; and Dr. James J. Galdabini, Pathologist.

We also wish to recognize the contributions of our colleagues at St. Vincent Hospital: Drs. Peter Chen, J. Smith, Milton A. Weiner, and Harvey Wolfman.

We acknowledge with appreciation the help of our faithful and talented secretaries, Selma Surman, Lorraine Bolduc, and Cecile Fanti, as well as the dedicated photographic assistance of Stanley Bennett, Chief Photographer at the Massachusetts General Hospital, and of Phillip Ruderman and Jane Griesbach at St. Vincent Hospital.

Mrs. Ruby Richardson at The Williams & Wilkins Company has given us invaluable support and assistance.

Finally, we thank Dr. Alice Ettinger for a lifetime of teaching, encouragement and inspiration.

J.R.D.
M.L.J.

Contributors

Christos A. Athanasoulis, M.D.
Associate Professor of Radiology, Harvard Medical School; Head, Section of Vascular Radiology, Massachusetts General Hospital, Boston, Massachusetts

Karl T. Benedict, Jr., M.D.
Instructor in Radiology, University of Massachusetts Medical School; Radiologist, St. Vincent Hospital, Worcester, Massachusetts
Clinical Associate in Radiology, Massachusetts General Hospital, Boston, Massachusetts

Spencer Borden, IV, M.D.
Clinical Associate Professor of Radiology and Pediatrics, University of Pennsylvania Medical School; Radiologist-in-Chief, Children's Hospital of Philadelphia, Philadelphia, Pennsylvania

Jack R. Dreyfuss, M.D.
Associate Clinical Professor of Radiology, Harvard Medical School; Radiologist, Massachusetts General Hospital, Boston, Massachusetts

Joseph T. Ferrucci, Jr., M.D.
Associate Professor of Radiology, Harvard Medical School; Radiologist, Massachusetts General Hospital, Boston, Massachusetts

Murray L. Janower, M.D.
Physician-in-Chief, Department of Radiology, St. Vincent Hospital; Professor of Radiology, University of Massachusetts Medical School, Worcester, Massachusetts

Lecturer on Radiology, Harvard Medical School; Clinical Associate in Radiology, Massachusetts General Hospital, Boston, Massachusetts

Charles S. Langston, M.D.
Clinical Instructor in Radiology, Harvard Medical School, Boston, Massachusetts
Radiologist, Mount Auburn Hospital, Cambridge, Massachusetts

John A. Long, Jr., M.D.
Attending Radiologist, National Institutes of Health, Bethesda, Maryland

James J. McCort, M.D.
Clinical Professor of Radiology, Stanford University School of Medicine, Stanford, California; Chairman, Department of Radiology, Santa Clara Valley Medical Center, San Jose, California

R. Ted Steinbock, M.D.
Resident in Radiology, Massachusetts General Hospital, Boston, Massachusetts

Austin L. Vickery, Jr., M.D.
Professor of Pathology at the Massachusetts General Hospital, Harvard Medical School; Pathologist, Massachusetts General Hospital, Boston, Massachusetts

Jack Wittenberg, M.D.
Associate Professor of Radiology, Harvard Medical School; Radiologist, Massachusetts General Hospital, Boston, Massachusetts

Contents

Chapter 14. PATHOLOGY OF POLYPOID AND NON-POLYPOID TUMORS OF THE COLON

AUSTIN L. VICKERY, JR., M.D.

Chapter 15. POLYPS

JACK R. DREYFUSS, M.D.

Chapter 16. THE POLYPOSIS DISORDERS

JACK R. DREYFUSS, M.D.

Chapter 17. MALIGNANT TUMORS AND OTHER COLONIC NEOPLASMS

JACK R. DREYFUSS, M.D.

Chapter 18. THE APPENDIX

JOHN A. LONG, M.D.

Chapter 19. OBSTRUCTION, TRAUMA, AND SURGERY

JAMES J. McCORT, M.D.

Chapter 20. OTHER COLONIC DISORDERS

CHARLES S. LANGSTON, M.D.

1

History of the Radiologic Examination of the Colon

R. TED STEINBOCK, M.D.

THE MOMENTOUS DISCOVERY

On November 8, 1895, Wilhelm Conrad Roentgen, professor of physics at the University of Wurzburg, Germany, first noticed a greenish light emanating from a paper coated with barium platinocyanide (Fig. 1.1). The paper was several feet away from a Crooke's vacuum tube completely enclosed by cardboard and activated by an induction coil. Moving his hand between the hidden tube and paper, Roentgen was amazed to see a black shadow cross the fluorescing surface.

During the following weeks, Roentgen experimented with the new rays and their penetration of various substances. He substituted a photographic plate for the fluorescent screen and made the first roentgenogram using his wife's hand. On December 28, Roentgen made his first announcement of the discovery, and by January 6, 1896, the exciting news was cabled around the world.

The penetrating x-rays generated intense interest among scientists, physicians, and the general public. Within a year after Roentgen's amazing discovery, some 50 scientific books and over 1000 articles on x-rays were published—many concerned with the possibilities of the x-ray in medical diagnosis and therapy. By 1901, Francis H. Williams of Boston published his classic textbook entitled *The Roentgen Rays in Medicine and Surgery*. Of the 635 pages of text, only 5 brief paragraphs described the colon (Fig. 1.2).

At first the utility of the x-ray appeared limited to the skeletal structures, thorax, and metallic foreign objects. The organs of the abdomen and pelvis produced a uniform density on the x-ray plate, providing little diagnostic information (Fig. 1.3). Furthermore, the exposure time for such a view of the body required over 30 min

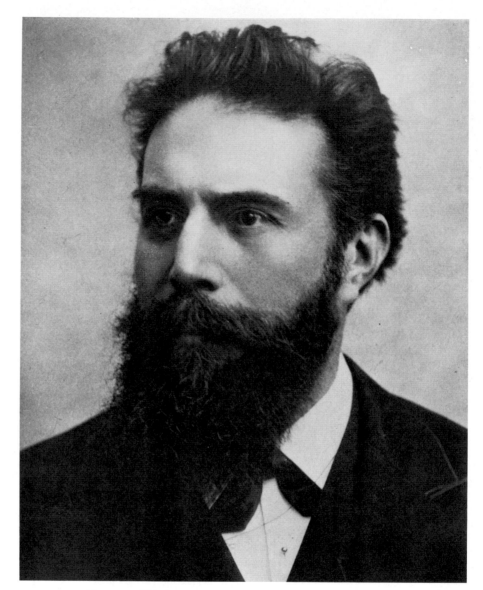

FIG. 1.1. WILHELM CONRAD ROENTGEN (1845–1923)
Discoverer of the x-ray in November, 1895.

compared with the 2 min needed for a radiograph of the hand. However, the development of improved equipment and pioneering research in roentgen techniques, particularly those utilizing radiopaque substances, quickly brought gastrointestinal examination to its rightful place in the forefront of radiology.

The exciting history of radiologic examination of the colon involves scientists and physicians on both sides of the Atlantic. The contributions of those early pioneers in radiology are reviewed in this chapter. The techniques of modern radiology are presented in Chapter 3.

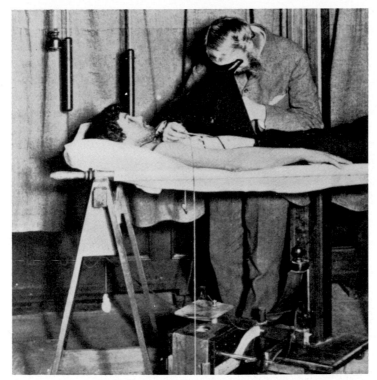

FIG. 1.2. FRANCIS H. WILLIAMS (1852–1936)
Dr. Williams is fluoroscoping a patient at the Boston City Hospital around 1900.
This illustration is from his classic textbook of 1901 and shows him outlining with
crayon the positions of the diaphragm in deep inspiration and expiration.

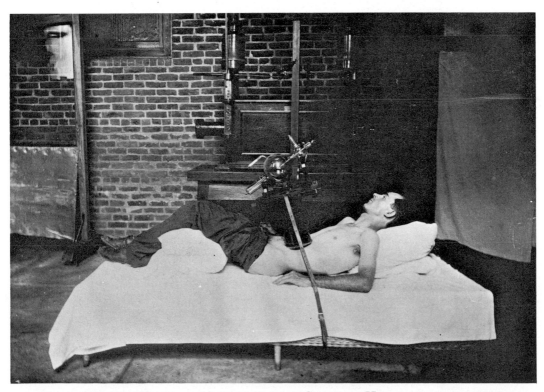

FIG. 1.3. X-RAY ROOM AT MASSACHUSETTS GENERAL HOSPITAL, ABOUT 1910.
Note that the x-ray tube and the cone are held steady against the patient by
means of a leather strap which passes under the wicker couch.

RADIOPAQUE STUDIES

The first endeavors to determine the form and position of the gastrointestinal tract were primitive (Fig. 1.4). Within months following Roentgen's discovery of the x-ray, Strauss in Germany gave patients gelatin capsules filled with ferrous oxide and bismuth subnitrate in an attempt to visualize the stomach. He was discouraged by the indistinct shadows that resulted, but the following year A. L. Benedict in the United States succeeded in locating lesions of the alimentary tract with similar capsules. Other workers tried metal coils, rubber tubes containing copper wire, and intragastric bags filled with lead acetate to outline the borders of the stomach and small intestine.

In the fall of 1896, while still a first-year student at Harvard Medical School, Walter Bradford Cannon began an important series of experiments in intestinal physiology utilizing the x-ray (Figs. 1.5 and 1.6). In December of 1896, Cannon fluoroscopically observed the mechanism of swallowing in the dog, frog, goose, and rooster using globular pearl buttons and capsules filled with bismuth subnitrate or barium sulfate. By April of 1897, Cannon and his classmate Albert Moser were feeding bismuth mixtures of varied consistency to study esophageal and gastric

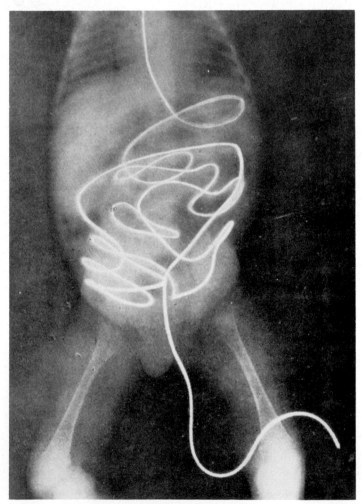

FIG. 1.4. METALLIC COIL CRUDELY OUTLINING THE POSITION OF THE INTESTINES
IN AN INFANT
From Archives of the Roentgen Ray, 1909.

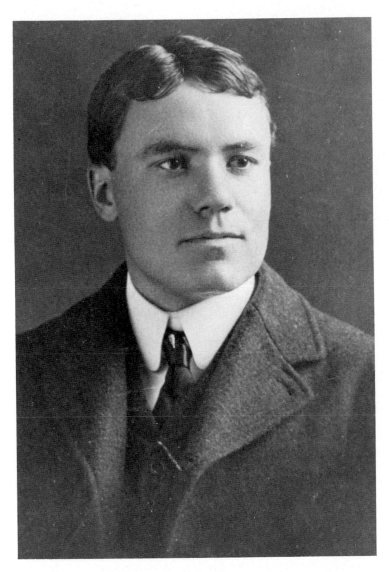

FIG. 1.5. WALTER BRADFORD CANNON (1871–1945)
Photograph of Cannon as a first-year Harvard medical student, about the time he
began his pioneering gastrointestinal investigations.

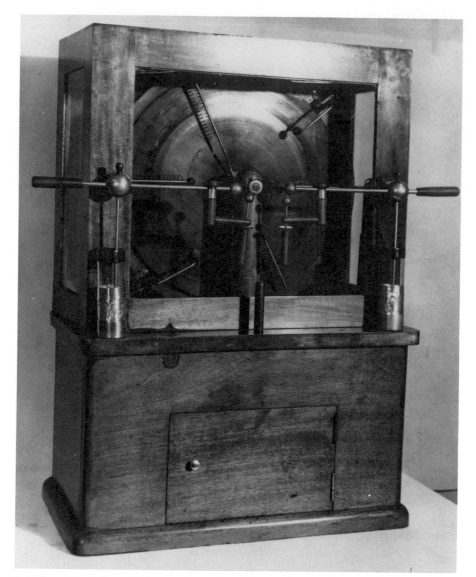

FIG. 1.6. ORIGINAL STATIC MACHINE USED BY CANNON AND MOSER TO GENERATE
THEIR X-RAY TUBE'S POTENTIALS

movements in cats and dogs. In the fall of 1897, the two students joined with Dr.
Francis Williams to extend their experiments to humans, and by 1902 Cannon
published an article concerning the physiologic movements of the colon as well as
the esophagus and stomach.

Workers on the other side of the Atlantic were also successful in using bismuth to
outline the colon. Rumpel in 1897 and Hildebrand in 1901 both fed bismuth orally
for several days and then injected air via the rectum to obtain radiographs of the
colon. However, only small amounts of bismuth were used, and the radiographs
could define only the grossest of lesions.

In 1904, Professor Herman Rieder of Munich made an important advance in
gastrointestinal radiology by standardizing the bismuth meal using 30 g of bismuth
subnitrate in 300 g of flour gruel and milk. He went further to define standard
positions and the intervals for obtaining radiographs. With the oral "Rieder's meal,"
an interval of 12–18 hr was required to obtain a radiograph of the colon.

Workers on both sides of the Atlantic quickly adopted Rieder's method, most notably Guido Holzknecht and Martin Haudek in Vienna, Franz Groedel in Germany, A. F. Hurst in England, and in the United States, George Pfahler, Henry Hulst, Auguste Crane, Ariel George, and James T. Case. Unfortunately, little attention was paid to the colon, perhaps due to the long interval required for the bismuth to reach the area. Although Rieder himself had advocated the use of a liter of fluid mixed with bismuth as an enema, its use for the colon examination was not widely accepted.

THE BARIUM ENEMA

The use of bismuth subnitrate soon fell into disrepute with reports of deaths caused by the substance or by toxic impurities in its preparation. Bismuth carbonate interfered with normal digestion. Bismuth oxychloride was too expensive. Finally, in 1910 Bachem and Gunter proposed the use of barium sulfate, which proved to be just as effective, safer to employ, and much less expensive than bismuth. It is interesting to note that Walter B. Cannon had employed barium sulfate in animal studies 12 years previously.

Although Schule performed one of the first opaque enemas in 1904, the method gained widespread acceptance only through the efforts of Fedor Haenisch of Hamburg. In 1910, Haenisch crossed the Atlantic from Germany to attend a meeting of the American Roentgen Ray Society. He presented his methods for properly cleansing the colon, the careful introduction of the opaque enema fluid under fluoroscopic control, and technical information on diagnosing carcinoma at an early stage. With his newly designed trochoscope, Haenisch could fluoroscope his patients in the horizontal position rather than use the awkward knee-chest position previously advocated (Fig. 1.7).

American radiologists at the meeting were enthusiastic about Haenisch's well-

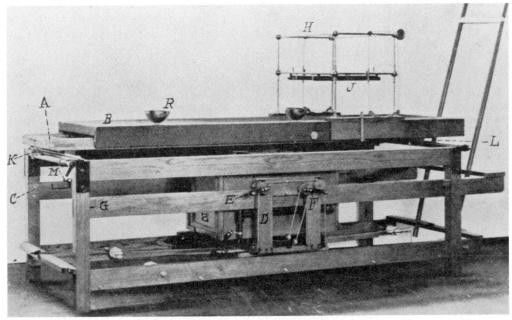

FIG. 1.7. TROCHOSCOPE

The trochoscope was designed by Fedor Haenisch of Germany. A mobile x-ray tube was mounted beneath the table, and a frame for holding a fluoroscopic screen or cassete was placed above the patient.

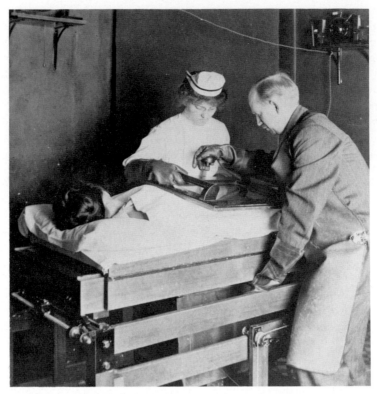

FIG. 1.8. JAMES T. CASE (1882–1960)

Dr. Case using a trochoscope to perform a barium enema on a patient at the Battle Creek Sanitarium in 1912.

formulated methods and quickly applied the new diagnostic technique in their own hospitals. This group included Eugene Caldwell and Lewis Gregory Cole from New York, Henry Pancoast and George Pfahler from Philadelphia, and James T. Case from Battle Creek (Fig. 1.8).

IMPORTANT EARLY TEXTBOOKS

Shortly after the widespread acceptance of the barium enema, several important textbooks on gastrointestinal radiology were published, further standardizing techniques, outlining new methods, and providing important sources of reference regarding the normal and abnormal appearances of the colon. In 1914, Franz Groedel of Germany edited a two-volume text which included 230 pages on the gastrointestinal tract (Fig. 1.9). Only 54 pages described the colon. Another German, Gottwald Schwartz, published a 153-page monograph on radiology of the colon, with 108 excellent illustrations. That same year, James T. Case issued an elaborate four-volume treatise on stereoroentgenography of the alimentary tract which included 36 uniquely developed stereograms of the colon (Figs. 1.10 and 1.11).

In 1915, Ariel George and R. D. Leonard of Boston published *The Roentgen Diagnosis of Surgical Lesions of the Gastrointestinal Tract* including 343 x-ray plates (Fig. 1.12). It provided an important atlas of normal and abnormal roentgen appearances, including illustrations of the gross specimens at operation and pathologic proof of diagnosis. That same year, Alfred Barclay of England published a 195-page monograph on alimentary tract radiology. This book formed the basis of his now classic textbook issued 18 years later.

In 1917, Russell D. Carman (Fig. 1.13A) and Albert Miller of the Mayo Clinic

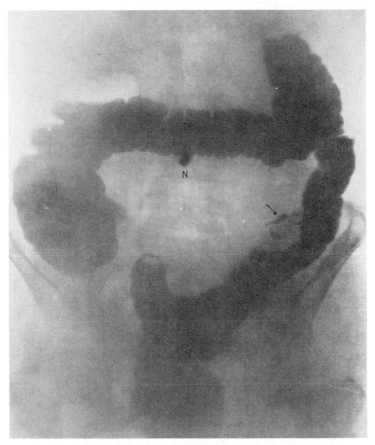

FIG. 1.9. CARCINOMA WITH FISTULA FORMATION OF THE DESCENDING COLON
Illustration from Franz Groedel's textbook of 1914. (A piece of metal marks the
position of the navel, "N.")

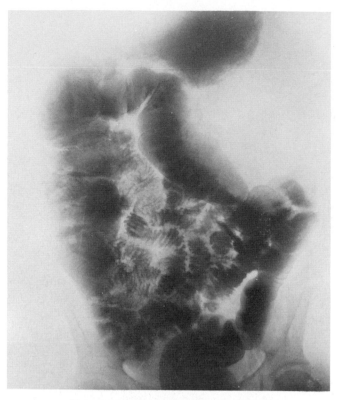

FIG. 1.10. SPLENIC ENLARGEMENT
Illustration from James T. Case's book on stereoroentgenography published in
1914 showing displacement of the colon by an enlarged spleen.

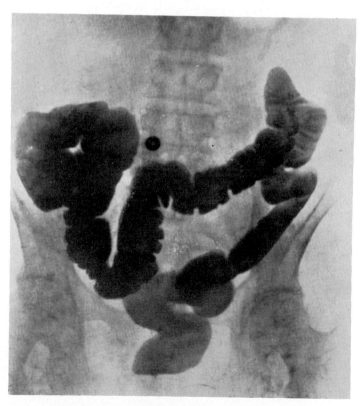

FIG. 1.11. NORMAL COLON
Illustration from James T. Case's book of 1914.

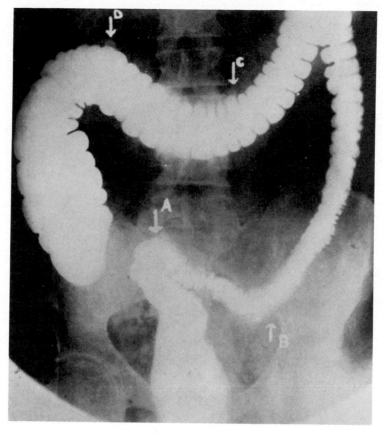

FIG. 1.12. DIVERTICULOSIS

Barium enema demonstration of four diverticula. Illustration depicted in George and Leonard's excellent gastrointestinal atlas of 1915.

published their classic textbook *The Roentgen Diagnosis of Diseases of the Alimentary Canal*. The 504 illustrations came from their study of thousands of patients at the Mayo Clinic. Over 100 pages of the book were devoted to techniques of colon examination, the normal colon, diverticulitis, appendicitis, colitis, stasis, cancer of the colon, and miscellaneous conditions.

With the onset of World War I, communication between radiologists in America and Germany came to a standstill. However, the use of the x-ray by the military in hospitals and induction programs greatly spurred further improvements in diagnostic technique and equipment.

THE DOUBLE-CONTRAST ENEMA

From 1910 to 1923 the barium enema was the method of choice for the colon examination and still retains this position today. Early investigators utilized it to correlate the roentgen signs with the pathologic findings so that diagnostic criteria could be established for various colon diseases. However, even this method had its shortcomings; small intraluminal lesions and polyps were difficult or impossible to identify.

As early as 1901, Francis Williams insufflated air into the colon, but could ascertain little more than its anatomic position. In 1910, Lewis Gregory Cole (Fig. 1.13B) and the gastroenterologist Moses Einhorn used air insufflation, and suggested that small mucosal lesions of the colon might be detected. Finally, in 1923 A. W.

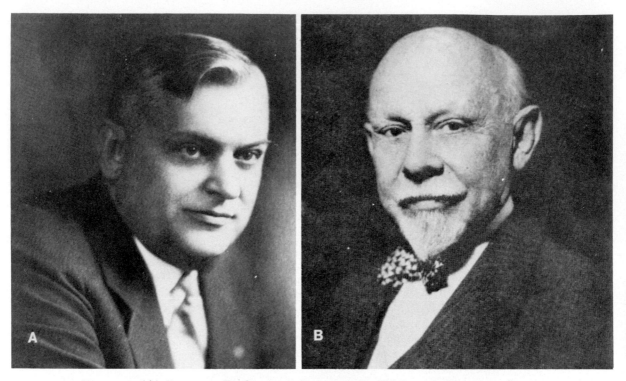

FIG. 1.13. **(A)** RUSSELL D. CARMAN (1875–1926); **(B)** LEWIS GREGORY COLE
(1874–1954)
Two of the American pioneers in gastrointestinal radiology. Carman emphasized
fluoroscopy while Cole utilized serial radiography to demonstrate gastrointestinal
lesions.

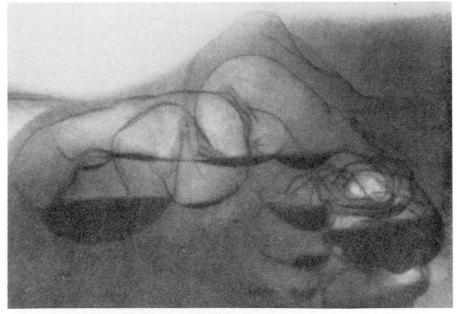

FIG. 1.14. DOUBLE-CONTRAST ENEMA
Right lateral decubitus view of the colon taken from A. W. Fischer's report of
1925.

Fischer of Frankfurt developed a method of examining the colon utilizing both barium and air to produce a double-contrast effect. He first experimented with surgically resected lengths of colon, employing various amounts and suspensions of barium sulfate followed by air injection (Figs. 1.14 and 1.15).

Fischer applied this method to many patients and presented a lengthy report in 1925. He laid the groundwork for detecting relatively small intraluminal tumors and stressed the value of air in visualizing stenosing lesions and enabling the examiner to "see through" overlapping loops.

In 1928, Kirklin of the Mayo Clinic visited with Fischer and was greatly impressed with the potential of the new method. He relayed these impressions to his associate, Harry Weber, who spent 2 years modifying and improving the double-contrast technique. By 1930, the American version of the double-contrast examination was established and Weber used it to contribute many classic reports on the radiologic diagnosis of various colon lesions.

The technical difficulties of achieving a proper double-contrast study dissuaded many from adopting the technique. Stevenson and his co-workers in Texas sought to standardize the examination with good success. Welin and his colleagues in Sweden later emphasized the importance of the double-contrast study for detecting small polyps.

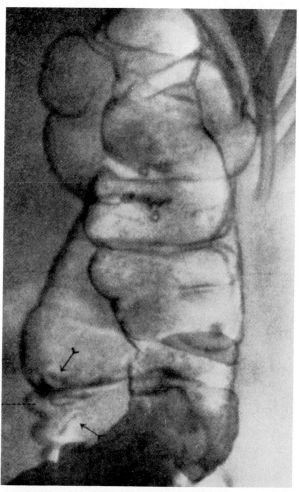

FIG. 1.15. TUBERCULOUS ULCERS OF THE DESCENDING COLON
Double-contrast study by A. W. Fischer, 1925.

IMPROVEMENTS IN THE COLON EXAMINATION

Technique

Over the years, various methods have been advocated and continue to be developed in an effort to improve the radiologic visualization of the colon. In 1933, several French radiologists used a dilute barium suspension transparent enough to demonstrate polypoid intestinal lesions. In 1936, Leo Rigler tried higher kilovoltage to penetrate ordinary barium suspension and reveal gastric polyps. This method was quickly applied to the colon by Gianturco in Illinois.

Chemicals

Various radiopaque chemicals were substituted for barium sulfate to achieve certain effects. In 1928, Bluhbaum, Frick, and Kalkbrenner used a thorium contrast agent to produce more even intestinal coating for the double-contrast examination. Less viscous organic iodides were introduced instead of barium in cases of dilated colon or suspected perforation.

In 1918, Gottwald Schwartz added tannic acid to the barium mixture and obtained superb mucosal detail on the evacuation films. However, the Food and Drug Administration banned the use of tannic acid in both cleansing and barium enemas in 1964 because of alleged hepatic toxicity.

Positioning and Projections

When Fedor Haenisch popularized the enema examination in 1910, he placed the patient in the supine position rather than the awkward knee-chest position previously employed. Haenisch relied mainly on the fluoroscopic image, taking a radiograph only in ambiguous situations or to record a finding. Later workers routinely made posteroanterior and left posterior oblique views of the entire colon a standard part of the examination and carefully moved the patient into various positions to insure proper filling of the colon. By 1925, Fischer was using a variety of positions and projections to obtain adequate air-contrast films.

In 1932, Stewart and Illick advocated stopping the inflow of barium and obtaining standard oblique views when the sigmoid colon was filled. The following year, Fricke emphasized the importance of the lateral view of the rectum based on anatomical and radiographic studies by Wolf in Germany. Still others such as Billing tried distending the urinary bladder with air or fluid to elevate and unfold the redundant sigmoid segment. In 1951, Rapp and later Moreton reintroduced the Chassard-Lapiné view, originally used for pelvimetry, and adapted it for studying the rectosigmoid and sigmoid. Ettinger and Elkin, in 1954, further stressed the value of special views of the colon as an aid in improving the accuracy of cancer diagnosis in the difficult to visualize distal segments of the large intestine.

Radiographic Equipment

Improvement in the primitive equipment first used by the early radiologists was crucial to the evolution of radiology as an independent branch of medicine and to its advancement as a science (Figs. 1.16 and 1.17). A radiograph of the colon, produced by the cantankerous Crooke's tube powered by a weak but noisy induction coil, required at least a 30-min exposure for the cumbersome glass x-ray plate. Clearly improvements were necessary in order to delineate more than the mere position and vague outline of the colon.

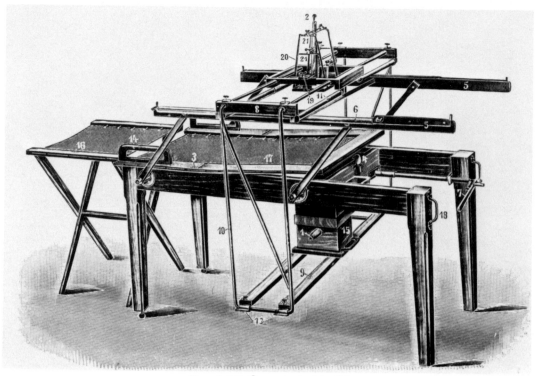

FIG. 1.16. ORTHODIAGRAPH
German horizontal orthodiagraph of 1913.

X-Ray Tubes

In the 1870's, Sir William Crookes designed many vacuum or gas tubes for the production of cathode rays, later known as electrons. In 1895, Roentgen discovered another type of ray emitting from these tubes which he termed the x-ray. From 1896 to 1912, a huge variety of gas tubes were designed for use in radiologic diagnosis and therapy, but all were limited by the easily damaged platinum anode and presence of gas within the tube as a source of electrons (Fig. 1.18).

Finally, in 1913 William D. Coolidge at the General Electric Laboratory developed the hot cathode tube using a heated tungsten cathode without the need for platinum or gaseous atmosphere. The first tube was used by Lewis Gregory Cole who arranged a special assembly to announce the tremendous advantages of the new Coolidge tube.

Power Sources

The early gas tubes were powered by static batteries or whirring induction coils (Fig. 1.19). Supplying proper current and amperage to the more powerful Coolidge tube was made possible by Clyde Snook's interrupterless transformer in 1907. A physicist and x-ray equipment manufacturer in Philadelphia, Snook made many contributions to x-ray technology. With the Coolidge tube and improved power source, the exposure time for radiographs was reduced to seconds or fractions of a second.

Bucky-Potter Grid

Another advance in producing better x-ray images was the introduction in 1921 of the Bucky-Potter grid to prevent secondary rays from reaching the film. This mobile grid was developed independently by Eugene Caldwell of New York, Gustav Bucky

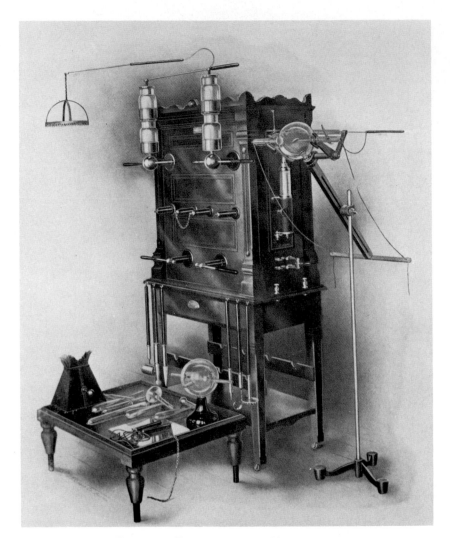

FIG. 1.17. RADIOGRAPHIC UNIT OF 1904
This typical unit consisted of a rotary coil generator, x-ray tubes, tube stand, and hand-held fluoroscope.

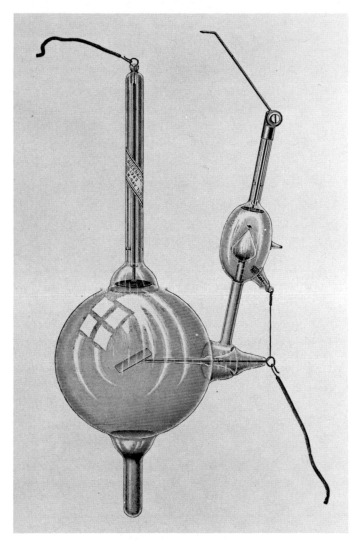

FIG. 1.18. SELF-REGULATING TUBE
This early gas tube designed by H. L. Sayen and manufactured by Queen and Co. was highly successful until supplanted by the Coolidge hot-cathode tube in 1913.

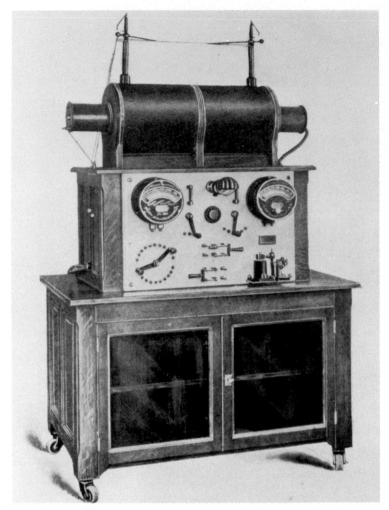

FIG. 1.19. INDUCTION COIL GENERATOR MADE IN 1905

of Berlin, and Hollis Potter of Chicago. The grid not only improved image clarity but enabled the use of larger x-ray plates needed for the colon examination.

X-Ray Films

From 1896 to 1920 radiographs were taken with glass plates covered with photographic emulsion. Although both photographic paper and celluloid films were available, they had a tendency to curl or crack. With the onset of World War I, however, the major American source of photographic glass from Belgium became unavailable. The logistics of supplying field hospitals with the fragile, cumbersome plates was nearly impossible, and the military spurred development of better radiographic film. Double-emulsion film, designed as early as 1897, was manufactured using a cellulose nitrate base. Because of its flammability and emission of poisonous fumes when burned, the base was changed to cellulose triacetate in 1929. With the advent of automatic film processing, the polyester base was developed in 1958 and remains in use today.

Intensifying Screens

The double-emulsion film had a further advantage of adapting well to the newly designed film-holder or cassette lined with intensifying fluorescent screens. In 1896,

Professor Michael Pupin of Columbia University had attempted lining his plate-holder with a fluorescing screen to intensify the photographic image, but the grainy fluorescent crystals produced further artifacts on the plates. By 1916, Carl V. S. Patterson of the Patterson Screen Company successfully produced satisfactory fluorescent screens for cassettes, which enhanced image clarity and significantly decreased radiation to the patient.

Fluoroscopy versus Radiography

The fluorescing paper used by Roentgen in 1895 was coated with barium platin-ocyanide. In his large research laboratory at West Orange, New Jersey, Thomas Alva Edison quickly tested a huge variety of substances and found that calcium tungstate fluoresced about 6 times more brightly. Within 4 months after Roentgen's discovery, Edison was manufacturing a hand-held fluoroscope utilizing his calcium tungstate screen (Fig. 1.20).

With the improved screen easily available, many early radiologists relied mainly on fluoroscopy, a term coined by Edison, rather than expensive x-ray plates requiring 30-min exposures. By the early 1900's, a controversy raged concerning the respective

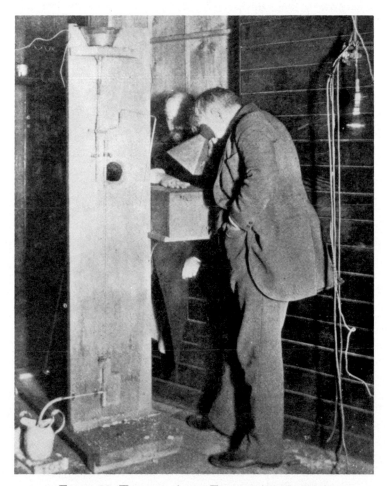

FIG. 1.20. THOMAS ALVA EDISON (1847–1931)
The great inventor is using a portable fluoroscope containing a calcium tungstate screen which he invented and began manufacturing within 4 months of Roentgen's discovery.

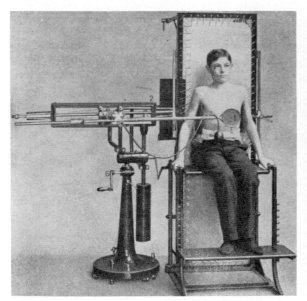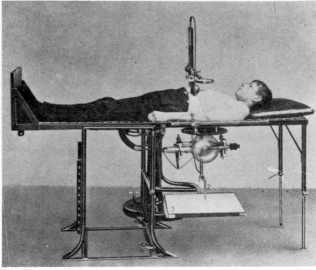

FIG. 1.21. ORTHODIAGRAPH FOR BOTH VERTICAL AND HORIZONTAL FLUOROSCOPIC
EXAMINATION
Designed by Franz Groedel in 1912.

merits of fluoroscopy and radiography (Figs. 1.21–1.23). Guido Holzknecht and other
distinguished Austrian and German radiologists advocated fluoroscopy to determine
the "symptom-complexes" necessary for a diagnosis of gastrointestinal disease.
Several radiologists such as Herman Rieder of Munich and Lewis Gregory Cole of
New York relied almost exclusively on x-ray plates to diagnose lesions of the
stomach, duodenum, and colon.

The controversy continued without a resolution. In 1910, Fedor Haenisch introduced the trochoscope, allowing greater ease in fluoroscoping the patient horizon-
tally while palpating the abdomen. In 1912, Eugene W. Caldwell built the first
motor-driven continuous tilting table. With the invention of the Coolidge tube the
following year, advocates of radiography could use much shorter exposure times,
decreasing radiation to the patient compared to the long fluoroscopy sessions.

Spot-Film Apparatus

The development of the spot-film apparatus provided not only an effective
compromise to the fluoroscopy-radiography debate but also a vital improvement in
the examination of the colon. In 1917, Gosta Forssell of Sweden and his student,
Ake Akerlund, designed an instrument for both fluoroscopy and radiography. It
contained a fluoroscopic screen which could be pressed against the patient and
locked in position maintaining any desired degree of pressure. For localized compression Akerlund inserted pads of cotton, wool, or cork between the patient and
screen. When the desired amount of pressure was obtained under fluoroscopic
observation, the carrier containing a rotary Bucky-Potter grid and cassette was
substituted for the fluoroscopic screen. The fluoroscopist then left the room completely while serial radiographs were taken. With such a procedure only the first
radiograph approximated what was seen at fluoroscopy. Subsequent films were
taken "blindly." Despite this time-consuming procedure, Akerlund achieved a great
advance in combining fluoroscopy and radiography. He also stressed the need of
compression to evaluate mucosal detail.

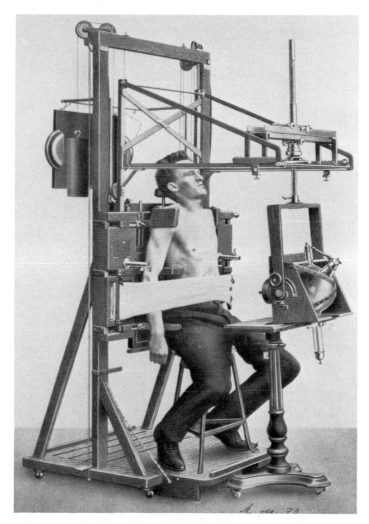

FIG. 1.22. ELABORATE RADIOGRAPHIC APPARATUS FOR GASTROINTESTINAL
EXAMINATION MANUFACTURED BY SIEMENS OF GERMANY IN 1911

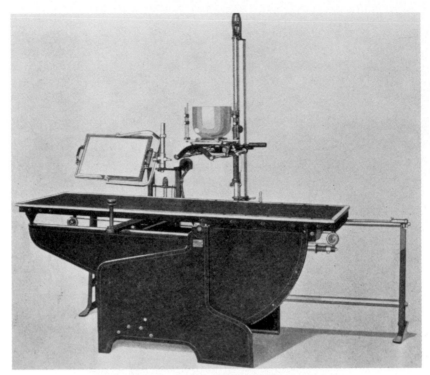

FIG. 1.23. KELLEY-KOETT MOTOR DRIVEN TILTING TABLE OF 1924, PARTIALLY
DESIGNED BY LEWIS GREGORY COLE
Note that the fluoroscopic screen could also be tilted.

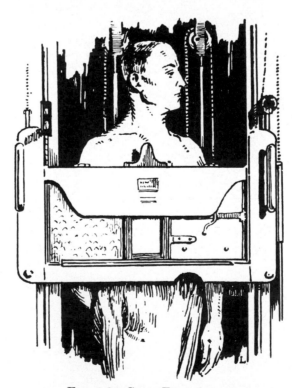

FIG. 1.24. SPOT-FILM APPARATUS
Illustration of the original spot-film apparatus designed by Hans Heinrich Berg in
1923.

In 1923, Hans Heinrich Berg of Berlin designed the first modern spot-film apparatus (Fig. 1.24). Berg applied local compression with a tube or padded cone mounted on the back of the fluoroscopic screen. With his apparatus, the transformer automatically switched to a higher power setting when the cassette slid into place. More importantly, Berg's spot-film device enabled the radiologist to intersperse a radiograph at any chosen moment during the fluoroscopic examination and instantly record what was seen, all with selected compression and optimal barium filling.

In the United States, Dr. Joseph H. Pratt at the Boston Dispensary heard of the diagnostic progress in gastrointestinal examination facilitated by Berg's technique and spot-film device. Dr. Pratt wrote Dr. Berg and requested that he send one of his pupils to Boston to introduce the new method. Dr. Berg sent Dr. Alice Ettinger and she brought with her the first Berg spot-film device to be used in this country. The Boston Dispensary later became a unit of the New England Medical Center and Dr. Ettinger the Radiologist-in-Chief.

With Dr. Ettinger's assistance and the Berg device as a model, Richard Dresser and Frank Scholz, an electrical engineer, designed a highly successful, light-weight, and inexpensive spot-film apparatus. By 1933 they described the improved device in the *New England Journal of Medicine*, and Frank Scholz soon began manufacturing them for widespread use (Fig. 1.25).

Image Amplification

In the 1930's radiologists experimented with cinefluoroscopy and radiography, but the low intensity light emitted by the fluoroscopic screen severely hampered progress.

Impetus for improving the fluoroscope was provided by Edward Chamberlain in his Carman Lecture of 1941. As early as 1938, Irving Langmuir designed an image tube to electronically amplify the fluorescent image. By 1948, John Coltman, an electrical engineer at the Westinghouse Laboratory, developed a working model of the fluoroscopic image intensifier. This important device banished the time-consuming requirement of dark adaptation and also permitted the use of practical cinefluorography.

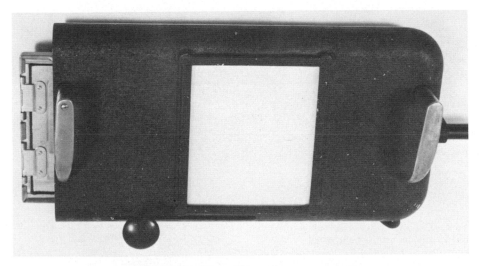

FIG. 1.25. SPOT-FILM APPARATUS

First production model of the spot-film apparatus manufactured by the Frank Scholz X-ray Corp. in 1935. By 1939, up to four spot films could be taken per cassette.

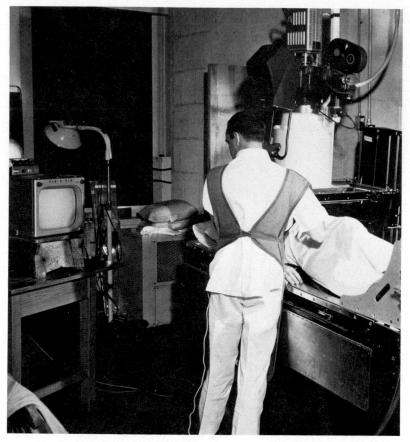

Fig. 1.26. First Massachusetts General Hospital Clinical Demonstration
of Televised Fluoroscopy, November 30, 1960

The examination was carried out with a unit designed by Webster and Wipfelder
and used under a grant for experimental evaluation between 1958 and 1962. The
image of this first intestinal study was also transmitted by coaxial cable to a group
of physicians in a nearby room.

Shortly thereafter, Ralph Sturm and Russell Morgan analyzed the limits of image
intensification and developed an alternative method involving direct television pick-
up from a fluoroscopic screen. In the 1950's the newly developed Vidicon television
camera was used successfully by Stauffer and others to display intensified images
and by the 1960's televised fluoroscopy had proven its practical advantages for
routine clinical use (Webster and Wipfelder; Fig. 1.26). The cumulative effect of
these electronic advances enabled gastrointestinal radiology to enter a new era of
sophistication and achievement.

BIBLIOGRAPHY

Akerlund, A.: Röntgenologische studien über den
bulbus duodeni mit besonderer berücksichti-
gung des ulcus duodeni. Acta Radiol. (Suppl.
I.), 1921.

Bachem, C., and Gunther, H.: Bariumsulfat als
schattenbildendes kontrastmittel bein rönt-
genuntersuchungen. Z. Röntgenk. Radium-
forsch., *12*: 369, 1910.

Barclay, A. E.: *The Alimentary Tract: A Radiographic Study*. Sherratt and Hughes, Man-
chester, 1915.

Barclay, A. E.: *The Digestive Tract: A Radiological Study of Its Anatomy, Physiology, and
Pathology*. Cambridge University Press, Cambridge, 1933.

Benedict, A. L.: Bismuth capsules—A new application for the x-ray. J.A.M.A., *30*: 565, 1898.

Berg, H. H.: Über engste verbindung von röntgen-durchleuchtung und aufnahmeverfahren (verfahren der gezielten momentaufnahmen). Fortschr. Röntgenstr., *33*: 25, 1925.

Berg, H. H.: Die direkten röntgensymptome des ulcus duodeni und ihre klinische bedeutung. Ergebn. Med. Strahlenforschung, *2*: 249, 1926.

Blühbaun, T., Frick, K., and Kalkbrenner, H.: Eine neue anwendungsart der kollöide in der röntgendiagnostik. Fortschr. Röntgenstr., *37*: 18, 1928.

Cannon, W. B.: The movements of the stomach studied by means of the Röntgen rays. Am. J. Physiol., *1*: 359, 1898.

Cannon, W. B.: The movements of the intestines studied by means of the Röntgen rays. J. Med. Res., *7*: 72, 1902.

Cannon, W. B.: Early use of the Röntgen ray in the study of the alimentary canal. J.A.M.A., *62*: 1, 1914.

Carman, R. D., and Miller, A.: *The Roentgen Diagnosis of Diseases of the Alimentary Canal.* W. B. Saunders, Philadelphia, 1917.

Carty, J. R., and Merrill, V.: Some essential considerations of the technic of gastrointestinal radiography. Radiology, *26*: 531, 1936.

Case, J. T.: The importance of stereoradiography, especially of the alimentary tract, with demonstration of plates. Proc. R. Soc. Med., *5*: 73, 1912.

Case, J. T.: *Stereoroentgenography of the Alimentary Tract*, 4 volumes. Southworth, Troy, 1914.

Case, J. T.: Fifty years of Roentgen rays in gastroenterology. Am. J. Roentgenol., *54*: 607, 1945.

Chamberlain, W. E.: Fluoroscopes and fluoroscopy. Radiology, *38*: 383, 1942.

Codman, E. A.: Study of cases of accidental x-ray burns hitherto recorded. Phila. Med. J., *9*: 499, 1902.

Cole, L. G.: Value of serial radiography in gastrointestinal diagnosis. J.A.M.A., *69*: 1947, 1912.

Cole, L. G., and Einhorn, M.: Radiograms of the digestive tract by inflation with air. N.Y. Med. J., *92*: 705, 1910.

Cole, L. G., Pound, R. E., Morse, R. W., Headland, C. I., Cole, W. G., and Naslund, A. W.: Roentgenologic exploration of the mucosa of the gastrointestinal tract. Radiology, *18*: 221, 1932.

Coltman, J. W.: Fluoroscopic image brightening by electronic means. Radiology *51*: 359, 1948.

Coolidge, W. D.: A powerful roentgen ray tube with a pure electron discharge. Phys. Rev., *2*: 409, 1913.

Dresser, R., and Scholz, F.: A device for making radiographs of the gastrointestinal tract. N. Engl. J. Med., *209*: 1343, 1933.

Ettinger, A., and Elkin, M.: Study of the sigmoid by special roentgenographic views. Am. J. Roentgenol., *72*: 199, 1954.

Fischer, A. W.: Früdiagnose des dickdarmkrebses, insbesondere seine differentialdiagnose gegen tuberkulose mit hilfe der kombinierten luft-und bariumfullung des dickdarms. Dtsch. Ges. Inn. Med., *35*: 86, 1923.

Fischer, A. W.: Aufgaben und erfolge der röntgenologischen diagnostik bösartiger und entzündlicher dickdarmgeschwülste. Ergebn. Med. Strahlenforschung, *1*: 1, 1925.

Fletcher, G. H.: An improved method of visualization of the sigmoid. Am. J. Roentgenol., *59*: 750, 1948.

Fuchs, A. W.: Edison and roentgenology. Am. J. Roentgenol., *57*: 145, 1947.

Fuchs, A. W.: Evolution of Roentgen film. Am. J. Roentgenol., *75*: 30, 1956.

Gary, J. E., and Schatzki, R.: Radiologic examination of the gastrointestinal tract. N. Engl. J. Med., *251*: 1052, 1096, 1954.

George, A. W., and Leonard, R. D.: *The Roentgen Diagnosis of Surgical Lesions of the Gastrointestinal Tract.* Colonial Medical Press, Boston, 1915.

Gianturco, C.: The comparative value of various methods in the roentgenologic examination of the colon. I.M.J., *71*: 67, 1937.

Gianturco, C.: High-voltage technic in the diagnosis of polypoid growths of the colon. Radiology, *55*: 27, 1950.

Glasser, O.: Technical development of radiology, 1906–1956. Am. J. Roentgenol., *75*: 7, 1956.

Groedel, F. M.: The roentgen ray examination of the digestive tract. Arch. Roentgen Ray, *12*: 122, 1907.

Groedel, F. M., ed.: *Gundriss und Atlas der Röntgendiagnostik in der Inneren Medizin*, 2 volumes. Lehmann Verlag, Munich, 1914.

Haenisch, G. F.: Ein neuer apparat zur orthophotographie, zugleich trochoscop und aufnahmetisch. Fortschr. Geb. Röntgenstr., *11*: 99, 1907.

Haenisch, G. F.: The roentgen examination of the large intestine. Arch. Roentgen Ray, *17*: 208, 1912.

Hamilton, J. B.: The use of tannic acid in barium enemas. Am. J. Roentgenol., *56*: 101, 1946.

Hildebrand, H.: Ueber den diagnostichen werth der röntgenstrahlen in der inneren medizin. Munch. Med. Wochenschr., *48*: 2008, 1901.

Janower, M. L., Robbins, L. L., Tomchik, F. S., and Weylman, W. T.: Tannic acid and the barium enema. Radiology, *85*: 887, 1965.

Ledoux-Lebard, R., and Garcia-Calderon, H.: Les techniques d'examen de la muqueuse du gros intestin. J. Radiol. d'Electrol., *17*: 429, 1933.

Morgan, R. H., and Sturm, R. E.: The Johns Hopkins fluoroscopic screen intensifier. Radiology, *57*: 556, 1957.

Moreton, R. D.: Double-contrast examination of the colon with special emphasis on studies of the sigmoid. Radiology, *60*: 510, 1953.

Morison, J. M. W.: X-rays and cancer diagnosis; including a note on the history of the opaque meal. Br. J. Radiol., *32*: 388, 1927.

Pfahler, G. E.: The diagnosis of the size, form, position, and mobility of the stomach and bowel by means of the x-ray. Trans. Coll. Phys., *27*: 79, 1905.

Potter, H. E.: Diaphragming roentgen rays: Studies and experiments. Am. J. Roentgenol., *3*: 142, 1916.

Potter, H. E.: History of diaphragming roentgen rays by use of the Bucky principle. Am. J. Roentgenol., *25*: 396, 1931.

Reynolds, R.: Cineradiography. Br. J. Radiol., *7*: 415, 1934.

Rieder, H.: Radiologische untersuchungen des magens und darmes beim lebenden menschen. Munch. Med. Wochenschr., *51*: 1548, 1904.

Rieder, H.: Beiträge zur topographie des magen-
darmkanales beim lebendem menschen über
den zeitlichen ablauf der verdauung. Fortschr.
Geb. Röntgenstr., *8*: 141, 1905.

Rigler, L. G., and Erikson, L. G.: Benign tumors of
the stomach. Radiology, *26*: 6, 1936.

Rigler, L. G., and Weiner, M.: History of roentgenology of the gastrointestinal tract. In *Alimentary Tract Roentgenology*, Vol. 1, edited by A.
R. Margulis and H. J. Burhenne. C. V. Mosby,
St. Louis, 1967.

Robins, S. A., and Altman, W. S.: Significance of
the lateral view of the rectum. Am. J. Roentgenol., *40*: 598, 1938.

Robinson, J. M.: Detection of small lesions of the
large bowel; barium enema versus double contrast. Calif. Med., *81*: 321, 1954.

Rumpel, T.: Die klinische diagnose der spindel
förmigen speiseröhrenerweiterung. Munch.
Med. Wochenschr., *44*: 383, 1897.

Schule, A.: Über die sondierung und radiographie
des dickdarms. Arch. Verdauungske., *10*: 111,
1904.

Schwarz, G.: *Klinische Röntgendiagnostik des
Dickdarms*. Springer, Berlin, 1914.

Sosman, M. C.: Medicine as a science: Roentgenology. N. Engl. J. Med., *244*: 552, 1951.

Stauffer, H. M., Oppenheimer, M., Stewart, G. H.,
III, *et al.*: Practical image amplifier techniques: Fluoroscopy, cine fluorography, spot-
film radiography and use with closed-circuit
television. Radiology, *65*: 784, 1955.

Stevenson, C. A.: Technic of the double contrast
examination of the colon. Surg. Clin. North
Am., *32*: 1531, 1952.

Stevenson, C. A.: The development of the colon
examination. Am. J. Roentgenol., *71*: 385, 1954.

Stevenson, C. A.: Clinical roentgenology of the
colon. Am. J. Roentgenol., *96*: 275, 1966.

Stewart, W. H., and Illick, H. E.: Method of more
clearly visualizing lesions of the sigmoid. Am.
J. Roentgenol., *28*: 379, 1932.

Strauss, F.: Beitrag zur wurdigung der diagnostichen bedentuung der Röntgen durchleuch-
tung. Dtsch. Med. Wochenschr., *22*: 161, 1896.

Sturm, R. E., and Morgan, R. H.: Screen intensification systems and their limitations. Am. J.
Roentgenol., *62*: 617, 1949.

Weber, H. M.: Roentgenologic demonstration of
polypoid lesions and polyposis of the large
intestine. Am. J. Roentgenol., *25*: 577, 1931.

Weber, H. M.: Carcinoma of the colon—Its roent-
genological manifestations and differential diagnosis. Am. J. Cancer, *17*: 321, 1933.

Webster, E. W., and Wipfelder, R.: The limitations
of combined image intensifier-television systems for medical fluoroscopy. I.R.E. Trans.
Biomed. Electronics, *9*: 150, 1962.

Welin, S.: Results of the Malmo technique of colon
examination. J.A.M.A. *199:* 119, 1967.

Williams, F. H.: *The Roentgen Rays in Medicine
and Surgery*. Macmillan, New York, 1901.

2

Anatomy and Physiology of the Colon

KARL T. BENEDICT, JR., M.D.

GROSS ANATOMY

The large intestine is a muscular tube, 120–150 cm long. Arching across the abdomen, it encircles the small bowel from which it receives the liquid products of digestion. It consists of seven anatomic subdivisions: cecum and appendix, ascending colon, transverse colon, descending colon, sigmoid colon, rectum, and anal canal (Fig. 2.1). On external inspection, the colon is characterized by three longitudinal muscle bundles, the tenia coli, between which balloon varying-sized sacculations termed haustra (Fig. 2.2). The tenia originate at the base of the appendix and extend to the rectum where they fuse into a single, circumferential band. When contracted they shorten the colon. Numerous fat-containing, peritoneal tags, the appendices epiploica, are attached to the surface of the colon mainly along the course of the tenia. They are more numerous distally and occasionally calcify.

On the internal surface of the large bowel are transverse ridges, the plica semilunares, which represent infoldings of the colonic wall between the haustra (Fig. 2.2, magnified area). Since they generally extend only between two rows of tenia, they can usually be distinguished from the spiraling or encircling plica circulares of the small bowel on plain radiographs of the abdomen. (Fig. 2.3).

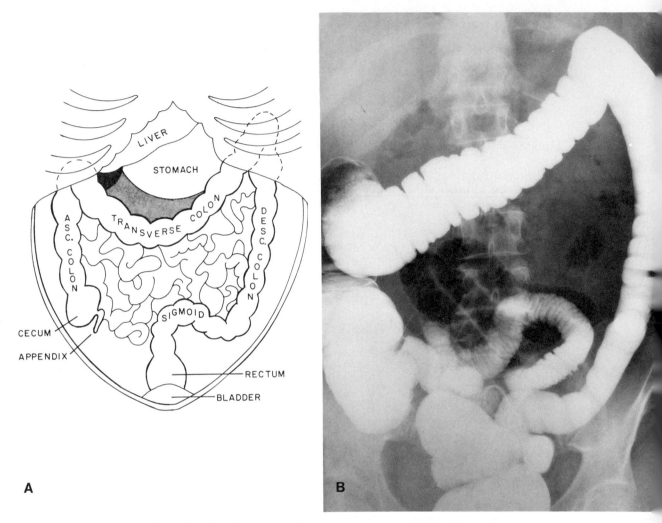

FIG. 2.1. POSITION AND DIVISIONS OF THE LARGE INTESTINE.
(A) Anatomic [greater omentum and gastrocolic ligament have been removed exposing the lesser sac and transverse mesocolon (shaded)]. Note gallbladder (solid black). (B) Radiographic.

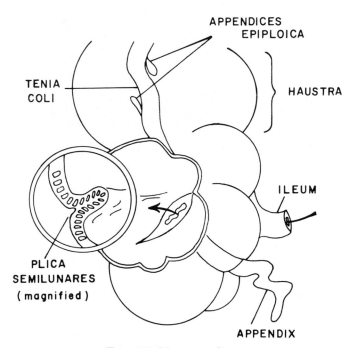

FIG. 2.2. NORMAL CECUM

A section of the wall is removed to expose the ileocecal valve (arrow). Note haustra, tenia coli, appendices epiploica, and the plica semilunares (magnified area).

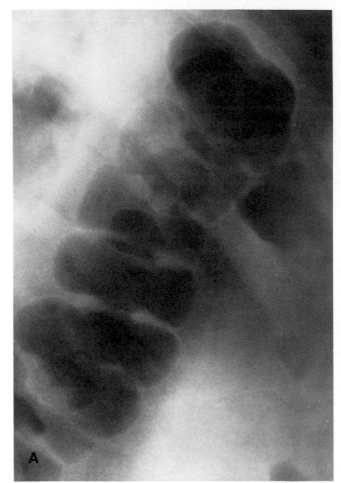

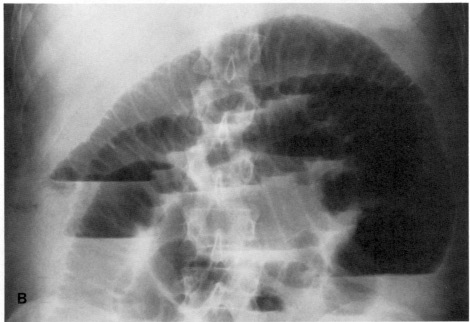

FIG. 2.3. GAS PATTERNS
(A) Plica semilunares between the haustra (normal colon). (B) Plica circulares (dilated small bowel).

HISTOLOGY

The colonic wall contains the same four layers found elsewhere in the alimentary tract: mucosa, submucosa, muscularis, and serosa. All four coats are found in the plica semilunares (the plica circulares of the small bowel contain only mucosa and submucosa). The colonic mucosa is flat, lined with columnar epithelium, and dotted by the tiny orifices of the colonic glands (crypts of Lieberkühn). There are shallow grooves in the mucosa which are known as innominate lines. These can be demonstrated on barium enemas and may mimic mucosal ulcerations (see Chapter 9).

The submucosa is loose connective tissue. It contains arterial and venous plexuses as well as Meissner's plexus, a collection of autonomic and sensory nerve fibers and neurons. The smooth muscle of the muscularis is arranged in an inner circular layer and an outer longitudinal layer. The latter is complete only in its thin inner portion, its outer portion being thickened into the three equally spaced tenia coli. The membranes of the smooth muscle cells are fused at points of contact termed nexuses. These are areas of low electrical resistance which may serve to integrate electrical events between the cells, permitting the smooth muscle to function as a syncytium. Within the muscularis is found a second autonomic nerve plexus, the myenteric (or Auerbach's) plexus. This plexus contains parasympathetic motor nuclei as well as autonomic and sensory nerve fibers.

The serosa is the visceral peritoneum and is absent in those portions of the colon which are extraperitoneal.

EMBRYOLOGY AND ANATOMIC VARIANTS

During embryologic development, the colon is initially left-sided but subsequently swings superiorly to the right, encompassing the small bowel. The cecum and ileocecal valve descend into the right lower quadrant. Sections of the primitive mesentery disappear as the ascending and descending portions of the colon become fixed to the retroperitoneum. The transverse and sigmoid portions of the colon retain their mesentery and remain mobile. In addition, the cecum usually is invested by peritoneum and may not be fixed in position.

Developmental variations include degrees of nonrotation (Figs. 2.4 and 2.11) and persistence of the mesentery to the ascending or descending colon. The latter is more frequent. When either mesentery is present, small bowel loops may lie between the abdominal flank stripe (lateral extension of the retroperitoneal fat) and the lateral wall of the colon (Fig. 2.5). If these loops are filled with liquid rather than gas, fluid in the paracolic gutter may be mimicked (Fig. 2.6). Colonic interposition (Fig. 2.7) and persistence of a juvenile cecum and appendix (Fig. 2.8) are other anatomic variants.

ANATOMIC RELATIONSHIPS

In its course around the abdomen and through the pelvis, the colon may be either intra- or extraperitoneal. Its anatomic relationships and peritoneal attachments are complex. During the following description, one should refer frequently to Figs. 2.1, 2.9 and 2.10.

Cecum and Appendix

The widest portion of the large intestine, the cecum, is a blind-ending pouch inferior to the ileo-cecal valve. It usually lies on the ilio-psoas muscle in the iliac fossa, but may be found in the true pelvis or in the right upper quadrant beneath

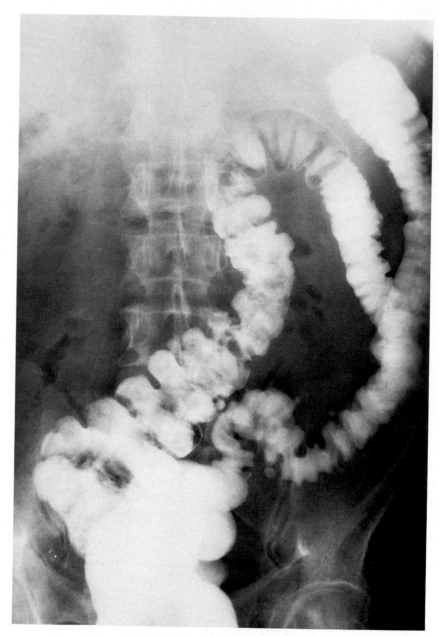

FIG. 2.4. NONROTATION OF THE COLON
The colon lies on the left.

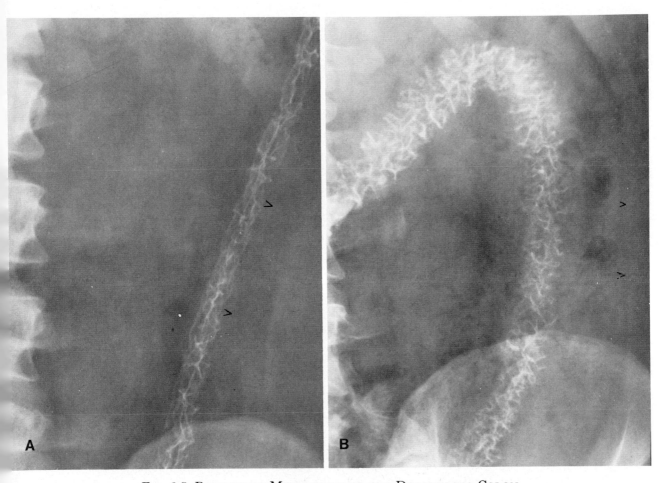

FIG. 2.5. PERSISTING MESENTERY TO THE DESCENDING COLON
(A) No mesentery present, lateral wall of descending colon adjacent to flank stripe (arrowheads on medial side of wide flank stripe). (B) Mesentery present, small bowel loops separate colon from thin flank stripe (arrowheads).

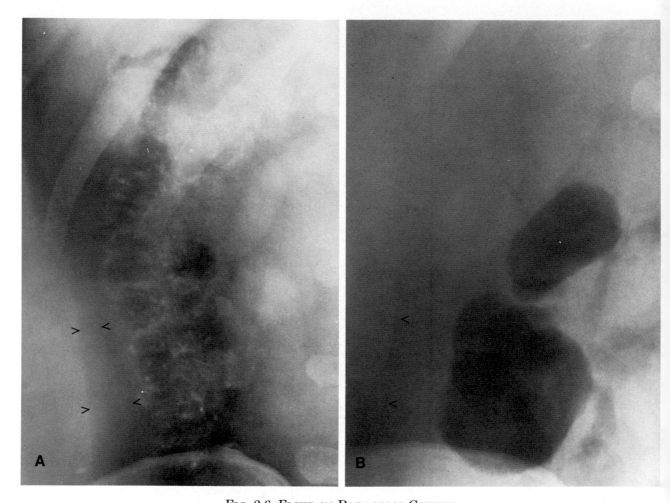

FIG. 2.6. FLUID IN PARACOLIC GUTTER

(**A**) Normal relationship of ascending colon and flank stripe. (Wide flank stripe
lies between arrowheads.) (**B**) Peritoneal fluid displacing colon medially (arrowheads
on thin flank stripe). This may be mimicked by fluid-filled small bowel when
ascending or descending colon is on a mesentery.

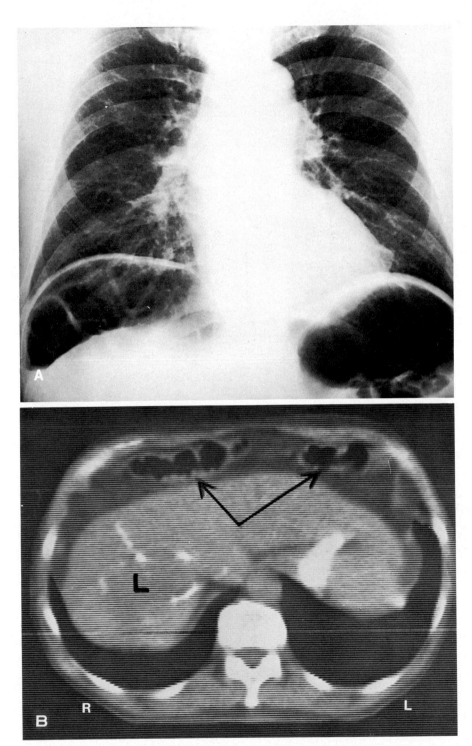

FIG. 2.7. COLONIC INTERPOSITION (CHILAIDITI SYNDROME)
(**A**) Upright chest radiograph (recognition of haustral pattern distinguishes colonic gas from a pneumoperitoneum). (**B**) CT scan showing transverse colon (arrows) interposed between liver (L) and anterior abdominal wall.

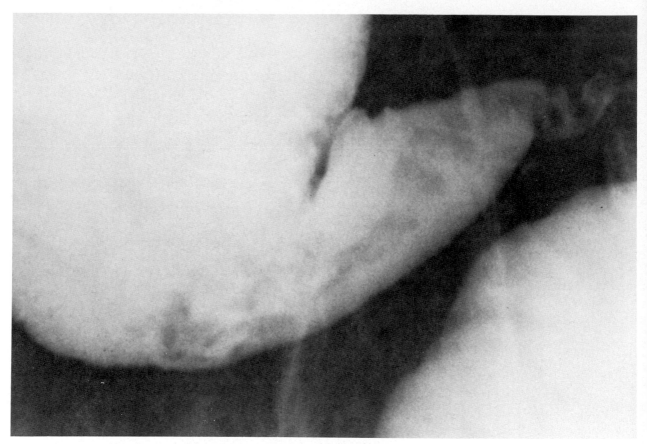

FIG. 2.8. JUVENILE CECUM AND APPENDIX IN AN ADULT (CONICAL CECUM)

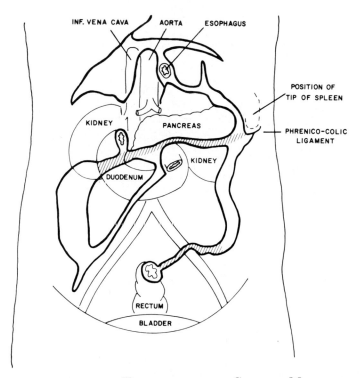

FIG. 2.9. ATTACHMENT OF THE TRANSVERSE AND SIGMOID MESOCOLONS TO THE RETROPERITONEUM

The lines of reflection of the peritoneum from the posterior abdominal wall are shown in bold line. The origins of the transverse and sigmoid mesocolons are shaded. Note the phrenico-colic ligament and the retroperitoneal organs.

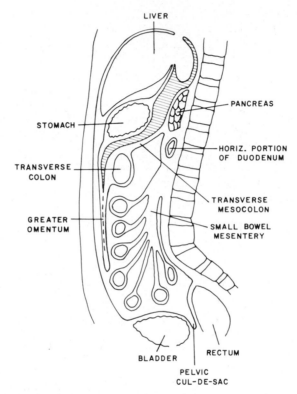

FIG. 2.10. MIDLINE SAGITTAL SECTION SHOWING THE RELATIONSHIP OF THE
ABDOMINAL VISCERA TO THE LESSER AND GREATER PERITONEAL CAVITIES
(MALE)
The lesser peritoneal cavity is shown crosshatched.

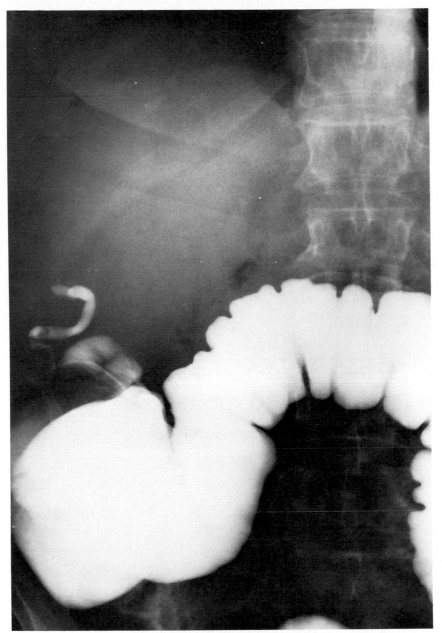

FIG. 2.11. SUBHEPATIC APPENDIX
The cecum has not descended into the right lower abdomen.

the liver (Fig. 2.11). Complete peritonealization of the cecum creates a retrocecal recess which frequently houses the appendix (65%). In 30% of persons the appendix lies within the true pelvis, at times extending to the left of midline.

Ileo-Cecal Valve

The ileo-cecal valve is an invagination of the circular muscle layer of the ileum. It is only partially effective as a one-way valve. During a barium enema, reflux into the terminal ileum can often be achieved. When outlined by barium, the valve has a characteristic appearance in profile, but may mimic a "mass" when viewed *en face* (Fig. 2.12).

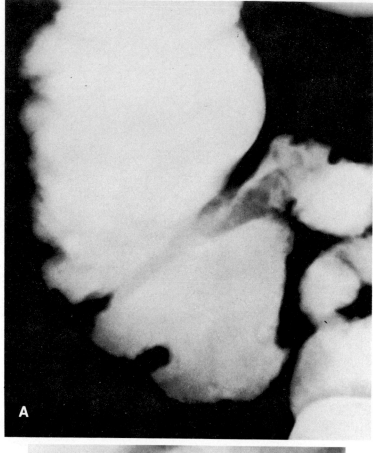

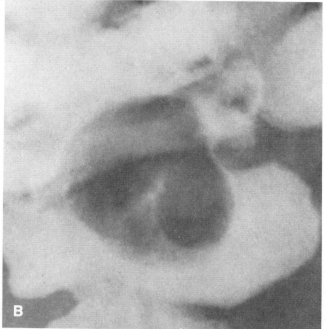

FIG. 2.12. NORMAL ILEOCECAL VALVE ON BARIUM ENEMA
(A) In profile. (B) *En face.*

Ascending Colon

Shorter than the descending colon, the ascending colon lies posteriorly in the right paracolic gutter, fixed to the retroperitoneum by the visceral peritoneum which covers its anterior surface. Laterally, it lies adjacent to the flank stripe and anteriorly is related either to the abdominal wall or to loops of small bowel. Superiorly, it reaches the lower pole of the right kidney, beneath the visceral surface of the liver, where it turns anteriorly and medially to form the hepatic flexure.

Transverse Colon

The transverse colon courses anteriorly and medially over the right kidney and duodenum where it acquires a mesentery, the transverse mesocolon. While the mesocolon is of variable length, at times permitting the transverse colon to descend into the pelvis (Fig. 2.13), its attachment to the retroperitoneum is quite constant (Fig. 2.9). Extending obliquely and superiorly from right to left, it crosses the inferior aspect of the descending duodenum and pancreatic head and lies along the inferior border of the pancreas throughout the remainder of its course. It terminates near the posterior aspect of the lower pole of the spleen.

The superior surface of the transverse colon is in relationship, from right to left, to the visceral surface of the liver, the gallbladder, and the stomach (Fig. 2.14). The intimacy of these relationships varies with body position, length of the mesocolon, and degree of distention of the stomach. Pathologic processes from the stomach can spread to the transverse colon along the gastrocolic ligament, and from the pancreas between the leaves of the transverse mesocolon (Figs. 2.15 and 2.16).

The attachment of the transverse mesocolon to the retroperitoneum divides the abdominal viscera into those which are supramesocolic (liver, gallbladder, stomach, pancreas, both adrenals, and all but the lower pole of the right kidney) and those which are inframesocolic (small bowel and mesentery, most of the left kidney, sigmoid colon and mesentery, and the female pelvic organs). Abdominal masses can be classified similarly, depending on the direction in which they displace the transverse colon. This concept is helpful in localizing masses on roentgen studies (Figs. 2.17 and 2.18).

The transverse colon lies anteriorly in the abdomen in contrast to the posterior position of the ascending and descending colon. The latter are located with the pancreas and descending duodenum in the anterior pararenal space of the retroperitoneum (Fig. 2.19).

Splenic Flexure

The anatomic splenic flexure (as opposed to what is conventionally called the "splenic flexure" on a barium enema), is one of the more firmly fixed and constant points along the course of the colon. It is located posteriorly, medial to the splenic tip. A fold of peritoneum, the phrenicocolic ligament, holds the flexure in position and helps support the spleen (Fig. 2.9). The "radiographic" splenic flexure is actually the distal transverse colon, and it usually lies along the antero-medial margin of the spleen, descending to reach the anatomic splenic flexure (Figs. 2.20 and 2.21). Since the radiographic splenic flexure is mobile, it may be seen inferior to the anatomic flexure but is usually the most superior portion of the colon as seen on a barium enema.

Descending Colon

From the anatomic splenic flexure, the colon descends retroperitoneally in the left paracolic gutter, reaching the pelvic brim where it again acquires a mesentery and becomes the sigmoid colon.

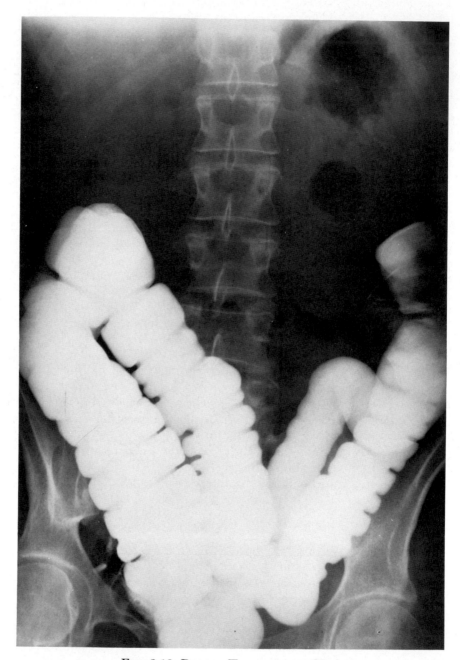

FIG. 2.13. PTOTIC TRANSVERSE COLON

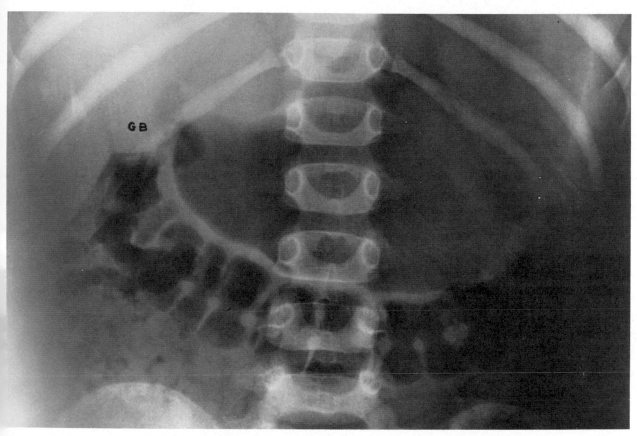

FIG. 2.14. ANATOMIC RELATIONSHIPS OF THE SUPERIOR SURFACE OF THE
TRANSVERSE COLON
Note gallbladder (GB) as well as stomach and right lobe of liver.

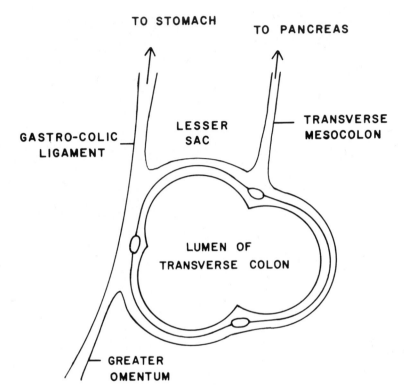

FIG. 2.15. TRANSVERSE MESOCOLON AND GASTROCOLIC LIGAMENT (LATERAL SCHEMATIC VIEW)

Pathologic processes from the stomach may spread to the colon via the gastrocolic ligament, generally involving the superior surface of the transverse colon. Processes from the pancreas may extend through the transverse mesocolon, generally involving the inferior border of the transverse colon.

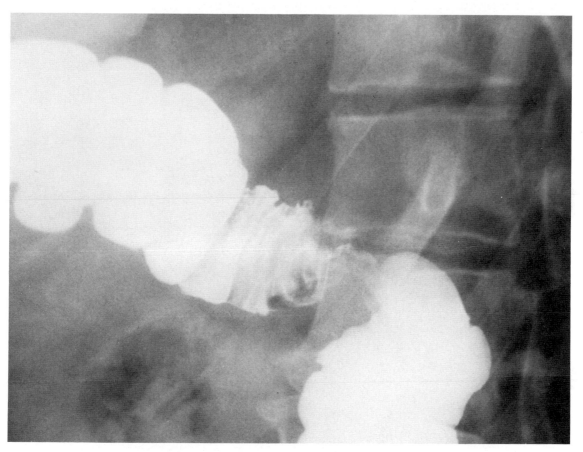

FIG. 2.16. CARCINOMA OF THE TAIL OF THE PANCREAS EXTENDING TO THE
SPLENIC FLEXURE

The transverse mesocolon ends at the splenic flexure (right posterior oblique
view).

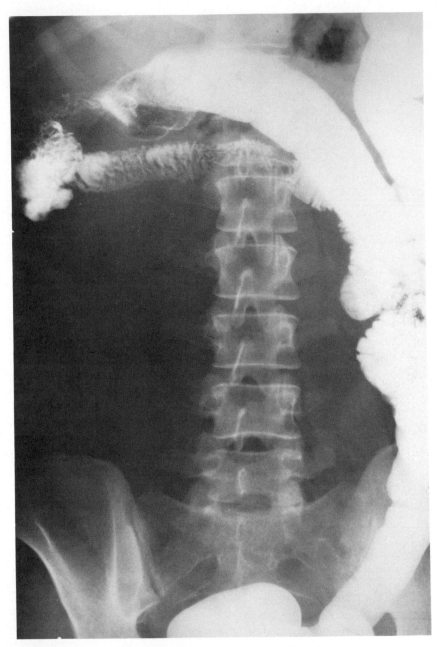

FIG. 2.17. INFRAMESOCOLIC MASS

Huge ovarian cyst elevating transverse colon and cecum (hepatic flexure is contracted).

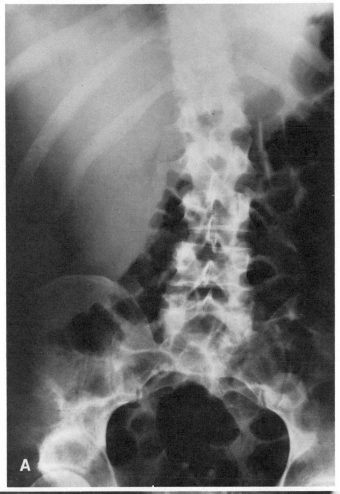

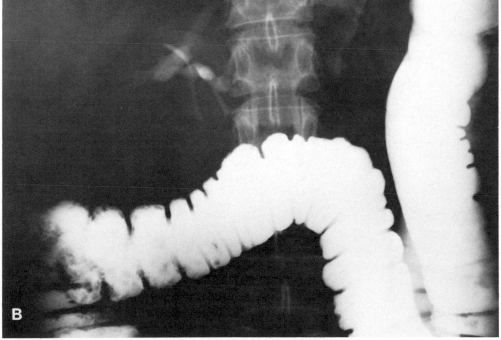

FIG. 2.18. SUPRAMESOCOLIC MASS

(A) Enlarged liver displacing colon inferiorly and medially. (B) Right renal cyst displacing proximal transverse colon inferiorly.

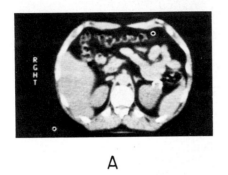 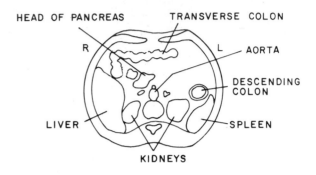

A

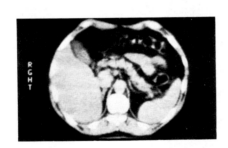 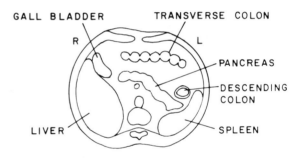

B

FIG. 2.19. NORMAL ANATOMIC RELATIONSHIPS OF THE COLON IN CROSS-SECTION (CT SCAN)

(**A**) The transverse colon lies anteriorly; the descending colon, posteriorly. (**B**) The descending colon and pancreas both lie within the anterior pararenal compartment of the retroperitoneum.

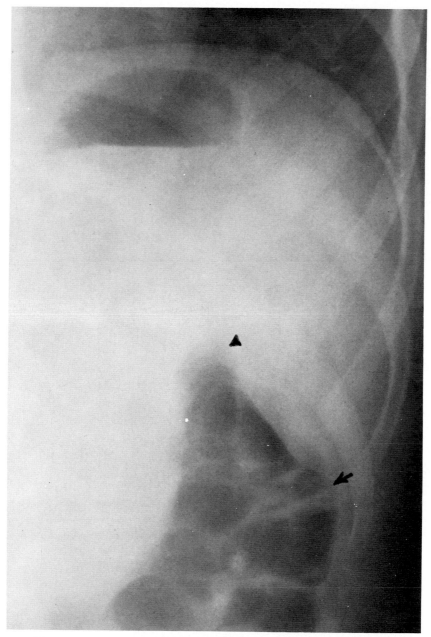

FIG. 2.20. SPLENIC FLEXURE, UPRIGHT CHEST RADIOGRAPH
Anatomic flexure, arrow; radiographic flexure, arrowhead.

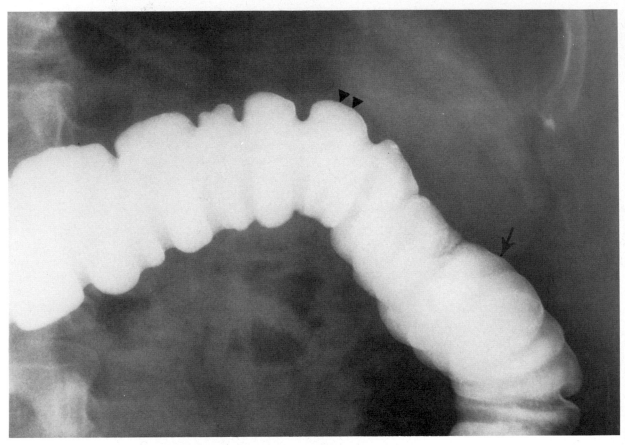

FIG. 2.21. SPLENIC FLEXURE, BARIUM ENEMA
Anatomic flexure, arrow; radiographic flexure, arrowheads.

Sigmoid Colon

Suspended on a V-shaped mesocolon attached to the posterior pelvic wall, the sigmoid colon may descend rather rapidly to join the rectum, or it may form one or two loops in the pelvis before joining it. When elongated (redundant), it is prone to twist (volvulus). The rectosigmoid is that segment of the colon on either side of the junction of the rectum and sigmoid; its exact boundaries cannot be defined on a barium enema.

Rectum

The peritoneum reflects off the anterior surface of the rectum to form the pelvic-cul-de-sac (Fig. 2.10). In the female, the uterus and vagina separate the recto-sigmoid from the bladder, which are adjacent structures in the male. Peritoneum covers the anterior and lateral aspect of the upper third of the rectum but only the anterior aspect of the middle third. The lower rectum is entirely extraperitoneal and bulges to form the rectal ampulla; thus, rectal perforations may be either intra- or extraperitoneal.

On lateral view of the barium-filled rectum, the presacral space (retro-rectal space) usually measures less than 1 cm in width. However, the range of normal is quite variable and this measurement is of limited clinical usefulness.

Anal Canal

The anal canal is approximately 4 cm long and extends through the muscular pelvic floor to the anus. It is capable of less dilatation than the more proximal ampulla. The internal anal sphincter is composed of involuntary smooth muscle. Fortunately, the external sphincter is striated muscle and under voluntary control.

BLOOD SUPPLY

The colon receives its blood supply from the superior and inferior mesenteric arteries.

Superior Mesenteric Artery (Fig. 2.22)

After a variable number of jejunal branches, the superior mesenteric artery gives rise to a constant right-sided branch, the ileo-colic artery. This vessel supplies the cecum, appendix, distal ileum, and variable portions of the ascending colon. Ileal arteries arise from the continuation of the superior mesenteric artery distal to the ileo-colic branch.

The right colic artery is variable in its origin, at times arising from the proximal superior mesenteric artery (38%), the middle colic-right colic trunk (52%), or the ileo-colic artery (8%). It is distributed to portions of the ascending colon and the hepatic flexure. The middle colic artery runs in the transverse mesocolon and supplies the transverse colon. It usually arises from the proximal superior mesenteric artery (44%) or the combined middle colic-right colic trunk (52%) and rarely from the celiac axis. In 3% of individuals, it is absent.

Inferior Mesenteric Artery (Fig. 2.23)

The inferior mesenteric artery gives off the left colic artery and one to three sigmoidal branches before continuing into the pelvis as the superior rectal or hemorrhoidal artery. The rectum also is supplied by the middle and inferior rectal branches of the internal iliac arteries. Abundant intramural anastomoses are present among the rectal arteries forming an important collateral network between the mesenteric and ilio-femoral circulations.

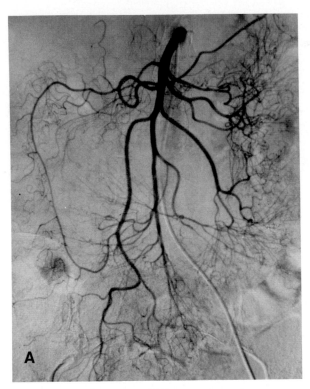

FIG. 2.22. SUPERIOR MESENTERIC ARTERY
(**A**) Arteriogram. (**B**) Schematic (J, jejunal branches; I, ileal branches).

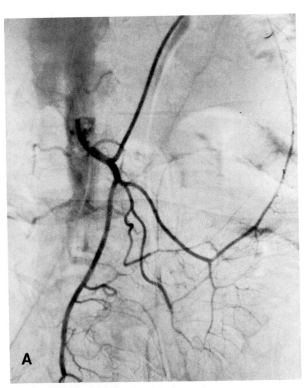

FIG. 2.23. INFERIOR MESENTERIC ARTERY
(**A**) Arteriogram. (**B**) Schematic.

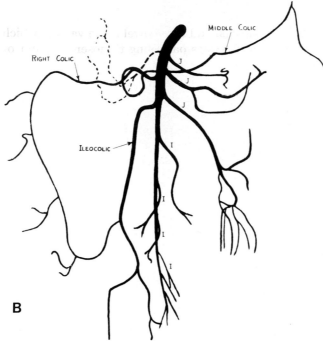

FIG. 2.22B.

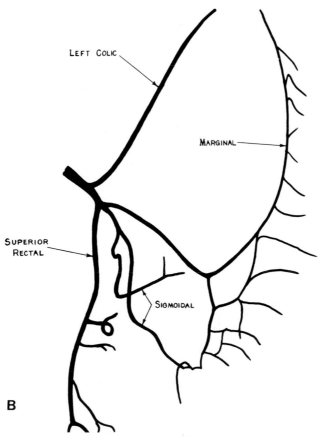

FIG. 2.23B.

Vasa Recta

The functional end-arteries of the small and large bowel are the vasa recta which arise perpendicularly from a series of arcades paralleling the mesenteric border of the intestines (Fig. 2.24). The vasa recta divide into two branches that nearly encircle the bowel wall. These two divisions and their branches penetrate the muscular layer near all three tenia to form a submucosal vascular plexus. The distribution of diverticula has been shown to parallel these sites of muscular perforation, and the domes of the diverticula have been shown to be related intimately to stretched penetrating arteries. These concepts are important in understanding both the formation of diverticula and their tendency to bleed.

Collateral Flow

A direct communication exists almost invariably between the ascending left colic artery and the left branch of the middle colic artery, providing one collateral route between the inferior and superior mesenteric circulations.

A second route is provided by the series of arcades along the mesenteric border of the intestines which form a more or less continuous pathway from the duodenum to the rectum. In the large bowel, this pathway is known as the marginal artery of Drummond; in the small bowel, it is known as the marginal artery of Dwight. Not really a single vessel, the marginal artery of Drummond is made up of portions of either the primary colic arteries themselves or the arcades arising from them, depending on the site of origin of the vasa recta (Fig. 2.24). The marginal artery is frequently absent or deficient at the splenic flexure (Griffith's point) (Fig. 2.25). When a segment is absent, a portion of the colon receives no direct vasa recta but is dependent upon the intramural vascular plexuses for its blood supply. Such

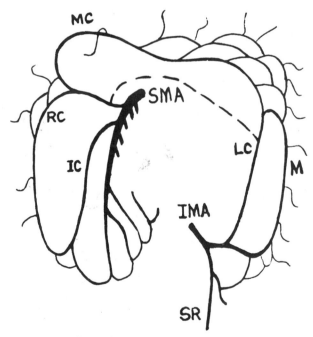

FIG. 2.24. MARGINAL ARTERY

The vasa recta arise perpendicularly from the "marginal" artery which is a more or less continuous series of arcades from the duodenum to the rectum (see text). The arc of Riolan (dashed line) is another, more centrally positioned, anastomotic pathway between the middle (MC) and ascending left colic (LC) arteries.

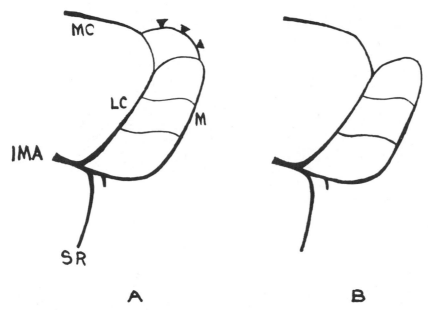

FIG. 2.25. GRIFFITH'S POINT, AT THE JUNCTION OF MIDDLE COLIC AND ASCENDING LEFT COLIC ARTERIES

(**A**) The marginal artery is intact at Griffith's point (arrowheads). (**B**) The marginal artery is absent (see text).

portions are prone to ischemic colitis when blood flow is reduced by obstruction or splanchnic vasoconstriction. The third collateral between the mesenteric arteries is the arc of Riolan, a retroperitoneal vessel which links the proximal portions of the superior and inferior mesenteric arteries (Fig. 2.24).

Mesenteric Veins

The venous drainage parallels the arterial supply. The right colic and middle colic veins empty into the superior mesenteric vein, and the left colic and sigmoidal veins drain into the inferior mesenteric vein. The superior mesenteric vein joins the splenic vein (which has received the inferior mesenteric outflow) to form the portal vein behind the head of the pancreas (Fig. 2.26). The hemorrhoidal venous plexus communicates with the inferior mesenteric and the systemic venous circulations.

LYMPHATIC DRAINAGE

The lymphatic vessels and regional lymph nodes of the colon are distributed along the course of the superior and inferior mesenteric arteries. Drainage from the right colon and transverse colon reaches the superior mesenteric and celiac pre-aortic lymph nodes; drainage from the left colon reaches the left para-aortic lymph nodes. Occasionally, lymphatic vessels from the splenic flexure empty directly into the lymph nodes along the splenic vein. Enlarged superior mesenteric pre-aortic lymph nodes may cause indentations along the superior surface of the horizontal portion of the duodenum; enlarged left para-aortic lymph nodes may compress the lateral aspect of the duodeno-jejunal flexure (ligament of Treitz).

Lymphatic drainage from the rectum is more complex. While the superior rectum may drain into inferior mesenteric or common iliac lymph node groups, most of the rectum is drained by lymphatics that parallel the middle rectal artery. These eventually empty into either internal iliac or presacral lymph nodes. The lower anal canal drains into the superficial inguinal nodes in the groin.

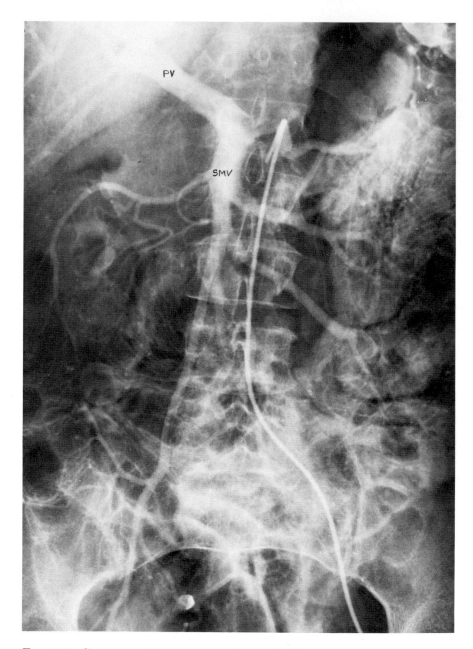

FIG. 2.26. SUPERIOR MESENTERIC VEIN (SMV) AND PORTAL VEIN (PV)
Venous phase of superior mesenteric angiogram.

PHYSIOLOGY

Function

The colon receives the liquid products of digestion (chyme), dehydrates them, and stores them prior to defecation. Dehydration occurs primarily in the proximal half of the colon, storage in the distal half. Approximately 500–1000 ml of chyme passes through the ileocecal valve each day, most of it derived from small bowel secretions. Only 100–200 ml is lost in stool. Chyme is dehydrated by the active transport of sodium across the colonic epithelium accompanied by the osmotic reabsorption of water. A small net loss of potassium results.

The colonic glands secrete an alkaline mucous but no digestive enzyme. A little digestion does occur due to the enzymatic activity of the colonic bacteria. Some of these bacterial fermentation products are absorbed in the colon. Vitamin K is perhaps the most important example.

Composition of Feces

In health the size and composition of the stool is largely dependent upon the diet. A person on a typical western diet passes 100–150 g of feces per day of which ⅔–¾ is water. The solid component is a mixture of dead bacteria, undigested roughage, cell debris, and bile pigment. Raising the intake of vegetable fiber (undigestable carbohydrates) increases the solid phase of the stool as well as the amount of water-soluble substances within it.

Colonic Gas

The normal intestinal tract contains 30–200 ml of gas, much of it found in the colon. Colonic gas is a mixture of swallowed air and variable amounts of carbon dioxide, hydrogen, methane, ammonia, and hydrogen sulfide produced by the intestinal bacteria. Some of these gases are explosive when mixed with oxygen, a potential hazard during colonoscopic polypectomy. Fortunately the colonic bacteria utilize oxygen, creating a relatively anaerobic environment. This coupled with proper pre-colonoscopic bowel preparation essentially eliminates this danger.

An estimated 7–10 liters of gas enters or is formed in the colon each day. Happily most of this is absorbed, an average of only 500 ml of flatus being expelled. Flatus production is increased by adding fiber to the diet, by conditions which reduce the colonic transit time, and by excessive air-swallowing.

Innervation

Colonic smooth muscle is innervated by the parasympathetic and sympathetic divisions of the autonomic nervous system. Classically, their actions are reciprocal: the parasympathetic (cholinergic) system stimulating and the sympathetic (adrenergic) system inhibiting muscle contraction. This is an oversimplification as there is now experimental evidence of the existence of both noncholinergic excitatory fibers and nonadrenergic inhibitory fibers to the colon. In addition, the sympathetic system contracts rather than relaxes the ileo-cecal valve and internal anal sphincter.

The cranial parasympathetic preganglionic motor fibers are distributed to the proximal half of the colon by the vagus nerve; the sacral parasympathetic fibers (S2, S3, and S4) are carried to the left colon, rectum, and anal canal by the splanchnic nerves. Preganglionic fibers synapse with motor neurons in the myenteric plexus from which postganglionic fibers emerge. A single motor fiber may innervate thousands of smooth muscle cells.

Preganglionic fibers of the sympathetic system (T8–L3) pass through the paravertebral ganglia to synapse within the celiac and superior mesenteric ganglia in the abdomen. The postganglionic fibers (adrenergic) are distributed rather uniformly with the mesenteric arteries. These synapse with neurons in the myenteric plexus and with smooth muscle cells directly. β-Adrenergic receptor sites are dominant and inhibit contraction. α-Adrenergic receptors may be excitatory.

Sensory nerves from the colon are distributed with both divisions of the autonomic system. While some of the afferent nerves have cell bodies within the posterior root ganglia of the spine, others have their bodies within the submucosal plexus and synapse within the myenteric plexus. Together the myenteric (predominantly motor) and submucosal (predominantly sensory) plexuses form an intramural nervous system which is capable of restoring colonic motor function following parasympathetic denervation. This process may require weeks or months to be completed. Sympathetic denervation has no appreciable effect on colonic function. Absence or destruction of the myenteric plexus abolishes coordinated motor function in the involved segment. Congenital absence of the plexus is seen in Hirschsprung's disease and results in a functional obstruction. An example of an acquired condition with a similar functional obstruction is Chagas' disease.

Motility

Colonic motor function has been studied by analyzing myoelectrical events (basic electric rhythm), measuring intraluminal pressure changes, and observing patterns of motion with time-lapse cinefluorography. Two patterns dominate: segmentation and mass movement. Neither is exactly analogous to the moving contraction ring of small bowel peristalsis.

Segmentation (haustration) is a kneeding or mixing movement. Weakly propulsive if at all, it tends to oppose the analward progression of the fecal stream, providing time for water reabsorption to occur. It is the major motor activity of the colon, and consists of rather uniformly spaced, stationary rings of contracted circular muscle accompanied by shortening of the tenia. A single haustral pattern may last minutes to hours before being replaced by a new pattern halfway between the first. Segmentation is increased in constipation, decreased in diarrhea. The resistive nature of segmentation explains the apparent paradox.

Mass movement is a propulsive contraction which occurs only a few times a day, generally after meals. It consists of haustral relaxation, the development of a proximal constriction ring, and the nearly simultaneous contraction of a large segment of colon. Feces may be moved ⅓–¾ the length of the colon in seconds.

Excitatory and inhibitory motor reflexes exist, but their neural and humoral control mechanisms remain incompletely understood. Certainly the intramural nervous system, extending from the esophagus to the rectum, plays a central role. Both segmentation and mass movement are stimulated by eating: the gastro-colic and duodeno-colic reflexes. Neither "reflex" is abolished by destruction of the spinal cord, and they are probably mediated by a hormone rather than by the parasympathetic nervous system.

The sympathetic nervous system participates in several reflexes, frequently initiated by pain, which inhibit large and/or small intestinal motor activity. These include the peritoneo-intestinal, reno-intestinal, and somato-intestinal reflexes. Their existence helps explain the frequent occurrence of localized or generalized adynamic ileus in a number of pain-associated conditions.

The defecation reflex is initiated by distention of the rectal ampulla, generally by feces. The resulting afferent impulses stimulate mass movements in the left colon, initially through the intramural plexus but subsequently reinforced powerfully by the sacral parasympathetic system. Simultaneously, the internal sphincter relaxes. Defecation is completed if the voluntary external sphincter is relaxed as well.

EFFECT OF DRUGS AND HORMONES ON COLONIC MOTILITY

Drugs and hormones alter colonic motor function by acting directly on smooth muscle or by acting indirectly through the autonomic nervous system. Some affect the basal muscle tone of the colon as well as segmentation and mass movement; others act more selectively on one or two of these. The action of some drugs is variable depending on the presence or absence of normal muscle tone and the relative balance between the parasympathetic and sympathetic systems at the time of their administration. The development of diarrhea is not a good measure of an agent's effect on motility since it may be induced by excitation of mass movements or inhibition of segmentation. Conversely, constipation may result from generalized atony or excitation of segmentation.

Hormones

Cholecystokinin may be the mediator of the gastro-colic and duodeno-colic reflexes, but this remains unproven.

Gastrin directly relaxes the ileo-cecal valve while stimulating colonic motility. Since partial gastrectomy does not abolish the gastro-colic and dudoeno-colic reflexes, gastrin is not likely to be the mediator hormone. The role of gastrin in normal motility is unknown.

Glucagon (pancreatic) inhibits gastrointestinal motility, probably by direct action on smooth muscle. It has been shown to reduce slow wave electrical activity in the human colon, an effect not blocked by sympatholytic drugs such as propanolol. Radiologists frequently use glucagon to overcome colonic spasm during barium enemas.

Secretin, serotonin, vasoactive intestinal polypeptide (VIP), and prostaglandins all relax colonic smooth muscle, but their physiologic role in the normal colon is unclear. Excess production of any of these inhibitory hormones by tumors or hyperplasias may cause diarrhea, possibly by reducing normal segmentation.

Vasopressin (Pitressin, Pituitrin) stimulates gastrointestinal smooth muscle, particularly in the colon. Intestinal cramping and diarrhea may be observed when Pitressin is infused intra-arterially to control gastrointestinal hemorrhage.

Anticholinergics

Atropine and other anticholinergic drugs act primarily on the proximal colon to reduce segmentation. They are not powerful depressors of motility. Effects are variable as vagal stimulation is only partially blocked. Little if any blockade of the sacral parasympathetic outflow to the distal colon is achieved. Many therapeutic agents have anticholinergic side effects. These include the antihistamines, the antiparkinsonian drugs (excluding levodopa), the phenothiazines, and the tricyclic antidepressants.

Cholinergics

The parasympathomimetic and anticholinesterase group of drugs stimulate smooth muscle contraction. Bethanechol (Urecholine) and neostigmine (Prostigmin) are representative. Both may cause abdominal cramps and diarrhea. Neostigmine, an anticholinesterase, is a particularly powerful stimulant whose effects are only partially blocked by atropine.

Sympatholytics

α- and β-adrenergic blocking agents have a limited effect on colonic motility. Tolazoline (Priscoline), an α-adrenergic blocker, may cause diarrhea. It is administered intra-arterially for its vasodilating effect which promotes visualization of peripheral arteries and the portal venous system during arteriography. Because of its cardiovascular actions it should be used with caution in patients with cerebral-vascular disease, coronary artery disease, and mitral stenosis.

Sympathomimetics

In general the adrenergic drugs relax gastrointestinal smooth muscle. However, in the presence of β-adrenergic blockade, norepinephrine and epinephrine contract colonic smooth muscle, probably through stimulation of the excitatory α-adrenergic receptor sites.

Other Drugs

Morphine and other opiates contract most smooth muscle. In the colon, morphine enhances basal tone, increases the amplitude of segmentation, and constricts the anal sphincter. The frequency of mass movement is sharply reduced and constipation results. Glucagon abolishes these effects.

Cathartics

The cathartics and their use in preparation of the colon for radiographic studies are discussed in Chapter 3.

Table 2.1 summarizes the action of various drugs, hormones, and other stimuli on colonic smooth muscle.

TABLE 2.1
ACTION ON COLONIC SMOOTH MUSCLE

Excitatory	Inhibitory
Cholecystokinin, gastrin	Glucagon, secretin, serotonin, VIP
Parasympathetic nervous system	Sympathetic nervous system
Gastro-colic and duodeno-colic "reflexes"	Painful stimuli via sympathetic reflexes
Parasympathomimetics (cholinergics)	Sympathomimetics (β-adrenergics) and anticholinergics
Opiates (constipating) and vasopressin (diarrheal)	Therapeutic agents with anticholinergic side effects
Distention of colon	
Irritation of colonic mucosa	

BIBLIOGRAPHY

Christensen, J.: The control of gastrointestinal movements: Some old and new views. N. Engl. J. Med., *285:* 85, 1971.

Harvey, R. F.: Hormonal control of gastrointestinal motility. Dig. Dis., *20:* 523, 1975.

Goodman, L. S., and Gilman, A., eds.: *The Pharmacological Basis of Therapeutics*, 5th ed. Macmillan, New York, 1975.

Gray, H.: *Anatomy of the Human Body*, 29th American ed., edited by C. M. Goss. Lea & Febiger, Philadelphia, 1973.

Guyton, A. C.: *Textbook of Medical Physiology*, 5th ed. W. B. Saunders, Philadelphia, 1976.

Hultén, L.: Regulation of colonic motility and blood flow. Nutr. Rev., *35:* 38, 1977.

Levitt, M. D.: Volume and composition of human intestinal gas determined by means of an intestinal washout technique. N. Engl. J. Med., *284:* 1394, 1971.

Meyers, M. A.: *Dynamic Radiology of the Abdomen*. Springer Verlag, New York, 1976.

Meyers, M. A., Volberg, F., Katzen, B., Alonso, D., and Abbott, G.: The angioarchitecture of colonic diverticula—Significance in bleeding diverticulosis. Radiology, *108:* 249, 1973.

Meyers, M. A.: Griffith's point: Critical anastomosis at the splenic flexure. Am. J. Roentgenol., *126:* 77, 1976.

Nebesar, R. A., Kornblith, P. L., Pollard, J. J., and Michels, N. A.: *Celiac and Superior Mesen-*

teric Arteries. Little, Brown and Co., Boston, 1969.

Ritchie, J. A.: Colonic motor activity and bowel function. I. Normal movements of contents. Gut, *9:* 442, 1968.

Sodeman, W. A. Jr., and Sodeman, W. A. Sr.: *Pathologic Physiology,* 5th ed. W. B. Saunders, Philadelphia, 1974.

Taylor, I., Duthie, H. L., Cumberland, D. C., and

Smallwood, R.: Glucagon and the colon. Gut, *16:* 973, 1975.

Whalen, J. P.: Radiology of the abdomen: Anatomic basis. Lea & Febiger, Philadelphia, 1976.

Vander, A. J., Sherman, J. H., and Luciano, D. S.: *Human Physiology—The Mechanisms of Body Function,* 2nd ed. McGraw-Hill, New York, 1975.

3

Techniques of Colon Examination

JACK R. DREYFUSS, M.D., AND MURRAY L. JANOWER, M.D.

INTRODUCTION

The radiologic literature is replete with variations on the theme of performing a barium enema. Much has been written about the superiority of certain laxatives, barium mixtures, apparatus, and the relative merit of using either a single-contrast barium technique or a double-contrast barium and air method. It should be emphasized that there is no one perfect technique. Experience and judgment eventually guide one to a choice of materials and procedures which are both flexible and rewarding for a given patient or problem to be evaluated.

The absolute key to a successful study, however, is preparation. Since most patients can be properly prepared if an effective regimen has been both prescribed and administered, the radiologist must adopt a strict program for bowel preparation and *insist* that it be carried out. Otherwise, the examination should not be performed. The bottomless pit into which an unwary radiologist may easily fall is the one filled with the residue of a poorly prepared colon and lined with unimaginative x-ray films from a mediocre examination (Figs. 3.1 and 3.2).

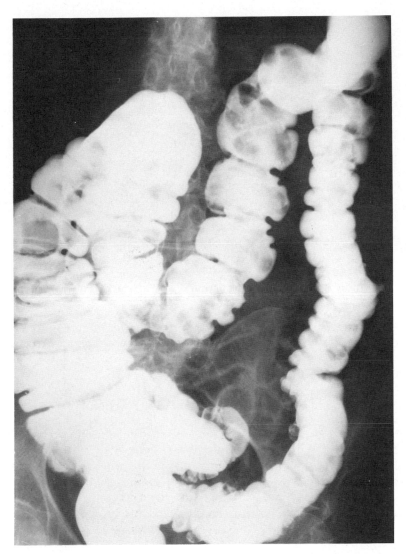

FIG. 3.1. FECAL FILLED COLON

Numerous filling defects, representing fecal balls, are present throughout the length of the colon.

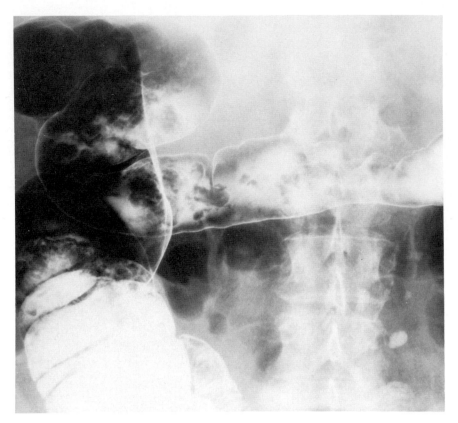

FIG. 3.2. APPEARANCE OF FECAL MATERIAL IN A PRIMARY AIR-CONTRAST ENEMA
The proximal transverse colon is studded with fecal debris of varying size and shape.

PREPARATION OF THE COLON

Until the recent past, the standard preparation for a barium enema was lax or marginal at best. It involved 24 hr on a low-residue diet, castor oil on the late afternoon before the day of examination, and a tap water enema in the evening. Numerous studies have shown that this type of preparation will not satisfactorily clean out even the majority of patients. Results from the more vigorous bowel preparations used for double-contrast examinations and colonoscopies have been so much better than the older 1-day preparation that it should now be abandoned. In its place, either a 48- or 72-hr castor oil preparation or a magnesium citrate preparation should be the standard. These will be discussed below.

Two-Day Preparation Using Castor Oil

For this or any other bowel preparation, the nursing and dietary services or the patient and his family should be provided with explicit, but understandable, written instructions, such as those given in Table 3.1. Whether the patient is to have a barium enema in a department of radiology of a hospital or in a radiologist's private office, the preparation should begin 2 days before the examination when a minimal residue diet is instituted (Table 3.2). Two nights before the enema examination, an adult patient should take 2 ounces (4 tablespoons) of milk of magnesia in half a glass of water before bedtime. On the day before the examination, the patient is instructed to have a clear liquid diet for all three meals and between meals (Table

TABLE 3.1

PREPARATION INSTRUCTIONS FOR EXAMINATION OF THE COLON (BARIUM ENEMA)

1. Two days before examination, have only a minimal residue diet for all three meals.
2. Two nights before examination, take 2 ounces (4 tablespoons) of milk of magnesia in half a glass of water, before bedtime.
3. On the day before the examination, have a clear liquid diet for all three meals, and between meals. No solid food should be eaten.
4. At 5:00 P.M. on the day before examination (unless otherwise directed by the patient's physician), take 2 ounces (4 tablespoons) of castor oil.
5. At about 10:00 P.M. on the evening before examination, take a cleansing enema. Use 1½ quarts of lukewarm water. (Patient should lie on the left side as the first 1/3 of the enema runs in, on the back for the middle 1/3, and on the right side as the last 1/3 runs in.)
6. Take a second cleansing enema on the morning of examination.
7. If examination is scheduled before noon, have only a clear liquid diet for breakfast.
8. If examination is scheduled in the afternoon, have only a clear liquid diet for breakfast and lunch.

TABLE 3.2

MINIMAL RESIDUE DIET

The minimal residue diet may be used in preparation for x-ray examinations of the large bowel when it is desirable to reduce fecal residue to an absolute minimum. The minimal residue diet is not adequate in vitamins and minerals and should not be used for more than several days at a time. This diet strictly limits the intake of milk, overcooked meat or eggs, and avoids fruit and raw or cooked vegetables.

Foods Allowed on Minimal Residue Diet	Foods Not Allowed on Minimal Residue Diet
MILK—Three-fourths to one cup daily, including that used in cooking	More than one cup of milk or milk beverages daily
BEVERAGES—Tea, coffee, decaffeinated coffee, powdered fruit drinks, carbonated beverages	
EGGS—Hard cooked	Raw eggs or soft cooked eggs
MEATS—Broiled, baked, roasted chicken, turkey, beef, lamb, veal, liver, white fish, crisp bacon	Fried or highly seasoned items such as prepared luncheon meats; cheese
BREAD—White bread and saltines	Dark breads and graham crackers; or breads containing bran, nuts, fruits, and seeds
CEREAL—Refined such as farina, rice, cream of rice, Rice Krispies, cornflakes; plain macaroni, noodles, spaghetti.	All other cereals; meat or tomato sauces
VEGETABLES—White potato without skin	All other vegetables
FRUITS—Juice only	All other fruits
DESSERT—Clear gelatin desserts without fruit, angel cake and non-milk sherbet	All others
FATS—Butter, margarine, crisp bacon (cream is part of milk allowance)	All others
SEASONINGS—Clear broth or bouillon, sugar, honey, pure sugar candy, jelly, corn syrup, salt; pepper in small amounts if desired.	All others

3.3). No solid food is allowed. At 5:00 P.M. on the day before the examination, an adult patient should take 2 ounces (4 tablespoons) of castor oil.

Three subjects that are poorly understood and require special attention are the taking of castor oil by the patient, the proper method of administering a preparatory enema, and the role of the radiology department in their administration.

Castor Oil

Castor oil can be made more palatable by mixing it with a carbonated beverage, fruit juice, or warm liquids with a strong flavor of their own, such as beef broth or

TABLE 3.3

CLEAR LIQUID DIET

A clear liquid diet may be used in preparation for x-ray examinations of the large bowel. This diet supplies fluids, but is inadequate in calories and all food elements and should be used only as specified in the Preparation Instructions for Examination of the Colon (Table 3.1).

Liquids Allowed
Water, ice, tea, coffee or decaffeinated coffee
Carbonated beverages
Clear bouillon, consomme, broth
Plain gelatin desserts, non-milk sherbet
Juices: apple, grape and lemonade
Sugar, salt

coffee, or by taking it several minutes after sucking on cracked ice to deaden the taste receptors in the tongue. The active principle in castor oil, ricinoleic acid, is released in the small intestine, and markedly stimulates the small bowel through mucosal irritation; the colon is stimulated very little. The rapid progress of small bowel contents through the colon prevents water resorption and semifluid stools result. There are no absolute contraindications to the use of castor oil other than suspected obstruction or perforation of the bowel, or in the case of patients with acute fulminating colitis who are bleeding or who have had recent major bleeding from the colon. It may be judicious to withhold castor oil when there is a question of acute diverticulitis, appendicitis, or in a severely debilitated patient. Even patients with chronic ulcerative colitis should be prepared.

How to Give a Preparatory Enema

On the night before the barium enema, additional bowel preparation is achieved by a tap-water cleansing enema at about 10:00 P.M., or after the castor oil has had its greatest effect. The prime purpose of this evening enema is to loosen particulate material and bring the remaining feces toward the lower bowel from whence it can be expelled during the night or the following morning.

Most patients, nurses, and doctors are totally unaware of the proper way to give a cleansing enema. If not given properly, it can be either miserably uncomfortable, worthless, or both. An enema bag with a good clamping device on the tubing is filled with 2000 cc of lukewarm tap water. With the patient lying supine in bed, or on the bathroom floor, the bag is hung no higher than 1 m above the level of the rectum. Initial inflow should be slow with several pauses so as not to overdistend the rectum or sigmoid and cause severe cramping which may prevent further filling of the colon. Patients should be advised that they may feel rectal pressure and cramps, and a definite urge to have a bowel movement during the enema. Patients should be instructed to breathe in and out through their mouth and attempt to retain the enema until the entire 2000 cc have been administered. The first third of the enema should be given with the patient turned to his left. The next third is given with the patient on his back, and the final third with the patient turned to his right. In this way, no one area is allowed to become overdistended and gravity is used to induce filling rather than hydrostatic pressure. The entire 2000 cc can be administered within a period of several minutes using this method.

The Role of the Radiology Department in Preparatory Enemas

On the morning of the barium examination, a second cleansing enema should be given. This second enema is best given in the department of radiology; a special enema aide can be trained in the technique of proper enema administration. A separate room should be set aside for the administration of these preparatory tap-water enemas. Although special tables and equipment are available to facilitate the administration of the preparatory enema, they can equally well be given on radiographic tables or stretchers. In those departments where special facilities or personnel are not available, the preparatory enema can be given by a trained x-ray technologist in the fluoroscopic room. It should be emphasized that a preparatory enema can be rapidly administered to most patients. However, adequate time must be allowed for the patients to completely evacuate their colon before the barium enema is performed. For some patients, this will take between 30 and 60 min. With the proper attention to scheduling of examinations, the fluoroscopy rooms can be used in such a manner that both preparatory and barium enemas can be administered in the same rooms without significantly delaying the fluoroscopic schedule.

Three-Day Preparation Using Castor Oil

For some patients, a 3-day bowel preparation should be carried out, particularly in the case of obscure intestinal bleeding, whenever a polyp study is done, or an examination for a "final decision." Many radiologists use such a meticulous preparation on a routine basis. The cleansing procedure and diet lists in Tables 3.1 and 3.2 may be used for this 3-day colon preparation. The only difference from the 2-day preparation is an additional day at the beginning, during which the patient will also follow a minimal residue diet and take 2 ounces of milk of magnesia before bedtime.

Magnesium Citrate Preparation

An entirely different sort of preparatory procedure using magnesium citrate has gained widespread acceptance in the last few years. This procedure has the advantage of requiring less time than the castor oil preparation; many radiologists claim it is more gentle on patients and the resulting bowel preparation is superior to that obtained with castor oil.

There are many modifications of the magnesium citrate preparation but a procedure in common use begins at noon on the day before the examination. The preparation is delineated in Table 3.4.

TABLE 3.4

MAGNESIUM CITRATE PREPARATION INSTRUCTIONS FOR EXAMINATION OF THE COLON (BARIUM ENEMA)

Time	Directions	Check as Completed
12 noon	LUNCH—Eat only a minimal residue diet	
1 P.M.	Drink at least one full glass or more or water, soda, or clear juice	
3 P.M.	Drink at least one full glass or more of water, soda, or clear juice	
5 P.M.	SUPPER—Eat only a clear liquid diet	
7 P.M.	Drink at least one full glass or more of water, soda, or clear juice	
8 P.M.	Drink one bottle of magnesium citrate (cold)	
10 P.M.	Take three *bisacodyl tablets** with at least one full glass or more of water	
	Do not crush or chew tablets. Swallow them whole. Do not take tablets within 1 hr of antacids or milk	
12 Midnight	Drink at least one full glass or more of water, soda or clear juice	
7 A.M.	BREAKFAST—Eat only a clear liquid diet and drink at least one full glass of water	

Prior to the x-ray examination, a cleansing tap-water enema is administered

* Brand name "Dulcolax."

In summary, preparatory regimes using either castor oil or magnesium citrate must not only be prescribed, but carried out. The single most effective step for ensuring proper bowel preparation is the administration of a tap-water enema in the department. There will still be some patients, however, whose colons will not be clean even if a tap-water enema has been properly given.

SEQUENCE OF SIGMOIDOSCOPY OR COLONOSCOPY AND THE BARIUM ENEMA

A question is frequently raised about the advisability of performing a barium enema on the same day that a sigmoidoscopy or colonoscopy is done. Ideally, the barium enema should not follow these procedures because a large quantity of air is introduced into the colon and spasm is frequently induced by instrumentation. However, from a practical point of view, the patients have already undergone rigorous preparation for either a sigmoidoscopy or particularly colonoscopy, and it may *not* be advisable to delay the patient's barium enema for an additional day. A 3-day delay is advised, however, if a biopsy was performed at the time of endoscopy.

SEQUENCE OF GASTROINTESTINAL AND COLON EXAMINATIONS

Traditionally, a barium enema examination has been performed prior to an upper GI series because residual barium in the small bowel or colon from any previous study is sufficient reason to cancel a non-emergency barium enema. However, with the advent of more widespread utilization of preliminary tap-water enemas in the radiology department, this is no longer the case. In fact, some radiologists prefer to do the GI series first so that the amount of residual barium in the colon can be used as a mark of the adequacy of colonic cleansing.

PRELIMINARY FILM OF ABDOMEN AND HISTORY

Both emergency and routine barium enemas should be preceded by a preliminary film of the abdomen, and the enema should not be started until this important film has been studied by the fluoroscopist. Not only is the adequacy of colonic preparation determined from this film, but the bones, soft tissue, air-filled structures, and areas of calcification that might later be obscured by barium are evaluated.

The fluoroscopist should insist on receiving a brief but pertinent history from the referring physician and should question and examine the patient before starting the enema, including the performance of a rectal examination, if indicated. The radiologist should then devise a plan for the examination including whatever special techniques and views seem appropriate for the patient and the problem presented. All too often, the same "routine" enema is performed on every patient regardless of physical findings or clinical presentation.

BARIUM ENEMA

Materials—Barium Mixtures and Additives

The formulation and manufacturing of commercial barium mixtures is a complex subject. Few radiologists take the time to investigate and understand the physics and chemistry of barium suspensions or their behavioral characteristics, much less to become familiar with the innumerable additives that may be present. With the availability of a number of standardized, effective products on the market, it is the rare radiologist who still uses a "homemade" barium mixture. The decision as to which barium to use is most often reached on the basis of current articles in the literature, product information provided by the manufacturer, and on one's own experience.

In the past, a satisfactory mixture was prepared by gradually adding 1200 cc of lukewarm water to 300 cc of U.S.P. barium. The mixture was then blended thoroughly in an electric blender. In order to stabilize the barium suspension and enhance mucosal coating, 300 cc of 5% carboxymethylcellulose was often substituted for 300 cc of the water. With thorough blending, this would result in an optimal 1% concentration of the suspending agent in the total 1500 cc of barium mixture for one colon examination. It was also the general practice to add sufficient tannic acid to the mixture for a 0.2–1.0% concentration. The tannic acid acted to precipitate protein from the surface of the bowel, thus improving the mucosal coating with barium. In addition, tannic acid acted as an astringent increasing peristaltic activity and causing a more complete evacuation of the enema. This all resulted in a more reliable postevacuation mucosal pattern. However, in March, 1964, the Food and Drug Administration issued a ban on the use of tannic acid in either cleansing or barium enemas following the reporting of alleged cases of liver necrosis and death secondary to the use of tannic acid. In spite of the lack of confirmation of these findings or the discovery of additional cases of such a complication, the Food and Drug Administration has continued its ban on the use of tannic acid. However, the FDA has sanctioned the use of a commercial preparation (Clysodrast) in which a strictly measured amount of tannic acid is the active ingredient. Accordingly, many radiologists add one or two packages of this preparation to the tap-water cleansing enema or the barium enema mixture.

In most departments and private offices, commercial barium mixtures are now used in which given amounts of barium and additives are supplied in bulk or liquid form as well as in plastic bags with attached tubing and a variety of enema tips for either single- or double-contrast enemas (Fig. 3.3). The amount of added water determines the concentration. For stability, fresh mixing and thorough blending or shaking are recommended before use.

Much has been written about barium sulfate suspensions and the advantages and disadvantages of the various brands available. There is a whole terminology applicable to the manufacture, testing, and performance of barium mixtures, such as grain size, density, film thickness, suspension, viscosity, foaming, flow, miscibility, adherence, agglutination, settling, flocculation, and sedimentation, among many others. It is sufficient in this age of multiple choices to become familiar with the characteristics of one or two commercial products.

Since the characteristics of each product differ, so will the recommended weight/volume or weight/weight concentration for various types of gastrointestinal examinations. For example, a 60% weight/weight concentration may be ideal for a primary air contrast examination with one brand whereas another brand may require a 30% weight/weight concentration for the same study. By personal experience, the radiologist can determine the ideal concentration to provide the suspension, density, flow rate, coating and absence of frothing, flocculation, and flaking which will consistently result in films of high diagnostic quality for single or double contrast examinations.

With regard to commercial barium preparations, it is, however, important to know that the manufacturers add various additives to their mixture which have a calculated effect on such factors as suspension, miscibility, coating, and even taste. (Most mixtures, depending on the amount of added water, are designed for use in either upper gastrointestinal or colon studies.) The specific additives in any given product

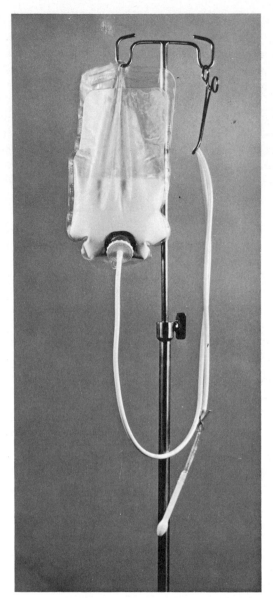

FIG. 3.3. DISPOSABLE PLASTIC ENEMA BAG AND TUBING READY FOR USE
The bag contains 1500 cc of an enema mixture.

are usually unknown to the radiologist since the Food and Drug Administration does not as yet require their listing on labels. Moreover, the manufacturers jealously guard their formulations as trade secrets. Among the known additives, some of which are surely in each company's barium mixture, are: carboxymethylcellulose, simethicone, acacia, tragacanth, polyethylene glycol, carragheenan, aluminum hydroxide gel, sodium citrate, polyoxethylene monooleate, colloidal silica, bentonite, artificial flavorings and, probably, many others.

The addition of such ingredients raises the possibility that a patient may have an unexpected topical or systemic allergic reaction of minor or major magnitude during the course of a barium enema, or shortly thereafter. While the proven occurrence of such reactions has not yet been reported in the literature, we are personally aware of one near fatal reaction and have heard of several others. The radiologist must, therefore, be alerted to this potential hazard and be prepared to render effective emergency treatment.

Single-Contrast Enema

Although there is a strong trend toward the double-contrast colon examination, most barium enemas performed in this country still utilize the single-contrast or single-column technique. Because it is the oldest technique and still in wide use, it will be described first. By definition, this method involves filling of the entire colon with barium under fluoroscopic control followed by the obtaining of a number of spot-films and large films of the barium-filled colon. The patient then expels the enema and postevacuation mucosal relief films are made. (If an air-contrast study is indicated, the colon of the patient is then partially refilled with a thicker barium mixture and this is distributed around the colon by air insufflation. Such a procedure is termed a secondary air-contrast examination.)

Fluoroscopic Examination

Barium enemas should only be done under fluoroscopic observation and with an assistant controlling the inflow of barium as directed by the radiologist. If properly done, the enema need not be an unpleasant experience for the patient. The secret is in controlled inflow and the use of position and gravity rather than force.

The enema tip should be carefully inserted either by the radiologist or by a well-trained and gentle assistant. If there are hemorrhoids, or if there is rectal spasm, the well-lubricated enema tip should be placed against the anus and held there with gentle sustained forward pressure until the anal ring relaxes enough to allow the enema tip to slip through. It can then be advanced toward the sacrum without discomfort. A very unhappy patient and an angry colon will be the certain results if an enema tip is used as if it were a meat skewer.

For elderly patients, or patients with a very lax anal sphincter, it may be necessary to use a catheter with an inflatable balloon tip. A variety of inflatable balloon tips are commercially available (Fig. 3.4). In general, a Bardex catheter is the prototype of such a dispensing tip. Fifty to 100 cc of air introduced from a syringe will usually be sufficient to prevent leakage. Because of the danger of bowel perforation, balloon catheters should not be used in patients with known rectal disease of any kind, diverticulitis, or ulcerative colitis. Inflation of the balloon should be done by the radiologist. The greatest danger of perforating a normal colon with a balloon retention catheter occurs when the balloon is overinflated while it is in the rectosigmoid rather than in the more distensible rectal ampulla. The rectosigmoid is fixed in position and narrowed by the peritoneal reflection. The rectal ampulla is not so constricted being surrounded only by pelvic soft tissues; it is also of larger diameter than the rectosigmoid. The insufflation of the balloon can usually be performed without fluoroscopic observation. To avoid malpositioning the balloon catheter, it should be pulled back against the anal sphincter after 50 cc of air have been instilled by syringe. Further inflation should then be carried out with the balloon safely seated in the rectal ampulla (Fig. 3.5). In general fewer than 10% of the patients will require a balloon catheter.

The use of a balloon catheter in a colostomy is not suggested, as colostomies have been lacerated by inflated balloons. One may, however, inflate the balloon of a Foley or Bardex catheter outside the patient and then insert the protruding tip of the catheter into the colostomy, the patient holding the balloon as an occluding mechanism by pressing it against the colostomy stoma from the outside. A more satisfactory, simple technique is to insert a thin catheter through the cut tip of a baby's nursing nipple as shown in Fig. 3.6. The advantage of this method is that the

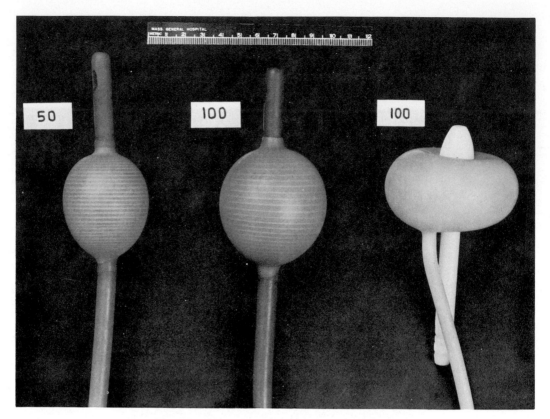

FIG. 3.4. BALLOON RETENTION CATHETERS

The amount of air in each balloon is indicated. The plastic enema tip and balloon on the right are disposable. When inflated with 100 cc of air, the center balloon measures 5.8 cm in transverse diameter.

catheter can be easily placed into the colostomy as far as required; the nipple tip easily fits inside the colostomy stoma and acts as an excellent tampon which the patient maintains in position with his hand.

The prime purpose of fluoroscopy during a barium enema examination is to control inflow, to spot-film any pathology demonstrated, and to study areas which may not be adequately recorded on overhead films of the filled colon. The enema bag should be hung about 1 m above the level of the table, never higher. Before starting the inflow of barium, the patient should be reassured that the examiner will be gentle and that there will be as little discomfort as possible. The patient should also be encouraged both to let the examiner know if there is discomfort and to do his or her best to retain the enema. This little extra explanation and reassurance is more valuable than a dozen retention catheters.

The patient, lying on his back, is then turned about 30° to the left. As soon as the rectal ampulla fills, it is wise to stop the inflow for a few seconds until the rectum adjusts to distention. The rectosigmoid and sigmoid may then be filled with similar pauses. As these segments of the lower bowel fill, it may be necessary to turn the patient slowly back and forth to uncoil loops and achieve uniform filling. With barium inflow stopped, fluoroscopic spot-films should be obtained of the filled rectosigmoid and sigmoid in whatever position best uncoils these segments.

Gradual filling may then continue with the fluoroscopist always watching the head of the barium column as it advances through the colon. As barium reaches the splenic flexure, the patient should be turned back into the supine position and, as barium begins to cross the transverse colon, the patient should be turned to his

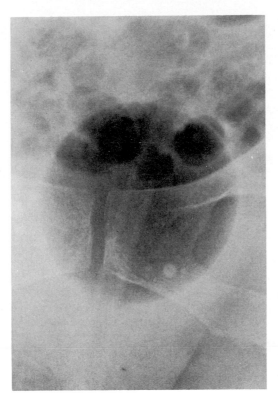

FIG. 3.5. BALLOON RETENTION CATHETER PROPERLY POSITIONED IN RECTAL AMPULLA
As radiographed, the balloon contains 100 cc of air, but it was first seated in the ampulla with only 50 cc of air in the balloon.

right to allow gravity to aid the flow of barium. At this point, it may also be helpful to ask the patient to take slow deep breaths in and out through the open mouth. This distracts the patient, enhances muscle relaxation, and utilizes the changes in intra-abdominal pressure to assist in passage of barium through the colon.

The filling of the cecum can be enhanced if the fluoroscopist uses his gloved hand for gentle ballottement over the cecal area. This acts to draw barium into the cecum; in other words, it is the release of pressure rather than the application of pressure which sucks barium into the cecum. Another helpful maneuver to fill the cecum is to turn the patient into the prone position or to move the table into the erect position. Since the cecum lies relatively anterior within the peritoneal cavity, this change in position more fully utilizes gravity. An attempt should be made to reflux barium into the terminal ileum (unless an air-contrast study is to follow) and in about 90% of patients, the ileo-cecal valve is sufficiently incompetent for this to occur. Occasionally, manual pressure on the filled cecum may assist in causing reflux.

Once the colon is filled, the cecal area and the flexures may be recorded on spot-films. At the same time, any areas of suspicion that were encountered during inflow of the barium should be rechecked. The fluoroscopist with his ability to visualize an abnormality directly is in a much better position to obtain appropriate films of a lesion than a technologist taking overhead films. Very rarely should a lesion be seen on a large film that has not been seen, appreciated, and documented at fluoroscopy. The well-trained fluoroscopist can perform a routine barium enema in 2 min of fluoroscopic time or less.

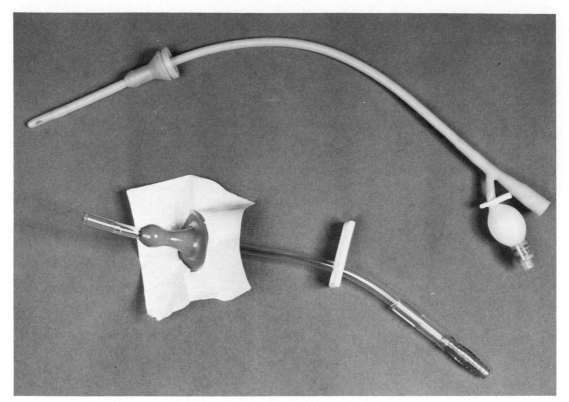

FIG. 3.6. COLOSTOMY ENEMA DEVICES

(Upper) This device was fashioned by passing the tip of a Foley catheter through the cut end of a rubber baby's nipple. (Lower) A manufactured device with plastic tubing and nipple. The square piece of plastic is coated with an adhesive which firmly seals the device to the skin around the colostomy stoma. With both devices, after the enema tube has been threaded into the colon, the nipple is inserted into the colostomy stoma as a plug to prevent leakage of the enema.

Roentgenographic Examination

Standard views

A number of relatively easy-to-achieve overhead views have been used over the years to record the basic facts of a barium enema examination. Of most value have been 14 × 17 inch films of the filled colon taken in the posteroanterior (Fig. 3.7) and left posterior oblique positions (Fig. 3.8) together with a posteroanterior film taken after evacuation (Fig. 3.9). These views will be adequate to demonstrate the entire colon in many patients but will fall short of the mark in patients with a redundant rectosigmoid and sigmoid and with flexures that are difficult to unravel.

Additional basic views which may be necessary to demonstrate the entire colon are: lateral rectal (Fig. 3.10), supine, and prone views in various degrees of patient obliquity, and the lateral decubitus view taken with a horizontal x-ray beam. Any of these films may be taken of the filled or evacuated colon. A judicious choice of one or two of them will complement the commonly used standard views to give a more thorough survey of the large bowel.

Special views

Since the rectosigmoid and sigmoid are the most difficult segments of the colon to see at fluoroscopy and the most awkward to radiograph, special views may be

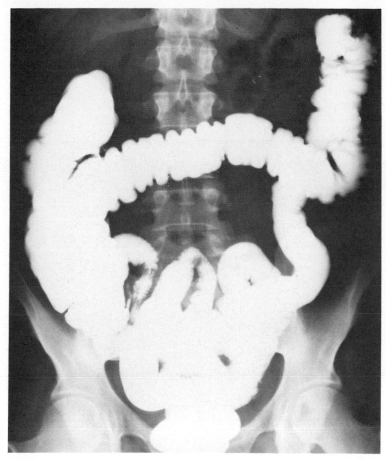

FIG. 3.7. POSTEROANTERIOR FILM

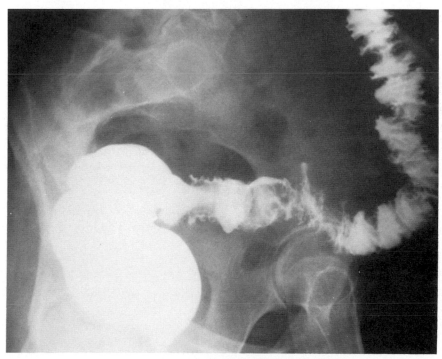

FIG. 3.8. LEFT POSTERIOR OBLIQUE FILM
This projection is particularly useful to demonstrate the sigmoid colon. There is a 3.5-cm polypoid tumor in the midsigmoid.

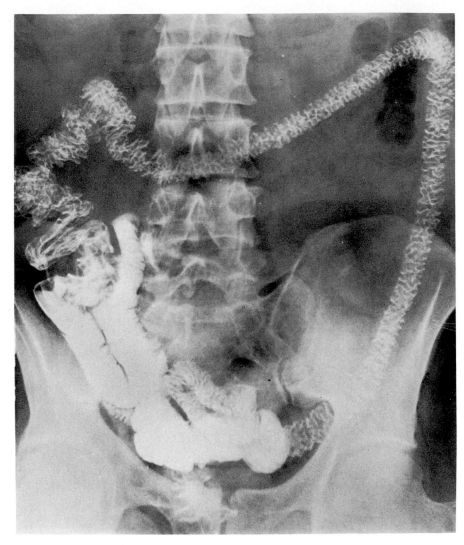

FIG. 3.9. POSTEVACUATION FILM

The bowel is contracted and without haustral markings. The mucosa has a finely crenated pattern.

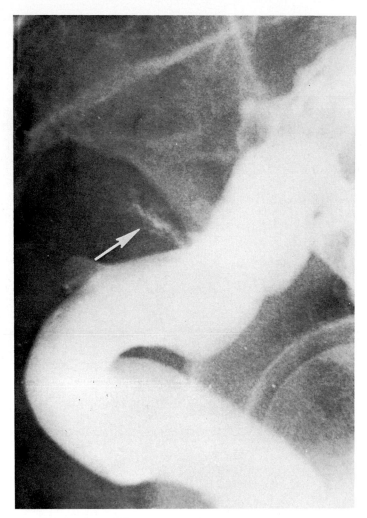

FIG. 3.10. LATERAL RECTAL VIEW

Diverticulitis with a microperforation (arrow) and an abscess in the presacral space.

necessary to uncoil the loops and to overcome foreshortening. Experience has shown that the angled oblique, Chassard-Lapiné, and the posteroanterior angled views are of great value. No one view is superior, but rather one or more of them should be selected as best suits the colon being examined and the lesion that has been shown at fluoroscopy or is suspected of being present.

An angled oblique view can be obtained with the patient turned 10–40° into either the left or the right posterior oblique position, depending on how the sigmoid loop was best uncoiled at fluoroscopy, and angling the central beam 35° toward the head.

The Chassard-Lapiné view is obtained by having the patient sit on the long side of the table with his feet resting on a stool and his buttocks as far back on the table as possible (Fig. 3.11). By bending forward and grasping his ankles, the pelvic outlet and the sigmoid colon are placed in a position parallel to the film. With a 14 × 17 inch film in the Bucky tray, its long axis in the long axis of the table, the central beam from the overhead tube is then directed through the sacrum and an exposure is made using factors for a lateral view of the pelvis (Fig. 3.12). Obviously, the enema tip must be removed prior to obtaining this view. A patient with a protruberant abdomen may be unable to assume the required degree of forward bending.

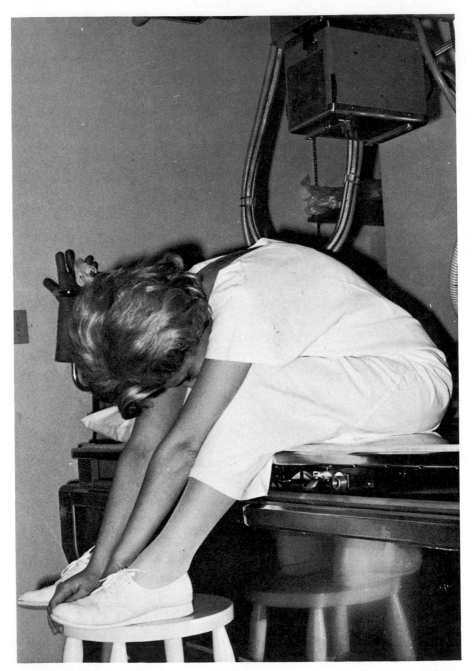

FIG. 3.11. POSITION OF PATIENT FOR OBTAINING THE CHASSARD-LAPINÉ VIEW

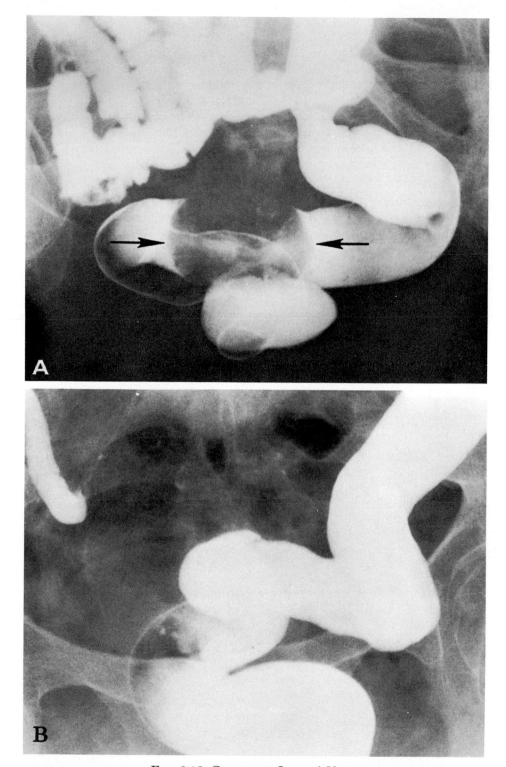

FIG. 3.12. CHASSARD-LAPINÉ VIEW
(A) Annular carcinoma of the sigmoid colon is well demonstrated on this special
view (arrows). (B) The lesion cannot be seen on routine posteroanterior view.

Finally, the posteroanterior angled view of the lower colon has proved so valuable that it should be a routine film in every barium enema examination. It may demonstrate small polypoid tumors of the rectosigmoid and sigmoid that were not seen at fluoroscopy or on any standard view. This film is obtained with the patient prone and the tube angled 35° toward the feet, the central beam passing through the symphysis pubis (Fig. 3.13). It is equally valuable in full or evacuation films as well as in air-contrast examinations (Fig. 3.14).

An angled view can also be made as an anteroposterior film for patients who cannot be placed in the prone position. For this variation, the tube is angled 35° toward the head, the patient lying supine on the table.

Double-Contrast Enemas

The double-contrast examination has been performed in as many ways as there have been radiologists writing on the subject. The major variables have included the preparation, the amount and type of barium used, the technique for filling the colon with a barium mixture, and the timing of insufflation.

Secondary Air-Contrast Technique

When an air-contrast examination is done following a single-contrast barium enema, it is essential that the patient be instructed to evacuate as much of the barium as fast as possible and return promptly to the fluoroscopy room. If this is

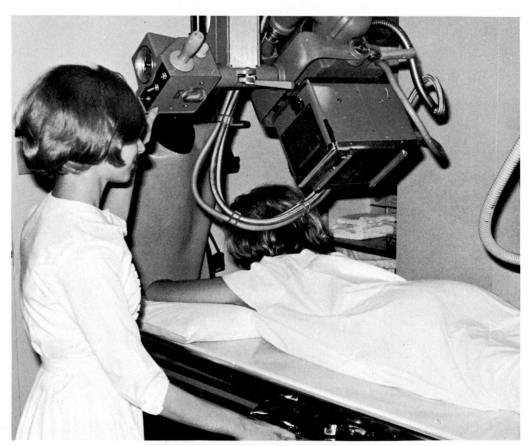

FIG. 3.13. POSITION OF PATIENT AND X-RAY TUBE FOR OBTAINING
POSTEROANTERIOR ANGLED VIEW
The tube is angled 35° toward the feet.

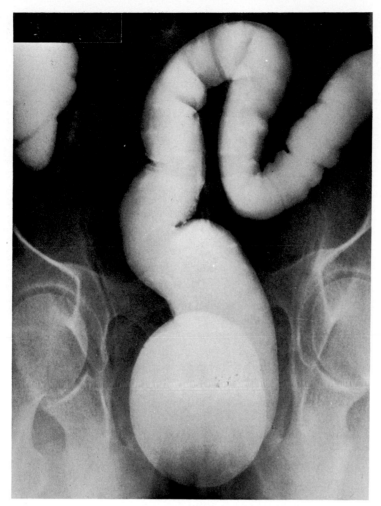

FIG. 3.14. POSTEROANTERIOR ANGLED VIEW
The rectosigmoid and sigmoid segments are projected without overlap.

not done, the barium tends to dry out against the mucosal surface. This drying results in a grotesque "cracked-paint" pattern with subsequent air distention (Fig. 3.15). Therefore, as soon as the patient is ready, a postevacuation film is obtained and the second part of the study is begun. After gentle reinsertion of the enema tip, a thick barium suspension blended to the consistency of light cream is allowed to flow into the colon as far as the midsigmoid. A sphygmomanometer bulb which has been attached to the enema bag tubing near the patient's anus is then used to insufflate the colon.

Air insufflation should be a painless procedure if it is started gradually and carried out slowly, and if no one segment of bowel is allowed to become overdistended. The fluoroscopist alone must control the inflow of air; it should not be done by an assistant or technician. To facilitate the smooth spreading of barium through the colon ahead of the advancing air, the patient is slowly turned from the supine position to his left, then prone, onto his right side and, finally, back to the supine position. Asking the patient to breathe deeply and using gentle manual ballottement will have the same favorable effect for easier filling as they do when a liquid enema is given. The colon, adequately filled with air, need not be more distended than for an enema done with liquid (Fig. 3.16). The transverse measurement across an

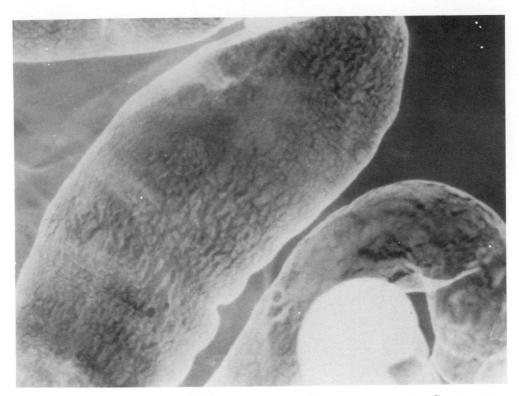

FIG. 3.15. "CRACKED-PAINT" APPEARANCE OF BARIUM ON AN AIR-CONTRAST
EXAMINATION

adequately filled segment of the average adult colon is about 7 cm for either liquid
barium or when adequately distended with air.

Before post-air films are made, and in order to enhance uniform coating and
distention, it is helpful to have the patient make one 360° rotation on the table.
This turning should obviously be reserved for those patients on whom such added
exertion will not be harmful.

The patient is now ready for overhead films of the air-filled colon. At an absolute
minimum, these films should include: posteroanterior, anteroposterior, left posterior-
oblique, posteroanterior angled view of the rectum and sigmoid, and a lateral view
of the rectum. The films should preferably be obtained in the above order to shift
the position of air and liquid. Other views that may be obtained are listed in the
following section on primary air-contrast technique.

With regard to the lateral film of the rectum, its chief value is in detecting an
intrinsic lesion (Fig. 3.17). Although considerable attention has been given to the
width of the retro-rectal space, it is so variable that the observation is of limited
value.

Primary Air-Contrast Technique

By definition, the barium and air studies are carried out simultaneously at "a
single sitting" in this technique of colon examination. A preliminary, single-contrast
enema is not performed. Instead, the colon is partially filled with a moderately thick
barium suspension which is immediately distributed throughout the entire length of
the colon by insufflation of large amounts of air. A primary air-contrast examination
may be performed on most patients except those with the possibility of obstruction
or perforation.

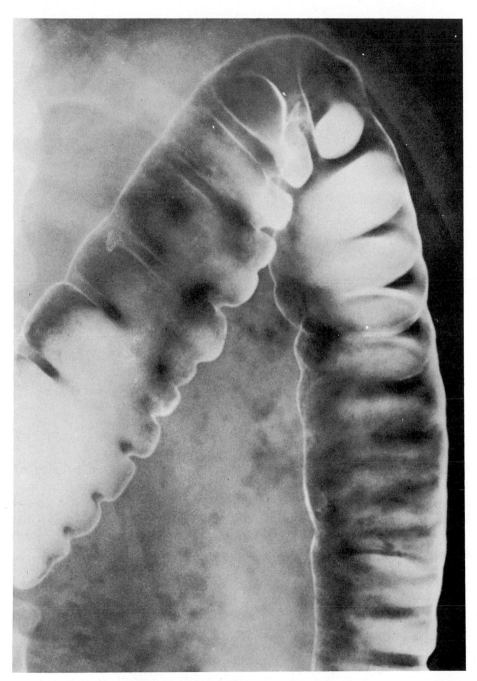

FIG. 3.16. AIR-CONTRAST ENEMA
Detail of splenic flexure adequately distended with air.

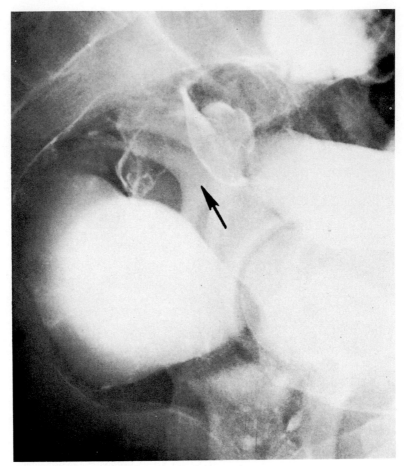

FIG. 3.17. LATERAL AIR-CONTRAST FILM OF RECTUM
A polypoid carcinoma of the rectosigmoid is well defined (arrow).

In order to enhance the coating of the bowel wall, a thicker barium, usually 60% weight to volume is used. Since only a portion of the colon will be filled, approximately 400 cc of solution will be adequate. Because of the increased viscosity of thick barium, a wide bore tubing, as wide as 1.25 cm, is used for administration of the enema. A balloon catheter is sometimes used to aid the patients in retaining the large amounts of insufflated air, unless rectal disease is suspected. In addition, 0.5–1.0 mg of glucagon may be given intravenously just before the start of the examination to aid relaxation of the colon.

The absolute prerequisite for a primary air-contrast enema is a meticulously prepared colon. The literature contains numerous intensive preparation regimens, but the two which have been most widely used are the 72-hr castor-oil method and the magnesium citrate (increased hydration) method, both described earlier in this chapter. Many radiologists believe that a preliminary tap-water cleansing enema is essential.

Specially designed enema tips and tubing are available which allow both inflow and drainage of the barium as well as insufflation. With the patient lying prone or supine, barium is allowed to flow as far as the splenic flexure or mid-transverse colon. Turning the patient so that the descending colon is dependent will assist passage of the somewhat thick barium mixture. It may be helpful to squeeze the plastic enema bag directly above the barium to assist in its smooth passage into the colon.

Before insufflation with air, as much of the barium as possible should be drained from the colon. If a wide bore tubing has been used, this can usually be accomplished by lowering the bag to the floor and releasing the clamp from the tubing. Placing the table in the near-erect position will also facilitate emptying. Another method for emptying the colon of nearly all the barium is simply to let the patient go to the toilet and evacuate as much as he can as rapidly as possible, then return to the fluoroscopic room for air insufflation.

Distention of the colon with air and the smooth spreading of the residual barium around the colon is best accomplished by first placing the patient in the left lateral or prone position. Manual insufflation by the fluoroscopist is then carried out until the entire colon is adequately distended as described in the earlier section on secondary air-contrast technique.

Overhead survey films

The number and sequence of air-filled films are critical for a complete study. There are many recommended views, but at least the following overhead films should be obtained: posteroanterior angled view of the rectosigmoid, the tube angled 35° toward the feet; a posteroanterior film (Fig. 3.18); a lateral rectum (Fig. 3.19) or a horizontal beam lateral rectum film with the patient in the prone position (Fig. 3.20); a left posterior oblique view; an anteroposterior film (Fig. 3.21); right and left lateral decubitus views (Fig. 3.22); and an upright film (Fig. 3.23). An anteroposterior or posteroanterior postevacuation film may also be of value.

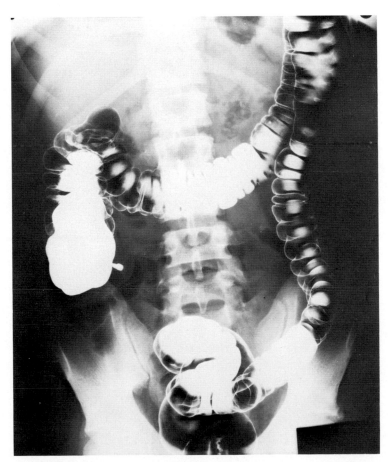

FIG. 3.18. AIR-CONTRAST ENEMA: POSTEROANTERIOR VIEW

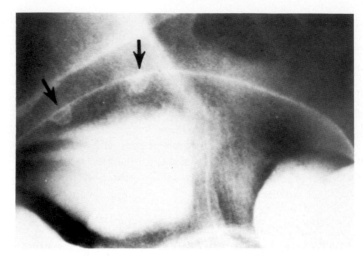

FIG. 3.19. AIR-CONTRAST ENEMA: LATERAL RECTUM
Detail from a lateral film of the rectum demonstrating two 4-mm polyps (arrows) arising from the superior wall of the rectosigmoid.

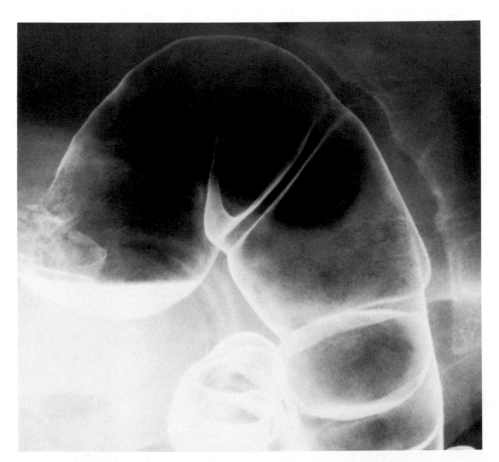

FIG. 3.20. HORIZONTAL BEAM AIR-CONTRAST LATERAL FILM OF THE RECTUM
The film was obtained with the patient in the prone position and the x-ray beam in a horizontal axis, parallel to the floor and the x-ray table.

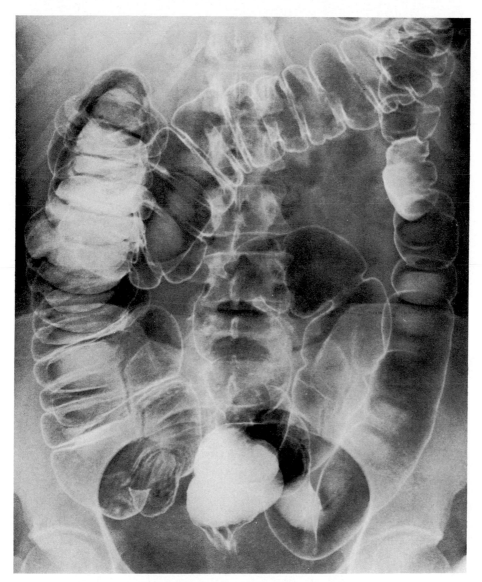

FIG. 3.21. AIR-CONTRAST ENEMA: ANTEROPOSTERIOR VIEW

The mucosal surface of the colon is elegantly demonstrated by a thin layer of barium as the lumen has been distended with air.

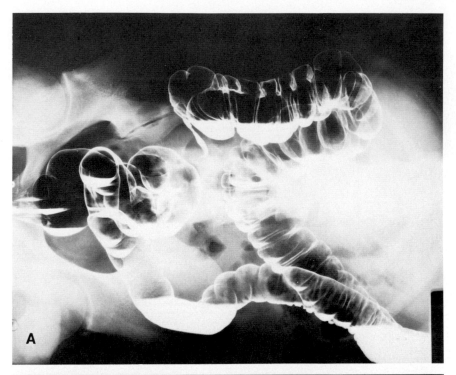

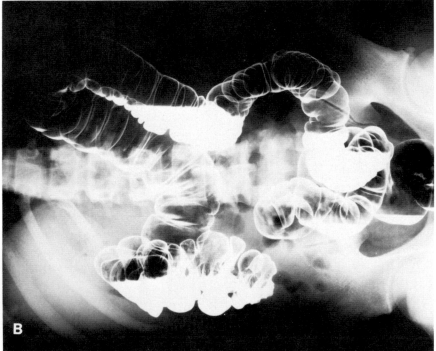

FIG. 3.22. LATERAL DECUBITUS AIR-CONTRAST VIEWS
(**A**) Left lateral decubitus. (**B**) Right lateral decubitus.

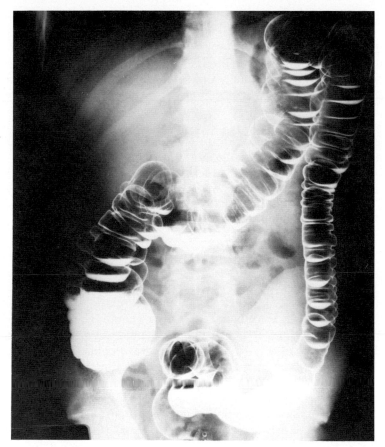

FIG. 3.23. AIR-CONTRAST ENEMA: UPRIGHT FILM
The flexures and transverse colon are particularly well demonstrated.

Single-Contrast versus Double-Contrast Controversy

One of the major controversies involving diagnostic radiologists concerns the role of the double-contrast enema in evaluating patients with possible colonic lesions. Statements have been made that the only acceptable method of examination is the double-contrast technique and that it is inexcusable to perform a routine single-contrast examination. As in many controversies, it would seem that there has been more heat than light in many of the published communications on the subject.

The proponents of the double-contrast enema (DCE) have been accused of comparing results in patients who have been enrolled in their own special studies with results from the literature on the single-column (SCE) enema. There are several differences in the series as reported. It must be recognized that the DCE patients have undergone meticulous preparation which certainly has not always been the case in the routine performance of a SCE. Furthermore, patients undergoing the DCE have received extraspecial attention (as patients in special studies so frequently do) as opposed to patients being routinely examined either in a hospital or office setting.

Proponents of the DCE feel that the performance of this examination is no more difficult than that of the SCE. They claim that the time required for the examination is the same or only slightly longer than for the SCE. Certainly, there are a greater number of maneuvers involved in the performance of a DCE. The larger number of overhead films obtained with the DCE also require additional room time. Furthermore, the radiation dose to the patient in the DCE technique will be considerably higher.

Proponents of the SCE place heavy reliance on the fluoroscopist and his ability to detect and demonstrate a colonic lesion and claim that the DCE technique leads to an assembly-line type of examination. Reliance on the individual radiologist to detect lesions during the performance of an examination has long been the cornerstone of gastrointestinal radiology. On the other hand, if one obtains a greater number of overhead films, most, if not all lesions seen at fluoroscopy, will be detected and there is the added possibility that small lesions not seen at fluoroscopy may be identified on the larger air survey films.

There is little controversy over the fact that certain patients should undergo air-contrast examinations. Included among these are: patients who are asymptomatic but have guaiac positive stools and a negative uppergastrointestinal examination; patients with rectal bleeding; patients with a previous history of polyps or colon cancer, or who have a family history of these lesions, and patients with such potentially ominous symptoms as anemia, change in bowel habits or weight loss.

While the above discussion is pertinent in making a decision as to the type of examination to perform, the most important component of the decision-making process should be the quality of the radiologic image and the ability of the radiologist to detect an abnormality of the colon. In this area, there is the greatest controversy.

The DCE proponents claim ability to detect polypoid lesions in 10–15% of patients, which rivals the incidence of polyps in the general population as determined by autopsy studies. In most hospital settings using the SCE technique, the incidence of polyp detection is nowhere near this figure. However, the SCE proponents question the necessity of detecting polypoid lesions of 2–9 mm within the colon. They state that the incidence of malignancy in polyps less than 1 cm is about 1% and they point out the high incidence of false-positive "lesions" caused by small gas bubbles and bits of feces which may resemble polyps in the DCE technique. They also believe that many unnecessary colonoscopies and repeat barium enemas will be performed in an attempt to make a differentiation and that a certain number of patients cannot be properly prepared regardless of effort.

The SCE proponents stress that the ability to utilize compression is lost with the DCE technique. The DCE proponents counter with the statement that excellent distention of the colon obviates the need for compression. The SCE proponents further state that the most valuable film in a barium enema study is the postevacuation film with which they can study the texture and integrity of the mucosal fold pattern. The DCE proponents counter that in many SCE examinations, an adequate postevacuation film is rarely achieved.

As the reader can easily appreciate, there are many factors in favor of each technique. However, an appropriate comparison study has yet to be devised. The key element in the quality of either type of study is the prior preparation of the patient, an area in which radiologists have been delinquent in the past. Given a patient who is well prepared and a radiologist who is interested in the quality of the enema which he performs, the two types of examinations may well yield similar results except for polyps under 1 cm in size. Here, the double-contrast enema is superior and, in expert hands, can match the results of expert colonoscopy.

OTHER EXAMINATIONS

Although other techniques have been devised for examining the colon, only a few have stood the test of repeated application by many radiologists. Any single technique may be successful in the hands of its advocate, but the aura pales when others cannot apply it with ease or reliability. Some of the proved basic variations for colonic examination follow.

High Kilovoltage Barium Enema

Diagnostic x-ray machines capable of operating at 120 KV or higher were responsible for a technique which allowed increased penetration of a watery thin barium mixture (Fig. 3.24). Fluoroscopic visualization was adequate, but the use of an image amplifier permitted even thinner mixtures of contrast material to be used. The technique is rarely used today.

Water-Soluble Contrast Enema

In cases where there is a recognized risk of encountering a colon perforation, a communicating fistula, abscess cavity, or a point of near-complete obstruction, the use of barium mixtures may be contraindicated because of the danger of inspissation, trapping, or prolonged peritoneal contact. In these cases, the use of a water-soluble

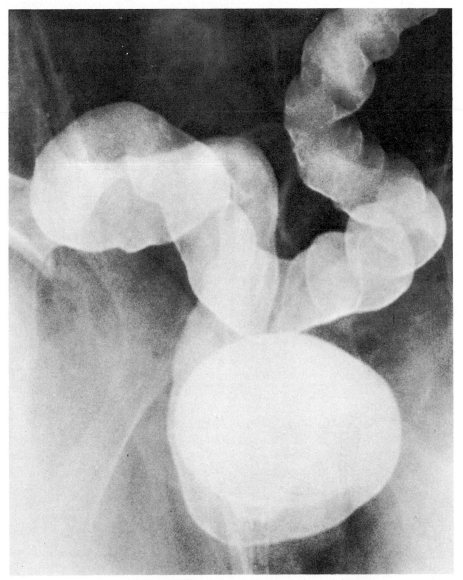

FIG. 3.24. THIN BARIUM, HIGH KILOVOLT FILM
Despite overlapping loops, this technique has demonstrated the interior of the rectosigmoid and sigmoid segments.

contrast material containing an iodine compound may be the agent of choice. Precautions similar to those used for intravenous studies should be followed. Other conditions in which a water-soluble contrast enema, rather than barium, may be used are examination of a defunctioned segment of bowel, and a catheter enema of a sinus tract connecting with the colon. Equal parts of water and the water-soluble contrast agent provide an adequate density on the x-ray films though fluoroscopic visualization may be only fair. The latter can be enhanced to more than optimal conditions by use of an image amplifier.

Oral Barium Meal

The value of following oral barium through the colon has lessened as techniques for a more thorough study of the colon by regular and air-contrast enemas have been developed. Where it is important to evaluate the status of the cecum and ileocecal valve, the oral study may still be helpful when good distention by retrograde examination is not achieved or where reflux into the terminal ileum did not occur. Therefore, the upper gastrointestinal route may be required for complete study in patients with suspected amebiasis, tuberculosis, ulcerative colitis, ileocolitis, and appendiceal disease. It should never be used in cases of suspected colon obstruction as impaction of the barium proximal to the obstruction may result. If it seems necessary to perform an upper gastrointestinal examination prior to a barium enema, and there is a question of possible colon obstruction, a water-soluble medium should be used rather than barium (Fig. 3.25). Although visualization of detail is not as good as with barium, the water-soluble material will quickly pass through the small bowel and may outline a colonic obstruction.

COMPLICATIONS AND PRECAUTIONS

A barium enema is a relatively safe examination if certain precautions are observed. It is an unwarranted procedure in toxic dilatation of the colon. Extreme caution should be used in unconscious or semicomatose patients or in patients with abdominal aortic aneurysms, severe coronary artery disease, recent myocardial infarction, or recent cerebrovascular accident. Caution must also be used in patients with suspected bowel perforation; there is no good evidence to indicate that a patient with a perforated appendix will be made worse by a barium enema.

Any foreign object placed in the rectum is a potential instrument of bowel perforation, and the thermometer, protoscope, sigmoidoscope, or enema tip have all been responsible for intramural and extraperitoneal perforations. An enema tip or catheter should always be inserted and advanced with caution, whether being introduced into the rectum or a colostomy stoma. Undue force may cause perforation, especially if there is localized disease, or sustained spasm. Perforation may also occur during the course of a barium enema at any point in the colon where the integrity of the bowel wall has been severely compromised by a disease process (Fig. 3.26). When perforation of the bowel occurs, it is the fecal contamination of the peritoneum that is the greater danger, rather than the barium itself. It has been suggested that barium and feces together are more damaging than either barium or feces alone.

A balloon catheter may cause rectal perforation. This complication has been discussed earlier. Fatal barium emboli may be one result of such a perforation. These emboli reach the lungs through breaks into the submucosal veins and then travel via pelvic veins to the inferior vena cava (Fig. 3.27).

The incidence of transient bacteremia secondary to a barium enema is extremely low, not differing statistically from that occurring during a diagnostic colonoscopy.

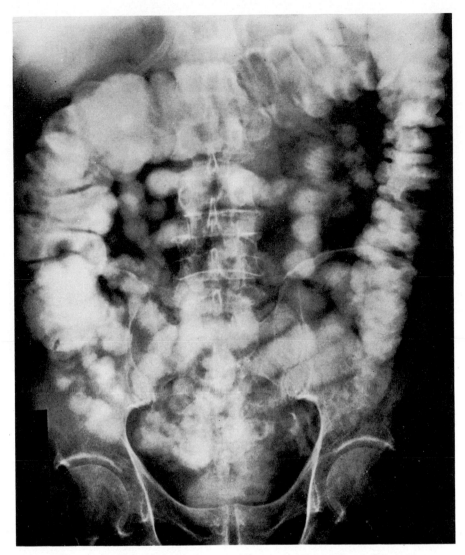

FIG. 3.25. DEMONSTRATION OF COLON BY THE ORAL ROUTE

Two hours after oral administration of a water-soluble agent, the entire colon is visualized.

The organisms are anaerobes and the bacteremia is most likely to occur during the enema as the rectosigmoid is fully distended and under maximum pressure. The route of infection is via the inferior hemorrhoidal veins. Prophylactic antibiotic therapy is not considered necessary in the average patient. Patients with valvular heart disease, intravascular prothesis, and compromised host defenses may need special consideration.

Excessive hydrostatic pressure may be a threat to the integrity of the bowel wall. If gravity and position are used to enhance filling, rather than increased hydrostatic pressure, there should be no danger of perforation. The bursting point of the colon is difficult to calculate and is dependent on more than the hydrostatic pressure used to perform a barium enema. It is related in part to the viscosity and rate of flow of the particular barium mixture used, the normal resting pressure of the lower colon, the added pressure caused by spasm or straining, and the physical fact that rupture is due to the product of the change in pressure across the wall times the radius of

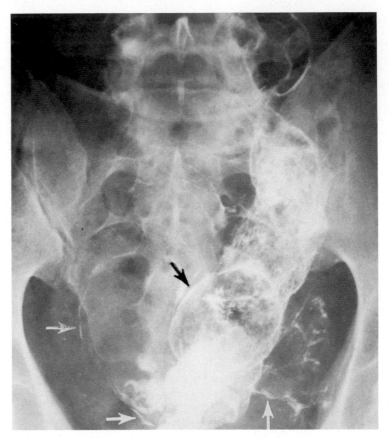

FIG. 3.26. PERFORATED COLON

This examination was performed 8 weeks following a sigmoid resection for volvulus and a protecting colostomy, in order to evaluate the sigmoid anastomosis prior to colostomy closure. A large fecal concretion (black arrow) was immediately encountered on initial inflow of barium. The examination was terminated and the patient allowed to evacuate. This postevacuation film shows barium streaks inside the peritoneal cavity (white arrows). Immediate surgery revealed a rock-hard, 7 × 10 cm fecal ball that had been retained in the rectum for 8 weeks and had eroded through the rectal wall.

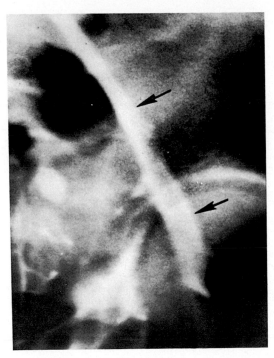

FIG. 3.27. BARIUM EMBOLUS

A fluoroscopic spot-film demonstrates a fatal barium embolus in the internal iliac vein (arrows), following inadvertent perforation of the rectosigmoid by a balloon catheter just prior to the start of a barium enema examination.

the intestine. It is advisable to keep the enema bag 1 m or less from the table top to lessen the chance of pressure combinations which might rupture the colon.

Another potential complication pertains to the heart. It has been well demonstrated in animals and man that distention of a hollow viscus may result in decreased blood flow to the heart. Not surprisingly, distention studies on humans where cardiac monitoring has been used have shown the development of cardiac arrhythmias including ventricular tachycardia, atrial tachycardia, and premature beats in almost half of the patients over the age of 60. ST-segment depression, indicating left ventricular ischemia has also been observed. There seems to be no correlation with age or with a history of previous heart disease. In view of these EKG abnormalities, it is rather surprising that myocardial infarction so rarely occurs during or following a barium enema examination.

Yet another potential complication of a barium enema is the possibility of an unexpected systemic allergic reaction to one of the many additives now present in commercial barium preparations. This subject has been discussed previously.

Common sense and judgment are essential to the performance of any diagnostic procedure, for there are no rules that will guarantee protection from accidents. The wise analysis of each patient and his problem, the performance of a planned and well-monitored examination—these are the requisites for a safe and rewarding evaluation of the colon.

BIBLIOGRAPHY

Brown, G. R.: The direct air contrast colon examination. A rapid simplified highly diagnostic procedure. Privately printed, Ft. Wayne, IN, 1968.

Butt, J., Hentges, D., Pelican, G., Henstorf, H., Haag, T., Rolfe, R., and Hutcheson, D.: Bacteremia during barium enema study. Am. J. Roentgenol., *130:* 715, 1978.

Canada, W. J.: Use of urokon (sodium-3-acetyla-mino-2,4,6-triiodo-benzoate) in roentgen study of the gastrointestinal tract. Radiology, *64:* 867, 1955.

Cove, J. K. J., and Snyder, R. N.: Fatal barium intravasation during barium enema. Radiology, *112:* 9, 1974.

Dodds, W. J., Scanlon, G. T., Shaw, D. K., Stewart, E. T., Youker, J. E., and Metter, G. E.: An evaluation of colon cleansing regimens. Am. J. Roentgenol, *128:* 57, 1977.

Dreyfuss, J. R., Robbins, L. L., and Murphy, J. T.: Disposable, plastic unit for barium-enema examination. Radiology, *77:* 834, 1961.

Eastwood, G. L.: ECG abnormalities associated with the barium enema. J.A.M.A., *219:* 719, 1972.

Ettinger, A., and Elkin, M.: Study of the sigmoid by special roentgenographic views. Am. J. Roentgenol., *72:* 199, 1954.

Fenlon, J. W., and Margulis, A. R.: Current concepts in cancer—Cancer of the GI tract: Radiologic diagnosis. J.A.M.A., *231:* 752, 1975.

Figiel, S. J., Figiel, L. S., and Rush, D. K.: Study of colon by use of high-kilovoltage spot-compression technique. J.A.M.A., *166:* 1269, 1958.

Gianturco, C.: High-voltage technic in the diagnosis of polypoid growths of the colon. Radiology, *55:* 27, 1950.

Goldstein, H. M., and Miller, M. H.: Air contrast colon examination in patients with colostomies. Am. J. Roentgenol., *127:* 607, 1976.

Janower, M. L., Robbins, L. L., Tomchik, F. S., and Weylman, W. T.: Tannic acid and the barium enema. Radiology, *85:* 887, 1965.

Land, R. E.: Colostomy enema. Radiology, *100:* 36, 1971.

Laufer, I: *Double Contrast Gastrointestinal Radiology with Endoscopic Correlation.* W. B. Saunders, Philadelphia, 1979.

Laufer, I.: The double-contrast enema: Myths and misconceptions. Gastrointest. Radiol., *1:* 19, 1976.

Margulis, A. R.: Is double-contrast examination of the colon the only acceptable radiographic examination? Radiology, *119:* 741, 1976.

Marshak, R. H.: The barium enema in the high risk carcinoma patient (Letter to the Editor). Radiology, *125:* 549, 1977.

Miller, R. E.: Examination of the colon. Curr. Probl. Radiol., *5:* 1, 1975.

Miller, R. E., and Lehman, G.: The barium enema—Is it obsolete? J.A.M.A., *235:* 2842, 1976.

Miller, R. E., and Skucas, J.: *Radiographic Contrast Agents.* University Park Press, Baltimore, 1977.

Noveroske, R. J.: Perforation of the rectosigmoid by a Bardex balloon catheter, report of 3 cases. Am. J. Roentgenol, *96:* 326, 1966.

Peterson, G. H., and Miller, R. E.: The barium enema: A reassessment looking toward perfection. Radiology, *128:* 315, 1978.

Rogers, C. W.: Method for double-contrast study of the colon. Med. Radiogr. Photogr., *51:* 30, 1975.

Salvo, A. F., Capron, C. W., Leigh, K. E., and Dillihunt, R. C.: Barium intravasation into portal venous system during barium enema examination. J.A.M.A. *235:* 749, 1976.

Seaman, W. B., and Wells, J.: Complications of the barium enema. Gastroenterology, *48:* 728, 1965.

Welin, S.: Results of the Malmo technique of colon examination. J.A.M.A. *199:* 119, 1967.

Welin, S., and Welin, G.: Experience with the Welin modification. In *The Double Contrast Examination of the Colon*, pp. 5–16. Georg Thieme Verlag, Stuttgart, 1976.

4

Congenital Diseases of the Colon

SPENCER BORDEN, IV, M.D.

NORMAL COLON

Size, Position, Contents

The pediatric colon is different from that of the adult in both health and disease. As compared to adult proportions, the abdominal cavity of an infant is small, the liver large, and the length and caliber of the colon large. The pediatric colon is redundant; the sigmoid is on a long mesocolon and swings into the right mid-abdomen while the hepatic and splenic flexures are depressed and often folded over. As the abdominal cavity elongates with linear growth of the infant, the colon becomes less redundant and approximates the adult position sometime after the age of 5.

The content of the colon also changes during infancy and childhood. Meconium, a soft, green, jelly-like material is expelled by normal newborns within the first day after birth. Stools formed on a diet of infant formula and foods are thick, light green or brown, putty-like, and frequent. By the age of 4 or 5 and when the child is on an adult diet, the stools become brown, solid and well-formed. The semisolid digested food, mixed with small bowel fluids and air in the right colon, becomes progressively dehydrated to form the lumpy stool of the left colon. Transit time from mouth to anus increases as the child grows older.

BARIUM EXAMINATION

Preparation

The degree of preparation prior to a barium enema in a child will vary with the indication for the examination. No preparation is required in emergency patients, in cases of suspected obstruction, or in acute inflammatory bowel disease.

Meticulous cleansing of the colon is not required in most pediatric patients. Mild catharsis begun on the preceding evening and clear liquids on the day of the examination are usually sufficient.

Air-contrast examinations are reserved for those few children with suspected polyps, and additional preparation is required. Infants and children without bowel control should have a low residue diet for 2 or 3 days with several cleansing enemas on the day of examination. Immediately prior to the study, a preparatory cleansing enema of thin barium and Clysodrast is fluoroscopically, advanced to the hepatic flexure and the patient is allowed to evacuate; the cecum should not be filled to avoid reflux into the terminal ileum. Fluoroscopically aided cleansing enemas are very effective and superior to "blind" enemas administered on the hospital floor; they are well worth the small investment of the radiologists' time and the slight additional radiation exposure.

Technique

A pediatric barium enema is guaranteed to be unsuccessful if attention is not given to details of technique. Complete immobilization of the infant and young child is mandatory. Children from age 4 onwards will cooperate without restraints if the procedure is explained to them in considerate, simple terms. Sedation with a mixture of Demerol, phenergan and Thorazine is occasionally required in older patients who are violently uncooperative, agitated, or severely retarded.

From the many types of rectal enema tips available, we prefer the large, straight olive-tipped rectal tube for use in both infants and children. Although the olive tip may seem to dwarf the neonatal anus, it can be passed on all babies except those with anal stenosis. A tight seal can be created by taping the buttocks firmly together around the enema tube. A pacifier or bottle nipple can calm the agitated baby and prevent crying and straining which increase intra-abdominal pressure and impede the flow of barium. We use balloon catheters only in patients undergoing hydrostatic reduction of previously diagnosed intussusception or who have an obstructing meconium plug. The fluid level in the enema bag is never raised more than 1 m above the table top.

Very premature infants require special techniques. The major threat to the premature child is hypothermia which may result following removal from the incubator. Loss of body heat is minimized by placement of the enema tube in the anus while the baby is still in the incubator, use of infrared heating lamps on the fluoroscopic table, and by rapid fluoroscopic study.

Once these details have been attended to, the enema may begin. The barium enema is a combination of fluoroscopic observation and spot-films, with overhead radiographs of the colon, both filled and postevacuation. The prone or Trendelenburg position is useful in filling the colon in patients with vigorous peristalsis, spasm, or inflammatory bowel disease. A tensely filled colon may be decompressed by lowering the enema bag to floor level, siphoning off some of the barium and then allowing the child to walk to the toilet in relative comfort. A posteroanterior evacuation film usually completes the study, but further fluoroscopy of the colon or refilling with air may help to further delineate a questionable finding on previous films.

If an air-contrast examination is indicated, the filling of the colon with thick barium and the insufflation of air must be controlled fluoroscopically (Fig. 4.1). Decubitus (Fig. 4.2) and upright films are also helpful. The same technical maneuvers described in Chapter 3 can also be used for the performance of this type of study on a child.

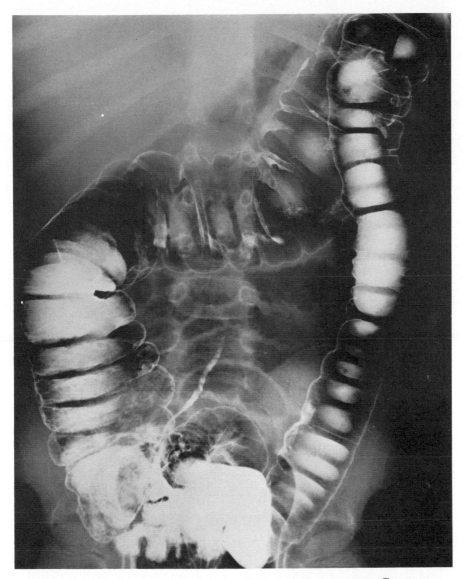

FIG. 4.1. NORMAL AIR-CONTRAST EXAMINATION OF THE COLON

Pharmacology

Pharmacologic agents have a limited use in the examination of the pediatric colon. Glucagon is a potent reliever of colonic spasm and is useful in helping a patient with an irritable colon to tolerate the barium enema examination. Proban-thine can also render the colon atonic and relieve spasm, but has greater systemic effects. Drug-induced hypotonia may be useful in children with inflammatory bowel disease, but not useful in patients with mechanical conditions, such as intussuscep-tion.

Although the usual barium enema suspension is mixed with water, some authors have suggested that water intoxication (the systemic absorption of large quantities of water with subsequent electrolyte abnormalities) can occur in a patient with a dilated or atonic colon and have recommended the use of saline for suspension of

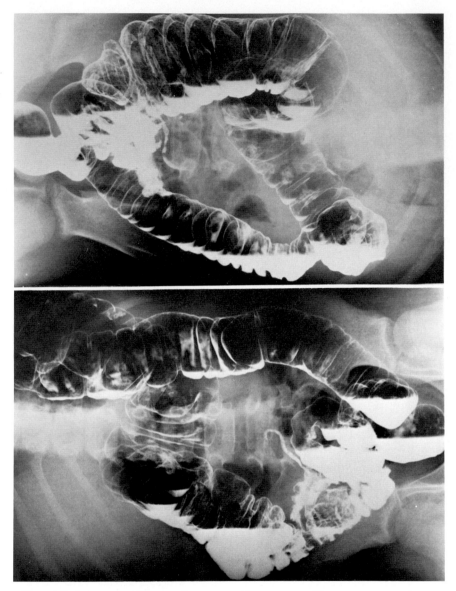

FIG. 4.2. LEFT AND RIGHT LATERAL DECUBITUS VIEWS OF THE COLON
Note deflation of the dependent and inflation of the elevated sides on these double-contrast enema films.

barium. The problem can be avoided by limiting the barium enema to the distal colon in patients with an obstructed or atonic large bowel.

Gastrografin and other hyperosmolar aqueous contrast materials draw large quantities of fluid into the bowel and can irritate the mucosa. We use these contrast materials in a dilution of 1 part contrast to 2 parts water and then only in cases of suspected perforation or for the hydrostatic dislodgement of meconium ileus or meconium plugs. The blood electrolytes should be carefully monitored.

NORMAL EMBRYOGENESIS AND ROTATION

The intestinal tract begins as a straight hollow tube suspended on a single mesentery and consists of the foregut, which extends from the mouth to the

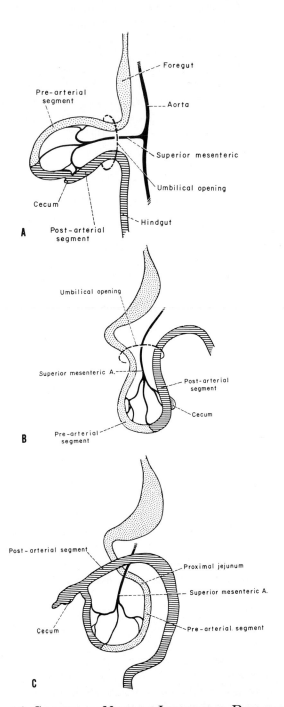

FIG. 4.3. STAGES OF NORMAL INTESTINAL ROTATION

(A) Fifth fetal week, lateral view. The prearterial segment lies superiorly to the superior mesenteric artery while the postarterial segment lies inferiorly. (B) Eighth fetal week, anteroposterior view. Following 90° of counterclockwise rotation, the prearterial segment lies to the right of the superior mesenteric artery and the postarterial segment on the left (C).

duodeno-jejunal junction; the midgut, which extends from the duodeno-jejunal junction to the mid-transverse colon and is supplied by the superior mesenteric artery; and the hindgut, which extends from the mid-transverse colon to the anus, and is supplied by the inferior mesenteric artery. About the 5th fetal week (Fig. 4.3), the intestinal tract grows rapidly in length and, because of the smallness of the abdominal cavity, the midgut herniates into the umbilical sac. The superior mesenteric artery acts as a dividing line between the prearterial segment, *i.e.,* the jejunum and proximal ileum which lie superiorly, and the postarterial segment, *i.e.,* the distal ileum and right colon which lie inferiorly. At about the 8th fetal week, the superior lying prearterial segment undergoes 90° of clockwise rotation so that it comes to lie in the horizontal plane to the right of the superior mesenteric artery with the postarterial segment on the left. Right and left refer to sides of the fetal abdomen. At about the 10th fetal week, an additional 90° of rotation occurs so that the prearterial segment now lies inferior to the superior mesenteric artery while the postarterial segment now lies superiorly; this is the exact opposite of the position of the segments when herniation occurred. Return to the abdomen begins as the proximal jejunum passes posterior to the superior mesenteric artery and comes to lie in the left upper quadrant. The ileum and colon follow, successively filling the left, middle, and right abdomen beneath the liver. The return of the midgut to the abdomen has been completed by the 12th fetal week. The mobility of the ascending and descending colon is lost as their mesenteries become fused w1th the posterior peritoneum. If there is faulty fixation at this stage, the cecum and ascending colon remain mobile. In summary, the process of intestinal rotation is initiated by herniation of the small intestine and the proximal half of the colon into the umbilical sac. The proximal jejunum which originally lies above the superior mesenteric artery rotates through a counterclockwise arc of 270° and retracts into the abdomen to lie posteriorly to the left of the artery. The rest of the small intestine and colon follow the jejunum into the abdomen and occupy the remaining space in the abdominal cavity, later with fusion of the mesenteries of the ascending and descending colons to the posterior abdominal wall.

ABNORMAL ROTATION AND FIXATION

In nonrotation, the proximal jejunum returns to the abdomen after having rotated only 90°. The small bowel, therefore, lies on the right side of the abdomen and the colon on the left.

In malrotation, the proximal jejunum returns to the abdomen normally and is followed by the remainder of the bowel; however, the cecum and ascending colon fail to migrate fully to the right lower quadrant. The cecum may lie on the left, in the center, or high on the right side of the abdomen.

In reverse rotation, the cecum returns to the abdomen first having reversed the counterclockwise rotation that has already occurred and comes to lie in the left upper quadrant wedged behind the superior mesenteric artery. This can result in partial or complete obstruction of the transverse colon.

Abnormal rotation results in an anomalous position of the cecum which frequently lies to the left of the duodenum. Peritoneal bands may run from the cecum across the second portion of the duodenum to the right posterior lateral abdominal wall. These bands may compress the duodenum and result in obstruction. A small bowel volvulus may occur if failure of fusion of the mesentery of the ascending colon and cecum to the posterior abdominal wall results in a faulty fixation of the small bowel mesentery.

Nonrotation of the colon and small bowel is frequently seen in patients with a congenital diaphragmatic hernia which occurs before the twelfth fetal week of gestation. Diaphragmatic hernias occurring later in gestational life or postnatally are not associated with nonrotation and nonfixation of the bowel. Nonrotation is associated with gastroschisis and omphalocele, where the abdominal cavity is decompressed sufficiently to accommodate the bowel, inhibiting the transfer into the umbilical sac. The colon, if sufficiently large, may also herniate into inguinal or femoral sacs. These are usually reducible, but occasionally become incarcerated and strangulated, causing bowel obstruction. The colon may fill the renal fossa in cases of congenital absence of the kidney or nephrectomy. Following partial hepatectomy, the right colon frequently rises to the right upper quadrant to fill the space occupied by the resected lobe of the liver.

During barium enema examination, attention should be given to fixation and mobility of the colon. Specifically, the mobility and position of the cecum, the orientation of the ileocecal valve, and the fixation of the ascending colon should be noted. The type of faulty fixation can be determined when the position of the ligament of Treitz, the jejunum, and the ileum are identified on an upper gastrointestinal examination.

NORMAL VARIANTS

Minor alterations in colon position can be considered as normal variants. The Chilaiditi syndrome (Fig. 4.4) applies to a patient whose right colon lies between the right hemidiaphragm and the dome of the liver. It can be an incidental finding on

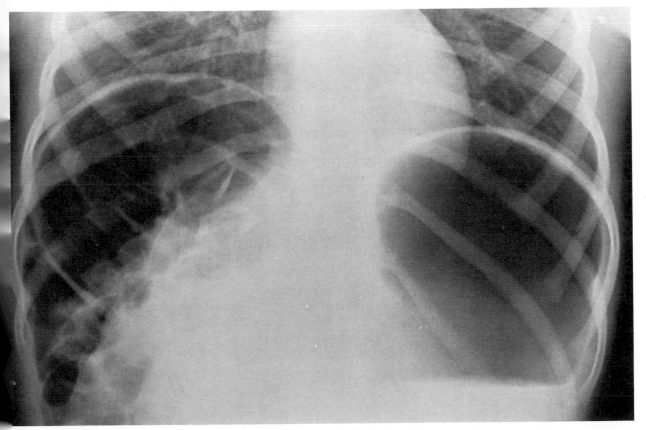

FIG. 4.4. CHILAIDITI SYNDROME
Interposition of the colon between the dome of the liver and diaphragm, a variant of normal position. This interposition may be inconstant and does not cause clinical symptoms.

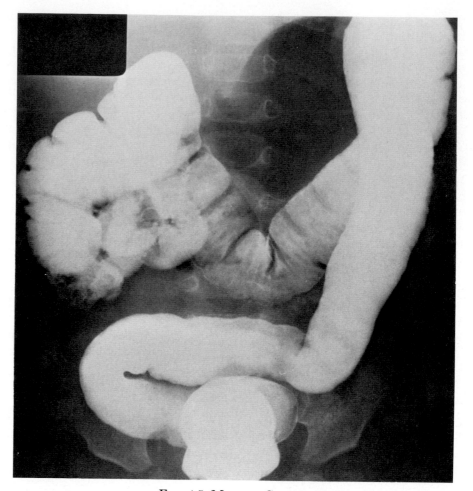

FIG. 4.5. MOBILE CECUM

The cecum is in the right mid-abdomen, a normal position for infants. A mobile cecum in older children may result from incomplete fixation of the ascending colon.

chest examination and causes no symptoms. Similarly, the cecum may be found to be quite mobile on barium enema examination (Fig. 4.5); it normally occupies the right iliac fossa when the colon is filled and distended with barium, but when faulty fixation leaves the cecum on its own mesentery, it may rise to the right mid-abdomen or upper quadrant with evacuation of the enema. The lymphatic follicles of the colon are often large in infancy and childhood. They may be found as uniform umbilicated filling defects in the right colon, or distributed throughout the colon, best seen on air-contrast examinations. Adherent feces (Fig. 4.6) should always be recognized for what it is. Finally, normal mucosal grooves, the innominate lines (Fig. 4.7), may be seen frequently on double-contrast enemas.

Ectopic anus refers to a ventral displacement of the anal opening on the perineum. There is shortening of the perineum between the anus and posterior margin of the vagina or scrotum. This condition may be recognized on clinical inspection, but has no specific roentgen features.

In some children, the transverse colon may be ptotic and drop into the lower mid-abdomen between normally placed splenic and hepatic flexures. Redundancy of the colon is a normal feature of infants, occasionally found in older children, and commonly associated with conditions that dilate and elongate the colon, such as aerophagia or chronic constipation.

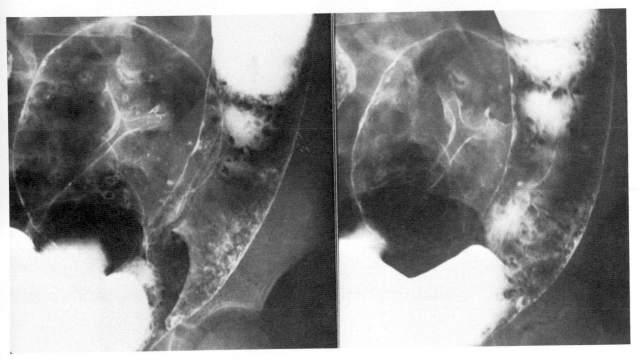

FIG. 4.6. FLECKS OF STOOL IN THE COLON

Adherent flecks of stool may mimic multiple polyps. The irregularity of contour and distribution are helpful signs; palpation at fluoroscopy or repeat enema examination may be required for differentiation.

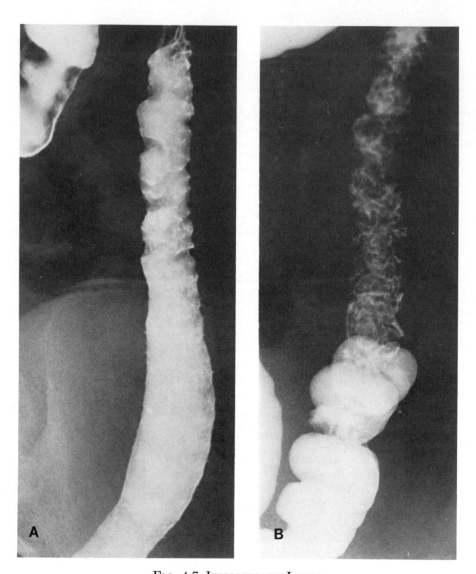

FIG. 4.7. INNOMINATE LINES
Normal mucosal grooves may appear as tiny spiculations along the margin of the barium-filled colon (**A**). The delicate crinkled appearance of the mucosa on the postevacuation film (**B**) helps to distinguish these normal structures from the ulcerations of inflammatory bowel disease.

CONGENITAL OBSTRUCTIONS

Atresia and Stenosis of the Colon

Isolated colonic atresia (Fig. 4.8) is rare, occurring approximately once in every 40,000 live births. The etiology is thought to be an intrauterine vascular insult with intestinal necrosis. Three distinct types of colonic atresia are described: an intraluminal diaphragm which completely obstructs the lumen; an atretic cord which joins the proximal and distal ends of the atresia; and a complete separation with a V-shaped gap in the mesentery corresponding to the area of earlier vascular insult. Congenital colonic stenosis is very rare; most stenoses are acquired lesions, the long-term sequelae of necrotizing enterocolitis.

The clinical presentation of colonic atresia in an infant who passes only one small-volume meconium stool. Abdominal distention progresses to an impressive degree. Vomiting is a late manifestation. Surgical correction of the atresia is mandatory; morbidity and mortality increase significantly after the fourth day of life.

The radiographic appearance is variable. Atresias involving the right colon may produce an abdomen filled with dilated loops of bowel with air fluid levels. The appearance may be identical to distal small bowel obstruction. With lesions in the transverse or left colon, a dilated air-filled loop of colon may be appreciated. In all cases of colonic atresia, no gas should be evident in the rectum unless introduced during digital examination.

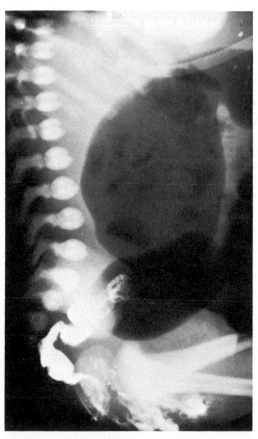

FIG. 4.8. SIGMOID ATRESIA

Barium outlines the atretic rectum and sigmoid colon. The dilated descending colon is outlined by gas proximal to the atretic segment.

The barium enema is usually diagnostic. A small caliber colon is filled until the obstructing lesion prohibits further retrograde flow of barium. Theoretically, the obstructing diaphragm, bulged caudally by stool, should indent the termination of the barium column, whereas mural atresia should cause the barium to terminate in one sharp point. However, this distinction is not always possible. In most cases, the air-filled colon proximal to the atresia will adequately localize the level of obstruction. In cases of colonic stenosis, conventional supine and upright films of the abdomen may be normal, or there may be a suggestion of obstruction with many dilated loops of bowel if the stenosis is severe. Air is usually present in the rectum and sigmoid, thus distinguishing colonic stenosis from atresia. A barium enema examination is usually definitive, demonstrating areas of fixed stenosis, occasionally at multiple levels, usually involving the left colon. Surgical treatment of colonic stenosis is mandatory in patients with high-grade obstruction or with formation of an enterocolic fistula. In cases of mild obstruction, some postinflammatory colonic stenoses have been shown to regress nearly completely without surgical therapy.

Imperforate Anus

Imperforate anus results from the failure of formation of the distal colon and anal canal. It is the most common cause of colonic obstruction in the newborn and occurs once in every 5,000 live births. This malformation is associated with many other complex anomalies including vertebral, tracheal, esophageal, renal, and radial anomalies (Vater syndrome). According to the classification of Ladd and Gross and modified by Santulli, there are four classifications of imperforate anus: type 1—anal stenosis at the level of the anal canal; type 2—solitary diaphragm at the level of the anal canal; type 3—anal atresia with no distal end identifiable (the Santulli modification classifies low rectal pouches, below the puborectalis sling, as type 3A and high rectal pouches, above the puborectalis sling, as type 3B); type 4—a distal rectal pouch at the anus and a focal defect in formation of the distal rectum, perhaps resulting from an intrauterine vascular insult.

Clinical manifestations of imperforate anus are usually obvious. A bulging diaphragm may occasionally be seen on inspection of the child's perineum if a type 2 atresia is present. Clinical inspection will show no anus in all babies with type 3 atresia. Type 4 atresia may be overlooked in the newborn, but is diagnosable by the inability to pass a rectal catheter proximally. Type 1 anal atresia presents with distal colonic obstruction. With type 3B anomalies, there is a very high incidence of fistulous connection to the bladder, urethra, vagina or a cloaca. Evidence of meconium in the urine is conclusive of a fistulous connection.

Radiographic evaluation is very important in defining the anatomy of patients with imperforate anus. Supine and upright films of the abdomen may show dilated loops of air-filled small and large bowel extending down to the lower rectum. In patients with atresia and terminal fistula, the dilatation may be absent as the colon decompresses into the urinary, genital, or perineal area. As first proposed by Wangensteen and Rice, inverted lateral films of the rectum were helpful in documenting the length of the atretic segment by allowing air to distend the rectal pouch and then measuring the distance from the pouch to the anal dimple (Figs. 4.9 and 4.10). However, crying by the baby may push the air-filled rectum caudally or, if the rectum is filled with meconium, air may not reach the caudal end of the pouch. Therefore, incorrect interpretation of both high and low type atresia may be made. Injection of aqueous contrast material through the rectal dimple into the distal rectal pouch has also been advocated. Occasionally a fistula may be demonstrated by this method and the accurate distance between the anus and distal rectal pouch

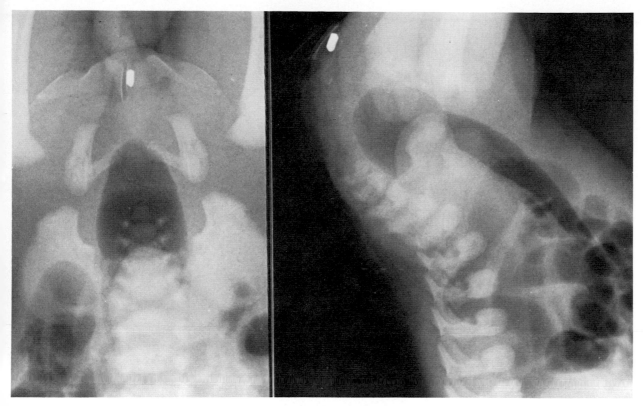

FIG. 4.9. INVERTED VIEWS OF THE RECTUM IN IMPERFORATE ANUS

As mentioned in the text, only an estimate can be made of the distance between the air-filled rectal pouch and the metal marker on the anal dimple.

visualized. Cystography and genitography should be undertaken in all patients with imperforate anus to search for fistulas.

Volvulus

Volvulus in the newborn is almost always associated with malrotation, partial rotation, and nonfixation. The failure of the mesentery to broadly attach along the duodeno-colic insertion leads to a shorter and narrower vascular pedicle allowing abnormal rotation. If the left and right colon mesenteries fail to fuse with the posterior peritoneum, the risk of volvulus increases dramatically.

The clinical presentation of infants with midgut volvulus is intractable vomiting, which rapidly becomes bilious; abdominal distention despite vomiting; hypovolemic shock; sepsis; and finally vascular collapse. If undiagnosed, the entire midgut may become strangulated and infarcted.

Radiographic examination in patients with obstructing volvulus may disclose only a dilated duodenum and stomach with no other air-filled loops of bowel visualized. Vomiting may decompress both the stomach and duodenum resulting in a gasless abdomen. In patients with incomplete obstruction or intermittent volvulus, swallowed gas may become trapped in the midgut and slowly be reabsorbed. In these cases, air seldom reaches the colon and, therefore, is almost never seen in the rectum. A barium enema will demonstrate the colon to be in an abnormal position, allowing a presumptive diagnosis of volvulus to be made (Figs. 4.11 and 4.12). An upper gastrointestinal series, preferably using air introduced by nasogastric tube,

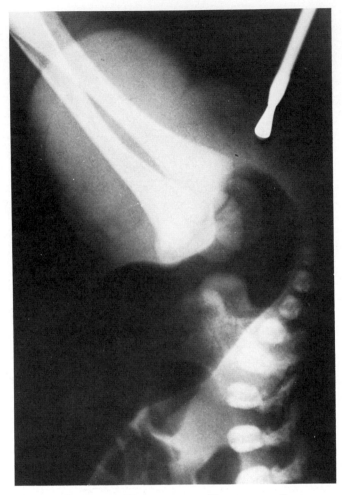

FIG. 4.10. INVERTED LATERAL VIEW OF THE RECTUM IN IMPERFORATE ANUS
   A glass thermometer is more hazardous than a metallic marker; pressure applied
to the anal dimple by the thermometer may falsely decrease the gap between the
colonic terminus and the anus.

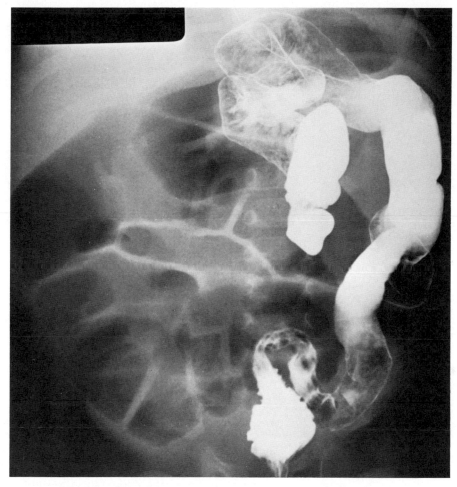

FIG. 4.11. NONROTATION OF THE BOWEL WITH VOLVULUS
The cecum is in the left mid-abdomen. Dilated loops of small bowel fill the right side of the abdomen.

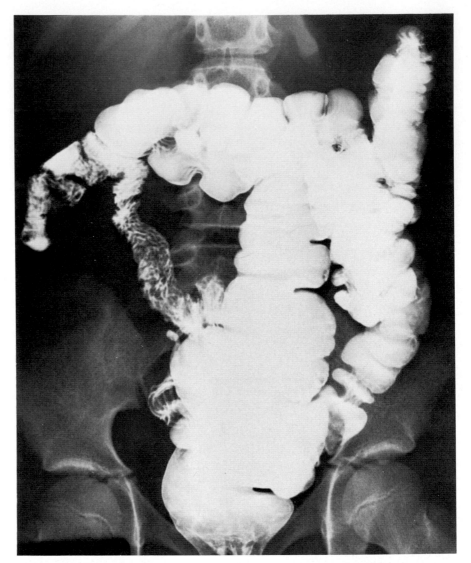

FIG. 4.12. NONROTATION OF COLON WITH MIDGUT VOLVULUS

This 10-year-old girl had episodes of bilious vomiting since birth. The cecum lies over the sacrum; the ileo-cecal valve faces right, and the ileum is in the right upper quadrant.

will reveal the site of obstruction proximally. Surgical treatment is required as an emergency procedure to untwist the volvulus and resect any necrotic areas of bowel. Perforation with free intra-abdominal air or peritonitis are ominous signs and indicate a less optimistic prognosis. Chronic intermittent volvulus may cause malabsorption and lymphangiectasia due to mechanical strangulation of lymphatics in the vascular pedicle.

Isolated volvulus with obstruction of the cecum or sigmoid colon has been reported in infants. However, it is not as common as would be expected considering the length of the sigmoid colon and its mesentery in the infant, and the incidence of incomplete fixation of the cecum. In both cases, radiographs of the abdomen will show massively dilated air-filled loops of small bowel and one large air-filled loop of colon. As in adults, a sigmoid volvulus may project into the right upper quadrant and a cecal volvulus into the left upper quadrant. No air is seen in the rectum if the volvulus is complete. Surgical correction is almost always required.

Hirschsprung's Disease

Hirschsprung's disease is the result of failure of development of mature ganglion cells in the myenteric plexus of the distal colon. Without ganglion cells, peristalsis ceases in the involved segment, but is hyperactive in the normally innervated colon. The proximal colon hypertrophies and dilates to accommodate the retained stool. (The term "congenital megacolon" is a misnomer, applying to the normal but dilated colon.) Obstruction to the flow of stool results in all cases, but may not exactly correlate with the length of the aperistaltic segment. In severe or fatal cases, enterocolitis of the proximal segment may supervene, perhaps secondary to a compromised vascular supply and to transmural infection.

For purposes of convenience, Hirschsprung's disease can be classified into three types: short segment disease of the most distal colon and rectum; long segment disease involving part or all of the left colon down to the rectum; and total aganglionosis of the entire colon from cecum to rectum.

The clinical presentation of Hirschsprung's disease may be variable. In severe cases, meconium may not be passed by 48 hr and abdominal distention rapidly develops. In other children, the onset is insidious with progressive constipation which may be transiently improved by enemas or digital disimpaction. As the constipation becomes more severe, vomiting, abdominal pain, cramps, and visible peristaltic contractions may be seen through the anterior abdominal wall. Progressive malaise, vomiting, and failure to grow may bring the child to medical attention. An untreated case may progress to death before puberty from inanition and intercurrent infection (Fig. 4.13).

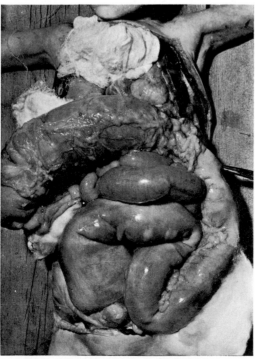

FIG. 4.13. HIRSCHSPRUNG'S DISEASE
Autopsy photograph of an 8-year-old girl with a hugely dilated large bowel.

Plain films of the abdomen will show signs of colonic obstruction in patients with short or long segment disease manifested by air-filled, dilated loops of proximal colon surrounding formed or semisolid stool. Lateral films of the abdomen generally show no air or stool in the rectum, except in those patients with very low segment disease. In patients with total aganglionosis, the radiographic pattern suggests distal small bowel obstruction, with little air or stool being identified within any portion of the colon.

The barium enema examination should be performed on the unprepared colon, without the use of prior cleansing enemas, digital exams, or balloon manometry. These manipulations may obscure the key radiographic feature: the transition zone between the nondilated, aperistaltic segment and the dilated, normally innervated proximal colon (Figs. 4.14 and 4.15). Care should be taken not to place the rectal tube beyond a low segment Hirschsprung's disease, thus bypassing the aperistaltic segment entirely. Delayed films of the abdomen 24 and 48 hr after examination may document slow passage of retained barium from the colon, a suggestive, but not diagnostic, sign of Hirschsprung's disease. Balloon manometry has been shown to be an effective adjunct to barium enema examination in Hirschsprung's disease and is especially valuable in patients with short aperistaltic segments.

The barium enema in patients with total aganglionosis shows a shortened colon of normal caliber, frequently with large amounts of reflux into a dilated terminal ileum. The 24- and 48-hr films will confirm poor passage of barium from the distal small bowel to the rectum.

Definitive diagnosis depends on biopsy of the colon and documentation of the absence of ganglion cells. Surgical treatment is proximal colostomy to decompress the obstruction, later followed by resection of the aganglionic segment. In the postoperative Hirschsprung's disease patient, the stooling pattern will return to normal, but some degree of dilation of the colon will remain.

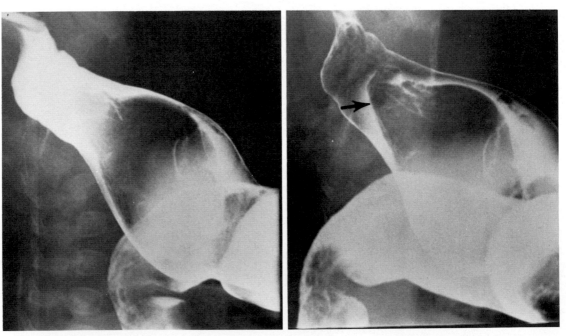

FIG. 4.14. LOW SEGMENT HIRSCHSPRUNG'S DISEASE IN A 4-WEEK-OLD INFANT WITH VOMITING

The distal colon is obstructed by a conical plug of stool. Failure of the lower rectal segment to distend is reflected in the contour of the stool plug (arrow).

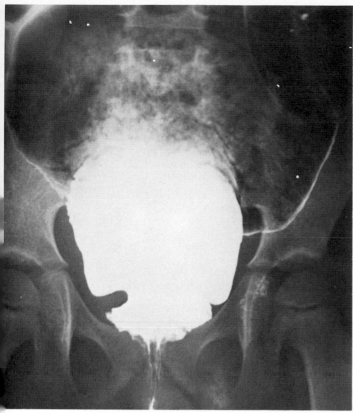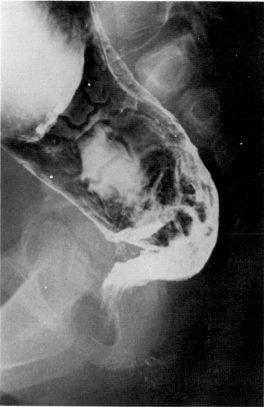

FIG. 4.15. LOW SEGMENT HIRSCHSPRUNG'S DISEASE

The distal rectum is nondilated as compared to the proximal rectum and sigmoid. Barium applied to the external surface of the anus is helpful in diagnosing low segment Hirschsprung's disease.

Meconium Plug Syndrome

The meconium plug syndrome is an obstruction of the colon caused by a large piece of solid meconium usually lodged in the left or sigmoid colon. The obstruction may be transitory and relieved by further straining by the baby or by mild saline enemas, or it may become complete with distention and vomiting. A barium enema examination will disclose a normal-sized distal colon with small pellets of meconium (Fig. 4.16). A large obstructing plug will be encountered when there is dilatation of the proximal colon. These plugs may be dislodged by using hydrostatic pressure and water-soluble contrast material to distend the luminal space, provide lubrication around the sides of the plug, and promote an influx of fluid into the colon assisting the passage of the plug. Meticulous care should be taken to prevent hypovolemia which can often result.

It is unfortunate that the entity of meconium plug syndrome is sometimes confused with meconium ileus. The latter condition, associated with cystic fibrosis, is completely unrelated although meconium ileus frequently results in a colon of markedly narrowed diameter (Fig. 4.17). Atresias of the ileum (Fig. 4.18) or jejunum (Fig. 4.19) can also result in a microcolon.

Small Left Colon Syndrome

As described by Davis, this syndrome affects children, most of whom are infants of diabetic mothers, who have a small colon from rectum to splenic flexure and a

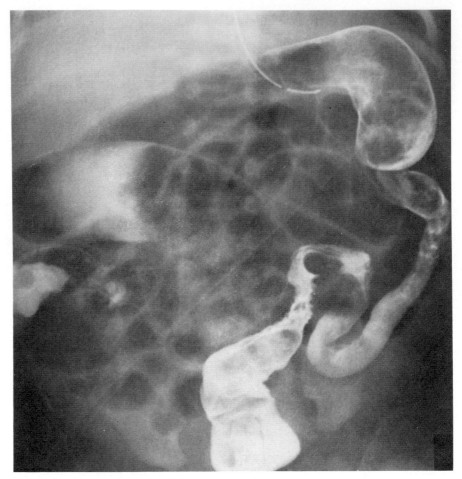

FIG. 4.16. MECONIUM PLUG SYNDROME
Water-soluble contrast enema in a newborn. The obstructing plug in the splenic flexure is outlined by contrast material. The proximal colon and small bowel are obstructed and dilated with air.

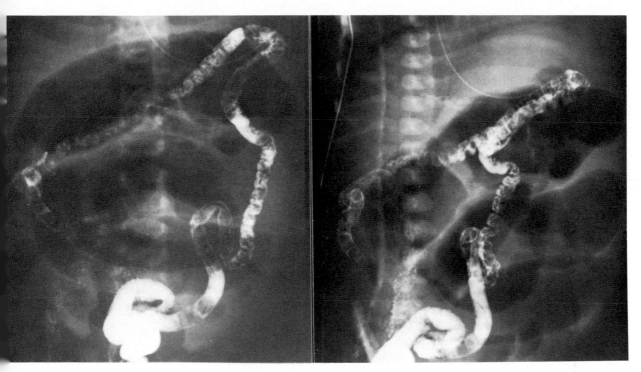

FIG. 4.17. UNUSED COLON IN MECONIUM ILEUS

Barium opacifies the small caliber colon and terminal ileum. Compare the multiple pellets of meconium seen in the transverse and left colon with the meconium in ileal atresia (Fig. 4.18).

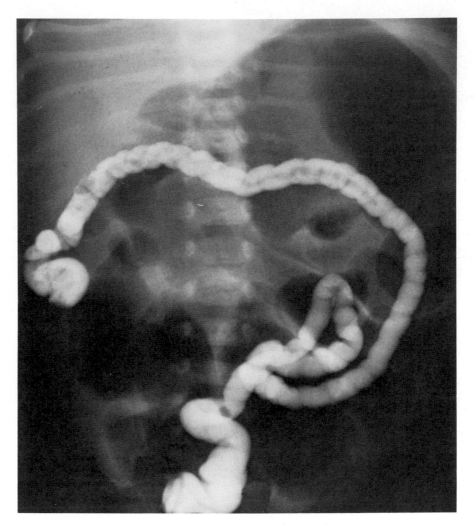

FIG. 4.18. MICROCOLON WITH ILEAL ATRESIA

The colon is unused and contains only one filament of meconium in the transverse segment. The multiple dilated loops of small bowel localize the obstruction to the ileum.

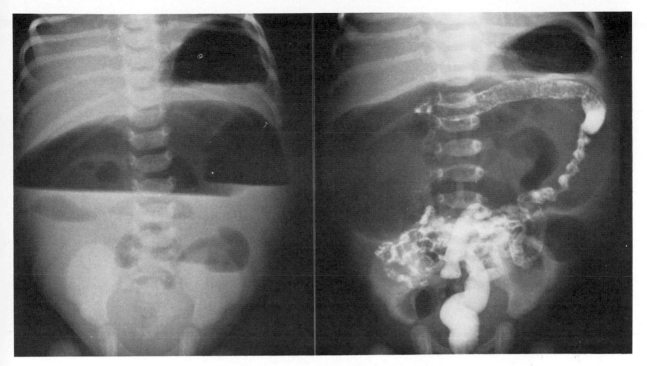

FIG. 4.19. MICROCOLON WITH JEJUNAL ATRESIA

A 24-hour-old baby presented with a protuberant abdomen. Barium opacifies the unused colon and ileum. Very distended loops of jejunum are partially filled with air and cause displacement of the hepatic flexure.

normal caliber colon proximally. There is a relative obstruction at the level of the splenic flexure which may require repeated barium enemas to dilate. Perhaps immaturity of the colonic neuroplexus plays a role in this syndrome, causing delay in normal peristalsis of the caudal end of the colon during infancy.

Bands

Peritoneal bands are adhesions or cords of fibrous tissue which may originate anywhere within the abdomen. While they are usually associated with malrotation, they may also occur in cases with complete rotation and fixation of the bowel. The usual level of obstruction is the duodenum or terminal ileum, although the colon may occasionally become obstructed.

Functional Obstruction in the Premature Infant

Functional obstruction is a condition in which the colon and small bowel do not normally maintain peristaltic activity. A transient obstruction of the colon has been described in premature infants which disappears within 4–7 days without therapy. Peristaltic activity may also cease in patients with hypovolemia and metabolic changes including hypokalemia, hypocalcemia, or acidemia. Septic shock, adrenal hemorrhage, and umbilical arterial catheterization all can cause a similar loss of peristaltic activity. In such cases, the child feeds poorly and may become distended. Vomiting is inconstant, and stooling may cease. Supine and upright films of the abdomen show distended loops of bowel throughout the abdomen from stomach to anus. Barium enema examination is normal, showing normal caliber and fixation of the colon. Expectant treatment and correction of any major metabolic disturbance is the treatment of choice.

DUPLICATIONS

Duplications of the colon, similar to stenosis and atresia, are thought to be the result of early intrauterine vascular insult. These duplications may be isolated from the cecum to the rectum, or may nearly duplicate the entire colon, even with a separate anus. Clinical symptoms depend on the degree of obstruction of the normal colon by the enlarging duplication. Barium enema examination will opacify those colonic duplications which communicate with the normal colon either at the proximal or distal end of the duplication. In duplications without communication, the barium enema will document a mass effect against the normal colon and small bowel by the large duplication mass. In such cases, the diagnosis is made by inference. Duplications of the right colon in the newborn frequently undergo intussusception (Fig. 4.20). The treatment in all cases of colon duplication is resection, once the diagnosis has been made.

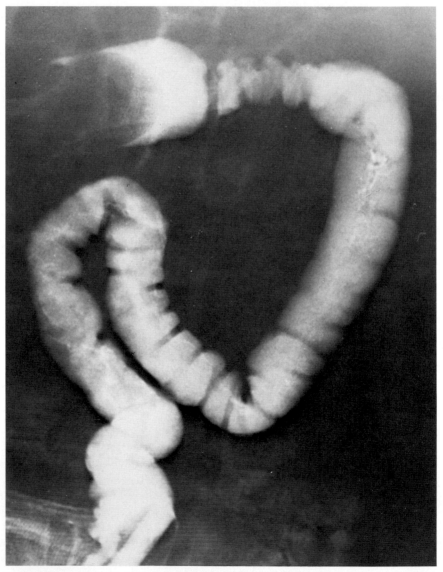

FIG. 4.20. CECAL DUPLICATION LEADING AN INTUSSUSCEPTION IN A NEONATE
Intussusceptions in newborn patients usually have a pathologic lesion as a lead point, frequently a cecal duplication.

BIBLIOGRAPHY

Bley, W. R., and Franken, E. A.: Roentgenology of colon atresia. Pediatr. Radiol., *1:* 105, 1973.

Campbell, J. R., and Blank, E.: Sigmoid volvulus in children. Pediatrics, *53:* 702, 1974.

Cremin, B. J.: The early diagnosis of Hirschsprung's disease. Pediatr. Radiol., *2:* 23, 1974.

Cremin, B. J.: Functional intestinal obstruction in premature infants. Pediatr. Radiol., *1:* 109, 1973.

Davis, W. S., and Campbell, J. B.: Neonatal small left colon syndrome. Occurrence in asymptomatic infants of diabetic mothers. Am. J. Dis. Child., *129:* 1024, 1975.

Frech, R. S.: Aganglionosis involving the entire colon and a variable length of small bowel. Radiology, *90:* 249, 1968.

Hope, J. W., Borns, P. F., and Berg, P. K.: Roentgen manifestations of Hirschsprung's disease in infancy. Am. J. Roentgenol., *95:* 217, 1965.

Houston, C. S., and Whittenborg, M. H.: Roentgen evaluation of anomalies of rotation and fixation of the bowel in children. Radiology, *84:* 1, 1965.

Kottra, J. J., and Dodds, W. J.: Duplication of the large bowel. Am. J. Roentgenol., *113:* 310, 1971.

Mahboubi, S., and Schnaufer, L.: The barium-enema examination and rectal manometry in Hirschsprung's disease. Radiology, *130:* 643, 1979.

Manzano, C., and Barrera, J. L.: Stenosis of the colon. Pediatr. Radiol., *5:* 148, 1977.

Mascatello, V., and Lebowitz, R. L.: Malposition of the colon in left renal agenesis and ectopia. Radiology, *120:* 371, 1976.

Noblett, H. R.: The treatment of uncomplicated meconium ileus by gastrografin enema. A preliminary report. J. Pediatr. Surg., *4:* 190, 1969.

Pochaczevsky, R., Ratner, H., Leonidas, J. C., Naysan, P., and Feraru, F.: Unusual forms of volvulus after the neonatal period. Am. J. Roentgenol., *114:* 390, 1972.

Sane, S. M., and Girdany, B. R.: Total aganglionosis coli. Radiology, *107:* 397, 1973.

Santulli, T. V., Kiesewetter, W. B., and Bill, A. H., Jr.: Anorectal anomalies: A suggested international classification. J. Pediatr. Surg., *5:* 281, 1970.

Singleton, E. B., Wagner, M. L., and Dutton, R. V.: *Radiology of the Alimentary Tract in Infants and Children,* 2nd ed., Chaps. 15 and 16. W. B. Saunders, Philadelphia, 1977.

Stephens, F. D., and Smith, E. D.: *Ano-Rectal Malformations in Children.* Year Book Medical Publishers, Chicago, 1971.

Swischuk, L. E.: Meconium plug syndrome: A cause of neonatal intestinal obstruction. Am. J. Roentgenol., *103:* 339, 1968.

Vanhoutte, J. J., and Katzman, D.: Roentgenographic manifestations of immaturity of intestinal neural plexus in premature infants. Radiology, *106:* 363, 1973.

Wagner, M. L., Harberg, F. J., Kumar, A. P. M., and Singleton, E. B.: The evaluation of imperforate anus utilizing percutaneous injection of water soluble iodide contrast material. Pediatr. Radiol., *1:* 34, 1973.

Wangensteen, O. H., and Rice, C. O.: Imperforate anus—A method of determining the surgical approach. Ann. Surg., *92:* 77, 1930.

Weber, H. M., and Dixon, C. F.: Duplication of the entire large intestine (colon duplex). Am. J. Roentgenol., *55:* 319, 1946.

5

Acquired Diseases of the Pediatric Colon

SPENCER BORDEN, IV, M.D.

Inflammatory Diseases	Vascular Insults to the Colon
Ulcerative Colitis	Benign Tumors
Crohn's Colitis	Juvenile Polyps
Appendicitis	Polyposis Disorders
Bacterial Colitis	Malignant Tumors
Amebic and Tuberculous Colitis	Lymphoma
Trichuriasis (Whip-Worm Infestation)	Carcinoma
Necrotizing Enterocolitis	Traumatic and Mechanical Lesions
Milk Colitis	Psychogenic Megacolon
Typhlitis	Intussusception
Pseudomembranous Colitis	Cystic Fibrosis

INFLAMMATORY DISEASES

Ulcerative Colitis

Ulcerative colitis first occurs in childhood in less than 20% of all cases. Although the disease can occasionally be found in the first 5 years of life, the usual age of onset is the teenage years. Pediatric patients tend to have a more severe disease than adults; moderate to severe activity is present in 90% of children, but in less than 50% of adults. Clinical symptoms of childhood ulcerative colitis include diarrhea with mucus or blood, rectal and abdominal pains which may be sharp and colicky, and episodic rectal bleeding. Systemic manifestations may include dehydration, hypoalbuminemia, anemia, weight loss, tachycardia, loss of appetite, and malabsorption. Complications include fatty infiltration of the liver, pericholangitis, chronic hepatitis or cirrhosis of the liver and arthritis. Cutaneous manifestations such as pyoderma gangrenosum and erythema nodosum may also occur.

The clinical diagnosis of ulcerative colitis may be strongly suggested by the history and confirmed by sigmoidoscopy, biopsy, and barium enema examination. The preliminary films of the abdomen may show thickening of the colonic wall suggestive of ulcerative colitis or may show toxic dilatation, which is a contraindication to barium enema examination. Most children are self-prepared by continuous diarrhea. To avoid the risk of perforation, we prefer not to give purgatives in cases of presumed ulcerative colitis.*

The earliest features of ulcerative colitis on barium enema examination are irritability and mucosal edema, the latter causing a longitudinal fold pattern best

---

* For a different point of view, see Chapter 9.

visualized on postevacuation films. Punctate ulcerations may be demonstrated in the distal colon. With more advanced disease, the contour of the colon becomes irregular and serrated. Pseudopolyps of residual or regenerating islands of mucosa are irregular in shape but similar in size (Fig. 5.1).

In chronic ulcerative colitis, the colon may appear short and rigid with loss of haustral pouches (Fig. 5.2). The normal mucosal pattern may be effaced or there may be scattered pseudopolyps.

The distribution of ulcerative colitis is characteristic and may serve to differentiate it from Crohn's colitis. The earliest areas to be involved with ulcerative colitis are the rectum and rectosigmoid. As the disease advances, the descending, transverse and ascending colon become progressively involved in a continuous manner. There are no areas of unaffected colon (skip areas). In many cases, these characteristic features sharply distinguish ulcerative colitis from Crohn's colitis, but in a small percentage of cases, radiographic differentiation is not possible.

Complications of ulcerative colitis are multiple and may be life-threatening. Toxic dilatation describes a very ill patient with severe mucosal destruction and atony of the colon. The patient is feverish, leukopenic, and frequently septic with a silent abdomen. Plain films of the abdomen in the supine position will disclose a markedly dilated transverse colon with little redundancy; pseudopolyps may be outlined by the intraluminal air. In this state, the colon is very friable and the risk of spontaneous perforation is great. Toxic dilatation is a contraindication to barium enema examination; prompt surgical treatment is required, particularly if a pneumoperitoneum has been documented.

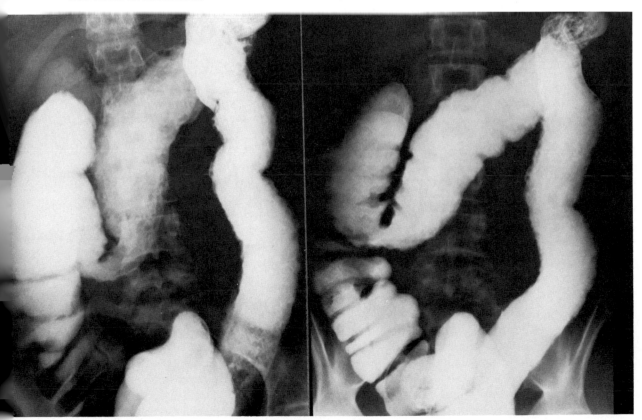

FIG. 5.1. EXTENSIVE ULCERATIVE COLITIS IN A 17-YEAR-OLD GIRL
The transverse and descending segments show diffuse mucosal ulceration with pseudopolyps. The involved colon is shortened and ahaustral; the cecum is spared.

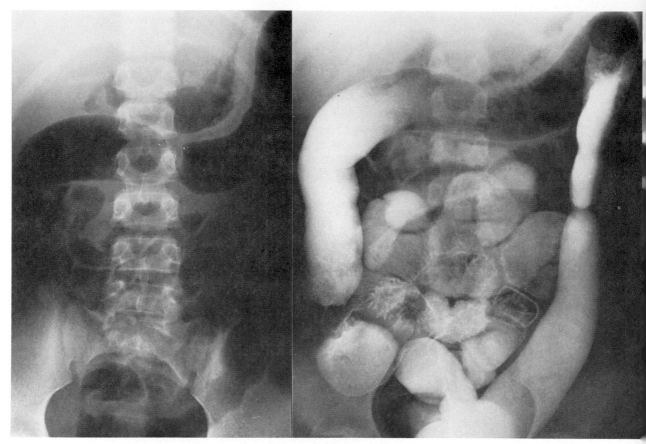

FIG. 5.2. CHRONIC ULCERATIVE COLITIS IN A 12-YEAR-OLD GIRL

The plain film shows the colon to be smooth, tubular, and shortened; there is an area of spasm in the transverse segment. The barium enema outlines the unchanging colon contour. Copious ileal reflux is common.

Backwash ileitis is a frequent finding in children with ulcerative colitis. The ileocecal valve may be widely patent, permitting easy reflux of barium. The terminal ileum may have an irregular contour with mucosal edema. Nodularity of mucosa and strictures, seen in regional enteritis, are not found.

Complications of long standing ulcerative colitis are failure of long term medical therapy, intractable hemorrhage, perforation, and the development of carcinoma.

Crohn's Colitis

The radiographic findings in Crohn's colitis are indistinguishable from those of regional enteritis of the small bowel with which it is usually associated, although a few children have disease limited to the colon. In children with regional enteritis, there is more frequent coexisting involvement of the colon than in adults.

The distribution of Crohn's colitis differs from ulcerative colitis; the ileum, cecum, and ascending colon are most frequently involved; anal disease with ulcerations leading to anal fissures, fistulas, and abscesses is 3 times more frequent. Normal segments of colon (skip areas) may be present between diseased portions, whereas the colon is always involved in continuity in ulcerative colitis.

Clinical manifestations of regional enteritis and Crohn's colitis in children are frequently more insidious and less obviously related to the gastrointestinal tract than those of ulcerative colitis. Weight loss, diarrhea, crampy abdominal pain, and anorexia are the most consistent features; failure to grow and delay in puberty and menarche are also common. Laboratory examination may confirm anemia from blood loss in the stool, hypoproteinemia from protein-losing enteropathy, and steatorrhea from malabsorption of bile salts.

Definitive diagnosis depends on barium studies or fiberoptic endoscopy. The yield from sigmoidoscopy is limited to those patients with rectal involvement. Preliminary films of the abdomen are usually nondiagnostic but may occasionally suggest a mass in the lower right quadrant. With early cases of Crohn's colitis, mucosal edema and thickening of the interhaustral folds in the right colon may be the only features (Fig. 5.3). With progressive disease, the colon may demonstrate multifocal areas of involvement with mucosal nodularity (Fig. 5.4), and rigid segments with thickening of the wall causing local strictures. Longitudinal ulcers may cause long furrows in the mucosa. Sinus tracks, fistulas, and abscesses are not uncommon. Total involvement of the colon, including the rectum, is unusual. In contrast to ulcerative colitis, nodularity and strictures of the terminal ileum and adjacent loops of small bowel are frequent. In cases of chronic Crohn's colitis, strictures may be documented at multiple levels with distention of unaffected, proximal portions of the colon.

The features of multifocal involvement of the colon and terminal ileum, nodularity and stricture formation, pericolic abscess and sinus track formation all serve to differentiate Crohn's colitis from ulcerative colitis. The rare case of isolated Crohn's colitis involving the entire colon may be difficult to differentiate from ulcerative colitis. Biopsy in these cases may be helpful.

Surgery is indicated in Crohn's colitis in the presence of obstruction, abscess formation, or fistulas. Local resections may be attempted, but the disease frequently recurs in previously unaffected segments (Fig. 5.5). Total colectomy is rarely indicated.

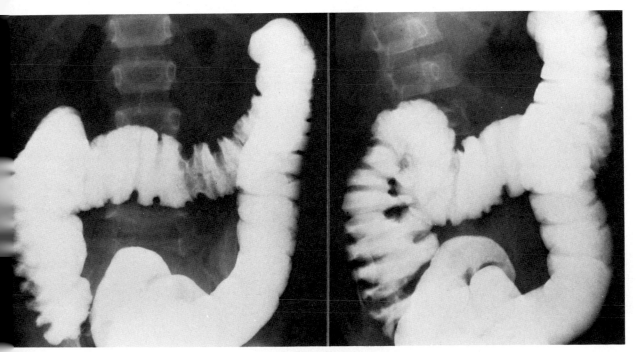

FIG. 5.3. CROHN'S COLITIS OF THE RIGHT AND TRANSVERSE SEGMENTS IN A
10-YEAR-OLD BOY

The interhaustral folds are markedly thickened in the cecum and transverse colon.

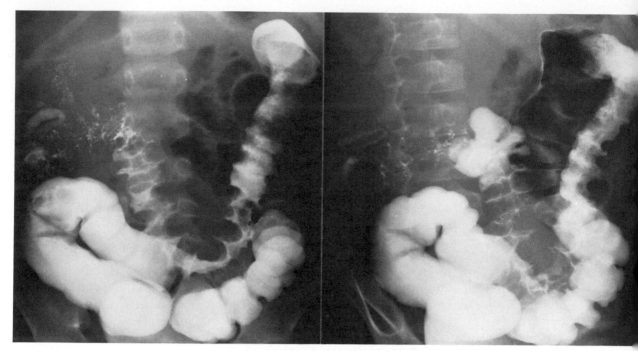

FIG. 5.4. CROHN'S COLITIS IN AN 8-YEAR-OLD BOY

The nodularity of the transverse colon wall is impressive and resembles intramural hematomas. The descending segment is also involved. Spasm prevents distention of the right colon.

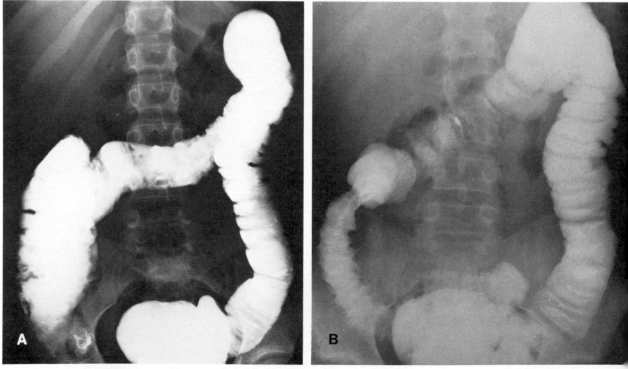

FIG. 5.5. CROHN'S COLITIS IN A 13-YEAR-OLD BOY

(A) Thickened haustral folds, ulcers, and nodularity of the right and transverse colon walls are present. (B) Twenty months after right colectomy, recurrent disease has involved the distal ileum proximal to the ileo-transverse colostomy anastomosis.

Appendicitis

The broad subject of appendicitis is treated in Chapter 18. Appendicitis in the debilitated child or neonate is very difficult to diagnose due to lack of specific symptoms. Lethargy, poor feeding, irritability, and a poor cry may be the only features in the neonate. Ruptured appendices with pneumoperitoneum or peritonitis are found in approximately 70% of neonates surgically explored for appendicitis.

Bacterial Colitis

The clinical manifestations of bacterial colitis may include fever, elevated white blood cell count, severe abdominal pain, and diarrhea with or without hemorrhage. Seizures may be present with shigellosis. Debilitated children and the very premature are predisposed to unusual pathogens, such as Candida. Plain film findings and barium enema examination are nonspecific. There may be severe spasticity and irritability of the colon, but ulcerations are rarely seen and the appropriate bacteriologic diagnosis is made by stool culture. The colon returns to normal in 10–14 days with appropriate antibiotic therapy.

Amebic and Tuberculous Colitis

The cecum is the portion of the colon most frequently involved by both tuberculosis and amebiasis; it will be irritable and fail to distend on barium studies. Small ulcerations may be demonstrated. Rectal ulcerations, hepatomegaly, and a right pleural effusion may also be present with severe amebiasis. Edema and irregularity of the terminal ileum are more frequent in tuberculosis, as are pulmonary or osseous lesions. The appropriate bacteriologic and parasitologic examinations will establish the correct diagnosis in most cases.

Trichuriasis (Whip Worm Infestation)

Whip worms may infest the colon, particularly in the tropical areas of the world. The eggs are ingested and hatch in the duodenum, forming larvae. The larvae pass to the colon where they become attached and grow to mature worms, measuring up to 3 cm in length. With severe infestation, anorexia and weight loss may progress to bloody diarrhea and rectal prolapse. Recovery of the whip worm from the stool provides the diagnosis. Radiologic demonstration of the whip worm is best accomplished by double-contrast technique. The worms may be seen as long, curvilinear radiolucencies attached to the bowel wall. A small area of mucosal swelling with central umbilication is found at the point of attachment. If the patient has been recently purged of the worms, the small umbilicated nodules may be the only radiologic feature of recent infestation.

Necrotizing Enterocolitis

Necrotizing enterocolitis is the most serious acquired disease of the colon in premature infants. The etiology is obscure, but important factors are prematurity and stress. Infants at risk are frequently gravely ill with cardiac, pulmonary, or hematologic disease which predispose them to hypoxia, acidosis, or infection.

The early pathologic changes consist of focal edema of the colon or small bowel, local inflammation with mononuclear cells predominating, and the presence of intramural gas. As the condition progresses, intramural hemorrhage, necrosis with sloughing of the mucosa, and greater amounts of intramural gas may be seen.

The clinical features of necrotizing enterocolitis include sepsis, irritability, leukopenia, and lethargy. Gastrointestinal features are abdominal distention, vomiting, and the passage of bloody material from the rectum.

Due to extreme friability of the colonic wall, radiologic diagnosis must depend on the plain abdominal film without a barium study. Supine and upright films of the abdomen are most useful; left lateral decubitus films are helpful to demonstrate small amounts of pneumoperitoneum. The earliest radiographic features are thickening of the bowel wall, sometimes associated with intramural gas and a rigid, unchanging segment of air-filled colon. When seen *en face*, small quantities of intramural air may simulate air mixed with stool; with progressive infiltration of the bowel wall by air, long, curvilinear, intramural radiolucencies may be seen (Fig. 5.6). Passage of air into venous structures of the colon wall leads to portal venous gas which is easily identified in the liver. Air trapped within the liver may be a transient phenomenon and be resorbed within 20 min. The presence of portal venous air implies a severe necrotizing enterocolitis and is associated with a high mortality rate. Small transmural ruptures into the peritoneal cavity may cause abscess formation, or a major rupture may cause pneumoperitoneum (Fig. 5.7); these are grave findings and require immediate surgical therapy.

While the presence of intramural air in the bowel wall is the most characteristic roentgen feature of necrotizing enterocolitis, it is not specific for this disease. Vascular occlusion of mesenteric arteries or veins by indwelling catheters may cause intestinal necrosis and the identical radiographic findings. Severe obstruction of the colon by atresia, Hirschsprung's disease, or severe colitis may also be associated with intramural air. Finally, intramural air may dissect from the mediastinal space in patients on positive pressure ventilation.

Complications of necrotizing enterocolitis are perforation, fistula and abscess formation, and the late development of a stricture. In patients with mild disease, successfully managed by antibiotics and nasogastric suction, strictures may be seen in the convalescent period, usually in the areas of most severe involvement by the necrotizing process. Such strictures may resolve spontaneously, but enterocolic fistulas require surgical treatment.

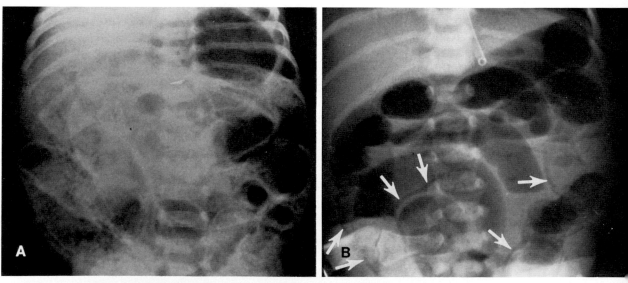

FIG. 5.6. WIDESPREAD INTRAMURAL AIR IN NECROTIZING ENTEROCOLITIS
(**A**) A supine film shows many air lucencies creating a bubbly texture. (**B**) On the upright film, the intramural air has assumed a curvilinear configuration (arrows). There is also air in the portal vein and small bowel dilatation.

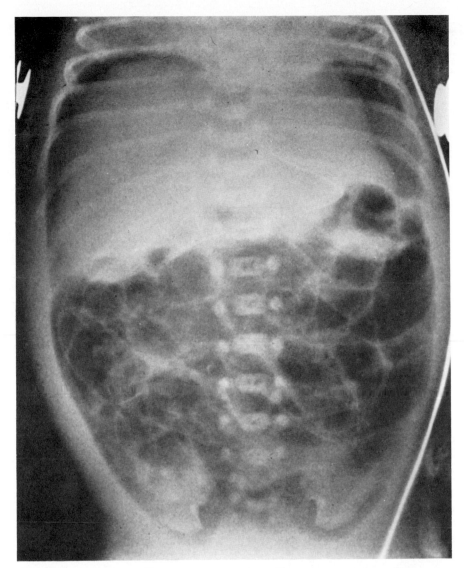

FIG. 5.7. NECROTIZING ENTEROCOLITIS WITH PERFORATION IN A PREMATURE
INFANT

The large pneumoperitoneum pushes the liver and spleen medially, distends the
abdomen, and elevates the diaphragm, further compromising the sick baby.

Milk Colitis

The diagnosis of allergy to cow's milk has been made infrequently on radiologic
grounds. Neonates may have abdominal distention and bloody diarrhea on a diet of
cow's milk, which subsides when the milk is removed. Subsequent challenges and
withdrawal of cow's milk to and from the diet provoke exacerbations and remissions
of the bowel symptoms. Barium enema examination will show multifocal areas of
mucosal edema and ulceration during the acute phase, which disappear when the
cow's milk is withdrawn. The findings are nonspecific.

Typhlitis

Typhlitis is a disease of children with leukemia or aplastic anemia in which the cecum undergoes hemorrhagic necrosis. The etiology is obscure, but may involve transmural inflammation and necrosis of the cecum. The clinical presentation is one of fever, progressive abdominal distention, and pain in the right abdomen. Radiographic studies may show a large soft tissue mass in the right lower or mid abdomen, signs of small bowel obstruction, and only a small quantity of gas in the colon. This condition is usually a terminal event in patients with severe underlying disease and may not be separable from ruptured appendicitis on clinical or radiologic grounds.

Pseudomembranous Colitis

Pseudomembranous colitis is a rare form of transmural colitis, frequently associated with staphylococcal infection. A diffuse yellow membrane is found on the inflamed and ulcerated mucosa. The membrane may be present on parts or all of the colon and may even extend into the small bowel. Children predisposed to this catastrophic illness are those on broad spectrum antibiotics and in a postoperative status. The clinical presentation is one of an acute, severe illness with abdominal distention and relentless diarrhea; vomiting and shock may rapidly develop.

Although the diagnosis may be made by identifying the yellow membrane at the time of sigmoidoscopy, barium examination will document the extent of involvement (Figs. 11.1 and 11.3). The radiographic features are mucosal edema, ulcerations, and irregular plaques of necrotic membrane separated from the mucosa. Supportive medical therapy including antibiotics, steroids, and fluid replacement may be curative.

VASCULAR INSULTS TO THE COLON

Ischemic insults to the colon can be produced by fibrin thrombi embolized from indwelling umbilical catheters. The embolization may be so severe that thrombosis of the superior and inferior mesenteric arteries occurs, causing necrosis of the large and small bowel which they supply. Umbilical venous catheters placed in the portal venous system for replacement of fluid or exchange transfusion may cause sufficient variation in intestinal venous pressure to cause intramural hematomas. If severe, perforation may result. There may also be an element of bowel ischemia in necrotizing enterocolitis.

Three additional diseases may cause intramural hematoma of the small and large bowel in the older pediatric patient. *Henoch-Schoenlein purpura* causes a diffuse skin rash, arthralgias, and hematomas frequently in the wall of the small bowel and occasionally in the large bowel. Intussusception may result with the intramural hematoma serving as a lead point. A barium enema may demonstrate either the thumbprinting of intramural hematomas or the intussusception. Intramural hematomas sometimes occur in patients with *hemophilia* following major abdominal trauma; these hematomas of the bowel may be documented by barium enema examination and may resolve with appropriate medical therapy in 10 days. Fifteen percent of patients with *hemolytic-uremic syndrome* may present with diarrhea, abdominal pain, and findings on barium enema which suggest an inflammatory process. However, intramural hematomas (Fig. 5.8) are commonly seen in addition to the ulcerated mucosa (Fig. 5.9). In several days, the other features of the disease—microangiopathic hemolytic anemia, thrombocytopenia, and uremia—may supervene. Sequential barium enema examinations during medical therapy will document disappearance of the intramural hematomas and resolution of the mucosal changes, although in some cases delayed strictures may develop.

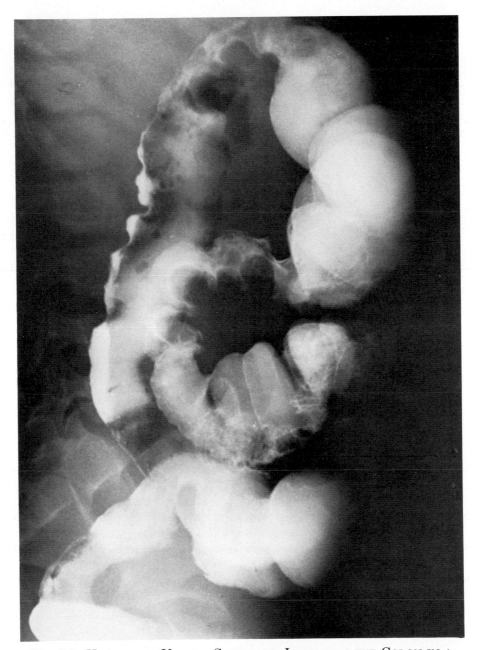

FIG. 5.8. HEMOLYTIC UREMIC SYNDROME INVOLVING THE COLON IN A
6-YEAR-OLD GIRL

Ten days after an attack of measles, this child presented with abdominal cramps and bloody diarrhea. Nodularity of the bowel wall is consistent with intramural hematomata.

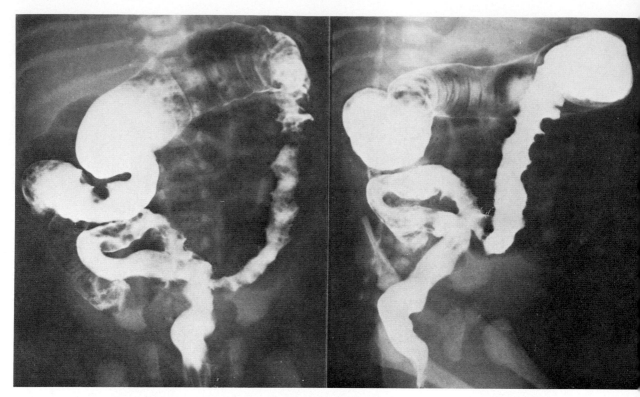

FIG. 5.9. NEONATAL HEMOLYTIC-UREMIC COLITIS IN A 4-DAY-OLD GIRL

An extensive colitis involves the splenic flexure and descending colon. The resected specimen showed mucosal ulceration, blood and gas in the submucosa and transmural inflammation.

BENIGN TUMORS

Juvenile Polyps

Juvenile polyps are the most common benign tumor involving the colon of children and are most frequently found in the rectum and sigmoid colon. Two or more polyps may be found in 25% of the cases. The peak incidence is between 2 and 5 years of age without sex predilection. The cardinal clinical manifestation is blood streaks on the stool in the absence of pain. An anal fissure should be excluded by direct visualization. Juvenile polyps may be as large as 2 cm in diameter, round or oval, and attached to the bowel wall by a broad or thin stalk. Rarely they may prolapse through the anus. Although juvenile polyps may reach 2–3 cm in diameter, they rarely obstruct the colon.

With appropriate clinical symptoms, the diagnosis of a juvenile polyp may be made by sigmoidoscopy and barium enema. Low-lying rectal polyps may be discovered by the examining finger. Barium enema examination (Figs. 5.10 and 5.11) is necessary to discover higher or multiple polyps. Double-contrast enema techniques after vigorous bowel preparation are required to demonstrate small polyps. Fluoroscopic palpation of the colon is frequently required to dislodge retained pieces of stool or to demonstrate the stalk tethering the polyp to the bowel wall. With the decreasing incidence of juvenile polyps as children grow older, it is likely that many polyps spontaneously undergo torsion and rupture of the stalk, passing in a bowel movement. There is no association of colonic carcinoma with isolated juvenile polyps. Treatment is therefore conservative; lesions within reach of the sigmoidoscope are snared and removed.

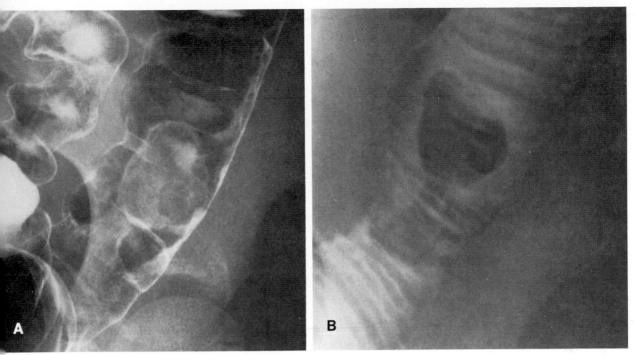

FIG. 5.10. A JUVENILE POLYP IN THE DESCENDING COLON OF AN 8-YEAR-OLD
BOY

The polyp is club shaped, 2 cm in diameter, and is shown outlined by air (**A**) and
by barium (**B**).

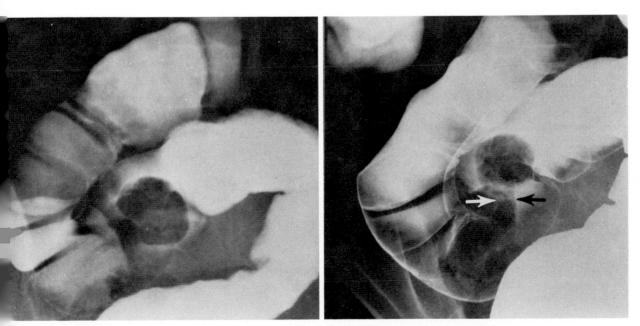

FIG. 5.11. A SIGMOID JUVENILE POLYP IN A 5-YEAR-OLD GIRL WHO HAD BLOOD-
STREAKED STOOLS

The lesion is lobulated and has a broad stalk (arrows).

Other benign tumors which may rarely arise in the colon are adenoma, villous adenoma, hemangioma, and hamartoma. The radiographic appearance of these lesions is nonspecific and an exact diagnosis may only be speculated radiologically unless there are additional clues, such as other hemangiomas, or electrolyte disturbances in cases of villous adenoma. Extracolonic lesions can also sometimes involve the colon (Fig. 5.12).

Polyposis Disorders

The presence of multiple polypoid tumors in the colon raises the possibility of a group of diseases including familial adenomatous colonic polyposis (Fig. 5.13), Peutz-Jeghers syndrome, the Gardner syndrome, juvenile polyposis of the colon, Cronkhite-Canada syndrome, and the Turcot syndrome. These multiple polyposis disorders are discussed in detail in Chapter 16.

Three other conditions should be excluded from consideration before a true polyposis disorder is considered. The first is retained stool which may mimic multiple small polyps. The irregular contours of these defects plus their variability in size may cause the fluoroscopist to repeat the barium enema or perform a double-contrast examination following evacuation in order to demonstrate the disappearance of adherent stool. The lymphoid follicular pattern of the colon is a normal condition in children. These multiple lesions are small, delicately umbilicated and should not be confused with polyps. The pseudopolyposis of ulcerative and Crohn's colitis should be distinguished from a polyposis disorder. The history and clinical findings are critical in such a differentiation.

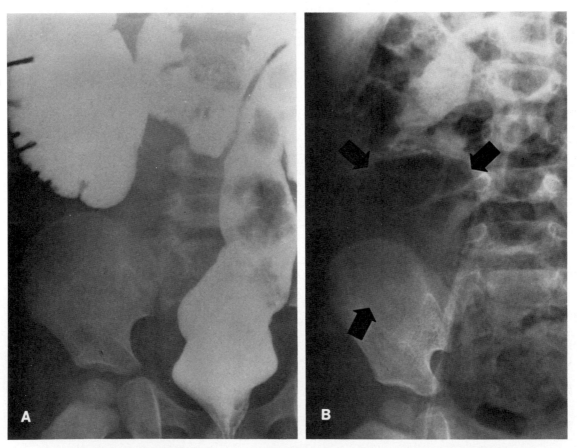

FIG. 5.12. LYMPHANGIOMA OF THE MESENTERY IN A 2-YEAR-OLD BOY
(A) The space between the cecum and sigmoid was not opacified by barium, yet no rounded contour indents the colon. (B) An avascular mass (arrows) is seen during the injection phase of a urogram. Nonpalpability is characteristic of these lesions.

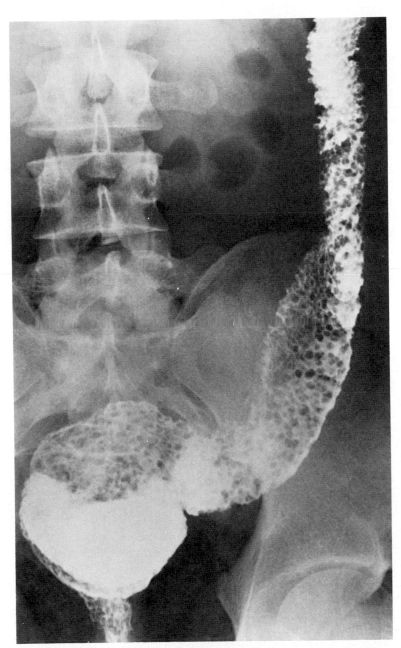

FIG. 5.13. FAMILIAL ADENOMATOUS COLONIC POLYPOSIS OF THE COLON IN A
17-YEAR-OLD BOY
The colon is carpeted with innumerable polyps.

MALIGNANT TUMORS

Lymphoma

Lymphomatous lesions of the pediatric colon include lymphosarcoma, Burkitt's tumor, lymphoma, and colonic involvement in acute lymphatic leukemia. These lesions tend to affect the ileocecal area, although lymphosarcoma may be widespread. Lymphomatous tumors not infrequently cause intussusception which may be the initial presenting complaint. Other patients may have clinical symptoms suggestive of appendicitis and the correct diagnosis may not be made until surgery. Additional clinical symptoms include a nontender right lower quadrant mass, iron deficiency anemia, and abdominal pain. A soft tissue mass may be detected on plain film examination, displacing adjacent loops of bowel. Barium enema study will show a nodular constriction of the right colon and ileum and inability to distend the lumen (Figs. 5.14 and 5.15). Unlike in Crohn's colitis, tuberculous colitis or amebiasis, spasm, perforation, and stricture are not radiographic features. Surgical excision of obstructing or intussuscepting tumors is required. Chemotherapeutic and radiotherapeutic treatment may be applied to widely disseminated lesions or to leukemic infiltrations.

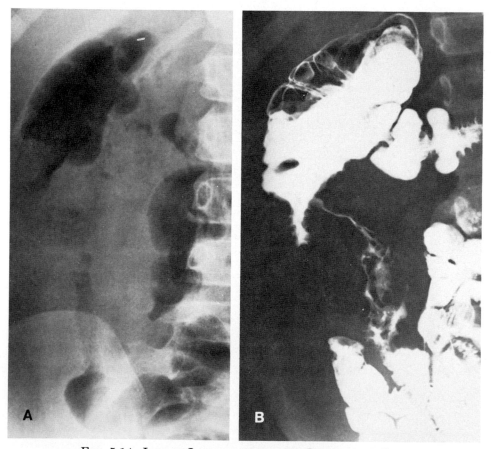

FIG. 5.14. LARGE LYMPHOMA OF THE ILEUM AND CECUM
(A) The plain film shows a large mass encircling a loop of small bowel and elevating the right colon. (B) The barium study shows marked nodularity and stenosis of the distal ileum together with constriction and infiltration of the cecum.

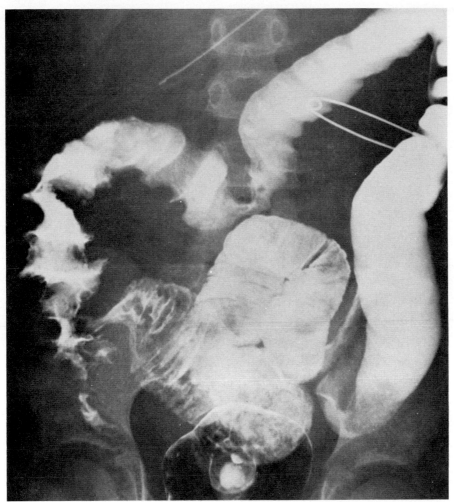

FIG. 5.15. LEUKEMIC INVOLVEMENT OF THE RIGHT COLON

This 6-year-old girl presented with acute lymphatic leukemia and a right abdominal mass. The wall of the right colon is infiltrated and nondistensible. The ileum is dilated.

Carcinoma

Primary carcinoma of the colon in children is rare, with some 200 cases being reported to date. The most common histologic type is a mucin-producing colloid adenocarcinoma which is most frequently found in the rectum and sigmoid. Both the primary tumor or secondary deposits may occasionally calcify (Fig. 5.16). The clinical manifestations include rectal bleeding, crampy pains, and constipation. Weight loss and anorexia may be a common feature if metastatic disease is present. Colloid carcinomas have the same radiographic features as colon carcinoma in the adult—large polypoid masses or constricting lesions with sharply defined shoulders. Such an appearance when combined with calcification in the tumor is considered diagnostic for colloid carcinoma of the colon.

Adenocarcinomas of the colon are more common in patients with chronic ulcerative colitis and familial adenomatous colonic polyposis. Carcinomas in patients with ulcerative colitis may be polypoid or small plaque-like lesions. Carcinomas in patients with familial adenomatous colonic polyposis may be indistinguishable

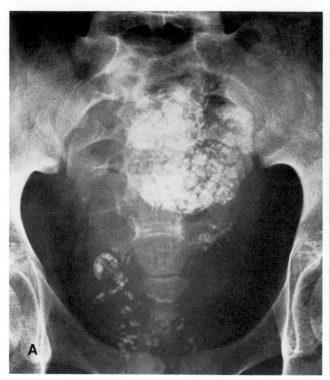
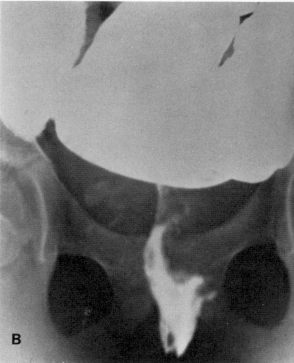

FIG. 5.16. PRIMARY COLLOID ADENOCARCINOMA OF THE RECTUM IN A
12-YEAR-OLD GIRL
(A) The preliminary film shows a densely calcified mass in front of the sacrum,
extending to the rectum. (B) A constricting mass with an intraluminal shoulder
encircles the barium-filled rectum. The child died with hepatic metastases which
were also calcified.

radiologically from nonmalignant polyps. Because the incidence of carcinomas in
these patients rises in the second and third decade, early colectomy is the only
definitive treatment.

TRAUMATIC AND MECHANICAL LESIONS

The wall of the colon in children may be damaged by changes occurring within
the wall, by perforations caused by sharp objects within the lumen of the colon and
by crushing and penetrating injuries from outside the colon. Vascular insults caused
by the hemolytic-uremic syndrome, indwelling umbilical venous catheters in the
portal system, and thrombi from indwelling umbilical arterial catheters have been
mentioned. Inflammatory lesions such as necrotizing enterocolitis may predispose
to perforation. Dissection of air within the bowel wall is frequently observed in
necrotizing enterocolitis, and occasionally seen in severe obstruction or in association
with the colitis proximal to Hirschsprung's disease. In all such cases, the appearance
of air within the wall means severe compromise of its integrity. Pneumatosis coli is
occasionally seen in asymptomatic patients with leukemia or collagen-vascular
disease. Although the etiology is unclear, these air collections resolve quickly,
causing no symptoms or complications. Dissection of air from the chest into the
colon wall is frequently seen in patients with an air block phenomenon in the chest.
Patients on positive pressure ventilators who develop a pneumomediastinum, asth-

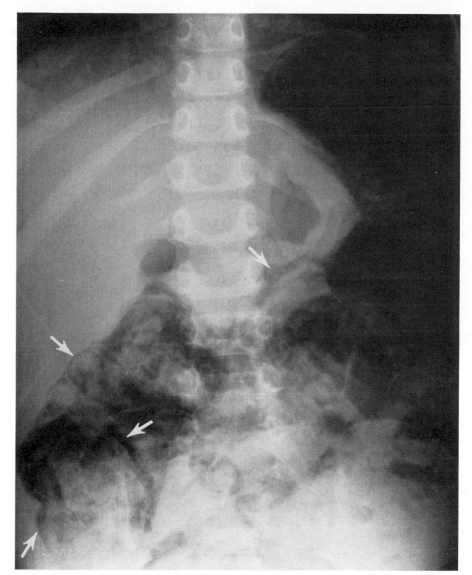

FIG. 5.17. PNEUMATOSIS COLI IN A 3½-YEAR-OLD BOY
This child was recovering from an acute asthmatic attack when curvilinear air densities in the wall of the colon were first suspected on a chest film and confirmed on a plain film of the abdomen (arrows).

matic patients (Fig. 5.17), or patients with cystic fibrosis may all show episodic pneumatosis coli which resolves spontaneously once intrathoracic pressure has been decreased.

Intraluminal foreign bodies in the colon rarely cause perforation. Round foreign bodies that reach the colon from above generally pass without consequence (Fig. 5.18). Even long sharp objects such as needles or nails may pass without difficulty. Occasionally, a sharp object such as a pin may perforate the rectum, presumably at the site of vigorous peristalsis and narrowing of the caliber of the lumen (Fig. 5.19). Foreign bodies inserted into the colon from below have a much greater likelihood of causing perforation or obstruction, particularly if they are bulky.

The colon may be perforated by a direct penetrating injury, such as a gunshot or

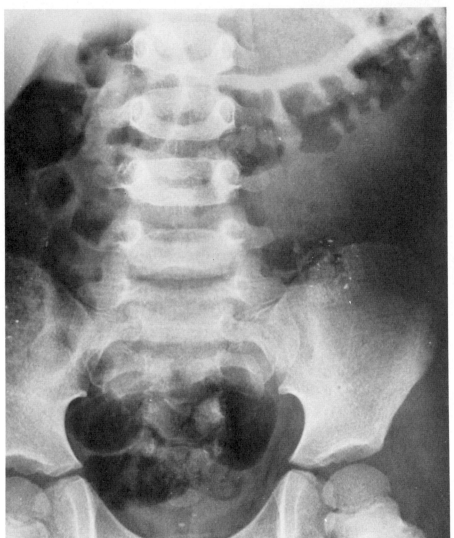

FIG. 5.18. LEAD PAINT INGESTION IN A 3-YEAR-OLD-BOY
Small flakes of radiodense material are scattered from the cecum to the rectum.
The colon should be cleansed of lead fragments before chelation is begun.

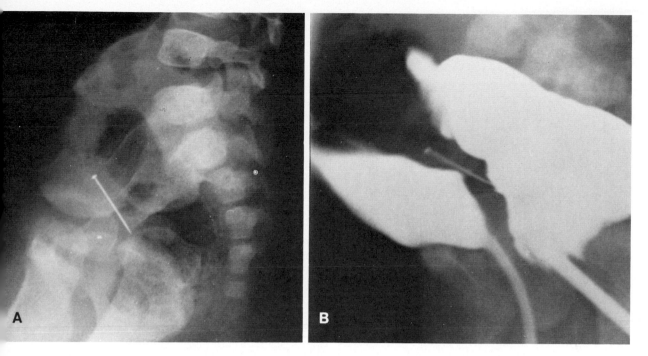

FIG. 5.19. SWALLOWED STRAIGHT PIN PERFORATING THE RECTUM IN A
12-MONTH-OLD BOY

A concern about the position of the pin (**A**) was caused by films 6 days apart
which showed the pin to be immobile in the rectal area. A combined cystogram and
barium enema (**B**) proved the extraluminal position of the pin.

knife wound. Major blunt trauma to the abdomen may cause rupture of the colon
in a small minority of cases, mainly at the splenic and hepatic flexures where the
colon changes from mesocolic to lateral abdominal fixation and is frequently associated with other visceral injuries such as duodenal rupture. Evisceration of the
bowel and partial avulsion of the mesentery may occur if the blunt trauma is
particularly severe (Fig. 5.20). Major crush injuries of the pelvis with fracture of the
pubic and ischial bones may occasionally cause low-lying extraperitoneal rupture of
the rectum or rectosigmoid. Spontaneous and idiopathic rupture of the colon may
be seen in the newborn infant, and the site of perforation is frequently the cecum.
The distinction between ruptured appendicitis and necrotizing enterocolitis is often
difficult in this age group. Immediate surgical intervention is required once a massive
pneumoperitoneum is documented on plain films of the abdomen. Iatrogenic injuries
of the colon include perforation of the rectum or rectosigmoid by malpositioned
enema tips, thermometers, or rectal tubes, or overdistended balloon catheters.
Hematoperitoneum or intramural hematoma may complicate transanal biopsies,
especially if above the peritoneal reflection. Finally, the colon may be injured by a
variety of medical procedures (Figs. 5.21 and 5.22).

Radiologic diagnosis depends on documentation of pneumoperitoneum, hematoperitoneum, extraperitoneal air, identification of intraluminal foreign bodies, or
identification of intramural hematoma from direct trauma or vascular insults.
Careful monitoring of initial inflow during barium examination is mandatory to
avoid massive intraperitoneal escape of barium from malpositioned enema tips.

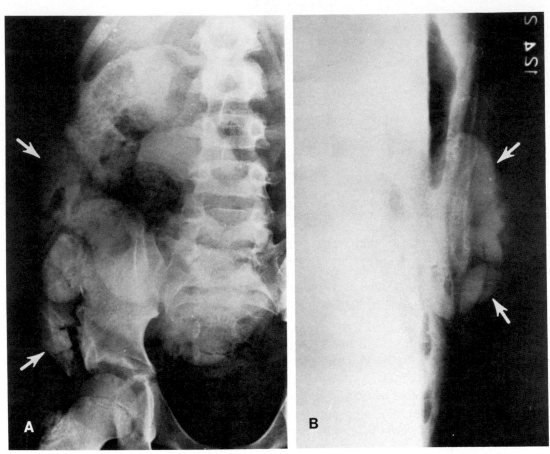

FIG. 5.20. TRAUMATIC EVISCERATION OF THE RIGHT COLON IN A 10-YEAR-OLD
BOY STRUCK BY A CAR

Supine (**A**) and horizontal beam (**B**) films show extra-abdominal loops of bowel
(arrows) and an open fracture of the iliac bone. The colon was transected at the
hepatic flexure, the transverse mesocolon partially avulsed, and the distal ileum
ruptured.

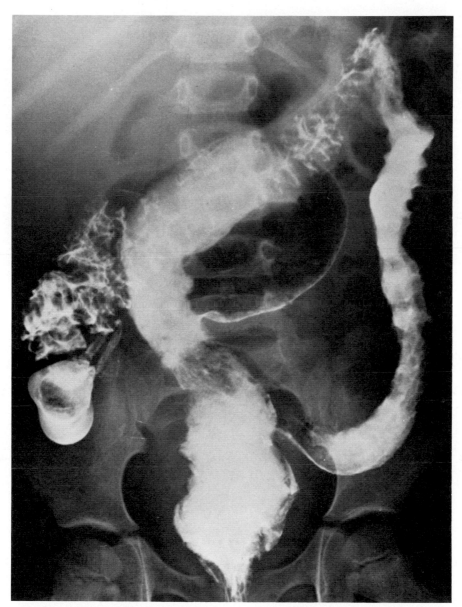

FIG. 5.21. IATROGENIC ALCOHOL COLITIS IN A 6-YEAR-OLD BOY

This patient received an enema of isopropanol instead of soap suds 2 days previously. He suffered a severe metabolic acidosis and 4 days of bloody diarrhea, but recovered with supportive treatment.

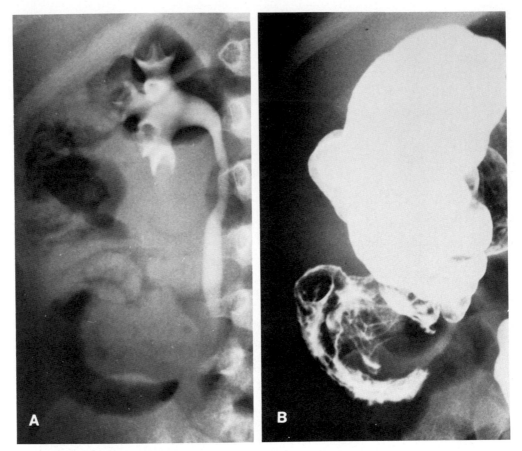

FIG. 5.22. STARCH GRANULOMATA SURROUNDING THE CECUM AND TERMINAL
ILEUM

This 13-month-old boy had an ileocolic intussusception reduced by surgery 3
weeks earlier. He developed fever and a right abdominal mass. The curvilinear air
shadows on the urogram (**A**) are shown by barium enema (**B**) to consist of a frozen
cecum and distal ileum. Starch granulomas were found in the specimen after ileo-
right colectomy.

PSYCHOGENIC MEGACOLON

Psychogenic megacolon describes a syndrome identified in children in the second
5 years of life who have extensive retention of stool and infrequent bowel movements.
Important historical components include a disturbed relationship of the child within
the family, and the onset of constipation from the time of toilet training or following
the death of an important family member. There may be frequent soiling of
underclothes, infrequent voluminous evacuation of stool, or even small amounts of
overflow diarrhea around a rectal impaction (Fig. 5.23). Attempts at disimpaction
by the patient, parents, or physician are usually unrewarding.

Plain film examination reveals massive quantities of stool in the rectum, sigmoid,
and left colon (Fig. 5.24). The colon frequently dilates up to 10–15 cm in diameter
and becomes redundant. Formed stool can be identified in one solid cast through
the colon to the anal verge. Barium enema examination, requiring no preparation,
and limited to the rectum will fail to disclose a nondilated segment above the rectal
verge (as might be seen in Hirschsprung's disease). The extensive mucosal edema

present in patients with psychogenic megacolon after disimpaction should not be confused with infiltrative diseases of the colonic mucosa.

The distinctive features of psychogenic megacolon as contrasted with Hirschsprung's disease include fecal soiling, a disturbed family relationship, the onset of symptoms during toilet training or other stressful events, and the presence of impacted stool in the rectum. Hirschsprung's disease may have more striking symptoms of obstruction and failure to thrive beginning in the earliest months of life, be associated with an empty rectum on digital exam, and unassociated with psychopathology in the family.

Other diseases or agents which may cause constipation include hypothyroidism, neurogenic bladders and rectums, and drugs, such as vincristine. Psychogenic, or functional megacolon, is also discussed in Chapter 20.

INTUSSUSCEPTION

Intussusception is the telescoping of one segment of bowel into the lumen of contiguous distal bowel, causing an intraluminal mass and, frequently, obstruction. In 90% of pediatric patients, the intussusception is ileocolic in type. Most patients are infants between 1–2 years of age; seasonal peaks occur in the spring and fall. The typical presenting clinical features are episodes of colicky abdominal pain, a palpable mass in the right lower or mid abdomen, and jelly-like bloody stools.

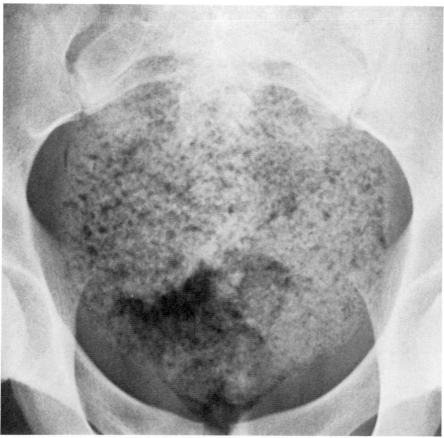

FIG. 5.23. FECAL IMPACTION IN A RETARDED 15-YEAR-OLD GIRL
The rectum is filled with particulate stool mixed with air which fills most of the pelvis. The stool abuts the anal verge.

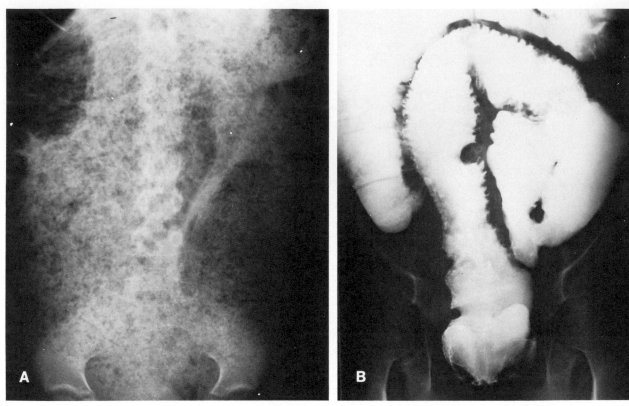

FIG. 5.24. MASSIVE PSYCHOGENIC MEGACOLON IN A 12-YEAR-OLD BOY
Symptoms began 6 years previously following death of a favorite relative. **(A)** A supine film documents an enormously dilated colon filled with feces. **(B)** Following disimpaction, a barium enema reveals that the mucosa of the sigmoid colon is markedly edematous.

Rarely, the intussusception will pass down the colon to reach the rectum and be discovered by the examining finger or prolapse through the anus. Ileocolic intussusception may spontaneously reduce and recur, so that a long chronology does not necessarily signify gangrenous bowel. The occurrence of vomiting depends on the degree of small bowel obstruction caused by the intussusception. Signs of peritonitis are presumptive evidence of necrotic bowel and preclude barium enema examination. Palpation of the abdomen should be minimized.

Plain film examination may disclose a mass in the area of the cecum or extending to the mid-transverse colon (Fig. 5.25). The tip of the intussusception may be outlined by air in the distal colon. The small bowel will be dilated in cases of small bowel obstruction. However, the abdomen may be largely airless in children with severe vomiting.

A barium enema examination is indicated in all infants without definite signs of peritonitis; the presence of radiographic small bowel obstruction does not contraindicate a barium enema. Maintenance of the fluid level within the enema bag at 1 m above the fluoroscopic table will avoid unphysiologic intraluminal pressures and the risk of perforation. The advancing column of barium within the colon will surround the intussusceptum confirming the diagnosis (Fig. 5.26).

A child with diagnosed intussusception, showing no signs of peritonitis, is a proper candidate for an attempt at hydrostatic barium enema reduction. Premedication with Demerol will diminish spasm and anxiety and relieve pain. A balloon catheter

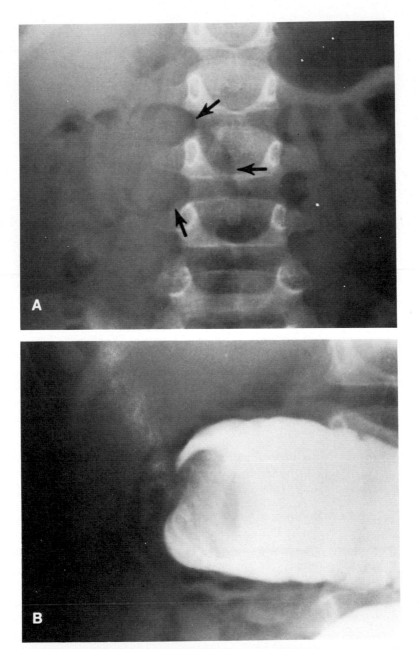

FIG. 5.25. ILEOCOLIC INTUSSUSCEPTION IN THE MID-TRANSVERSE COLON
(A) Plain film of the abdomen shows a tubular mass within the lumen of the right
transverse colon (arrows). (B) Barium replaces the air and defines the intussusceptum within the intussuscipiens, which is the mid-transverse colon.

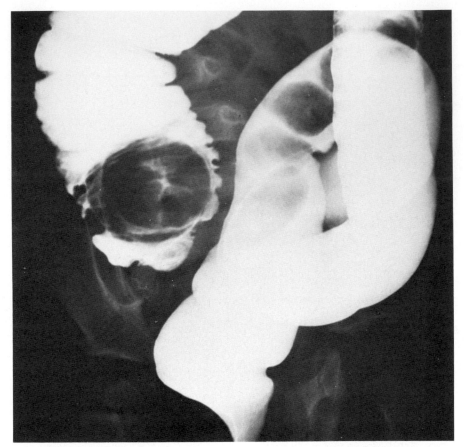

FIG. 5.26. A TYPICAL ILEOCOLIC INTUSSUSCEPTION IN A 3-YEAR-OLD GIRL
Barium surrounds the ileocolic intussusceptum as it advances into the ascending colon, the intussuscipiens.

is placed in the rectum and inflated under fluoroscopic observation. Three attempts at hydrostatic reduction, each lasting 15–20 min, will reduce most intussusceptions; the rest should be surgically reduced. Partial reduction of a long intussusception (Fig. 5.27) by barium enema will shorten and simplify a surgical reduction. The hydrostatic reduction of an ileocolic intussusception is considered complete when there is free reflux through a long portion of the ileum. Occasionally, a Meckel's diverticulum may be found as a mass within the ileum, the lead point for the original ileocolic intussusception. Hydrostatic reductions of intussusceptions caused by tumors are not indicated; surgical treatment is the method of choice. Occasionally, gangrenous bowel with adhesions between the intussusceptum and the intussuscipiens is the unexpected cause for failure to reduce an ileocolic intussusception (Fig. 5.28). The incidence of recurrent intussusception is approximately 5% in patients with surgical or hydrostatic reduction; another trial of hydrostatic reduction should be attempted in these patients. Success rates of hydrostatic reduction of uncomplicated ileocolic intussusceptions range from 30–80% and largely depend on the diligence of the examiner.

Intussusception in the newborn patient is usually caused by a mass lesion, frequently a duplication of the cecum. Once diagnosed, surgical exploration is indicated and hydrostatic reduction is to be avoided. In patients with cystic fibrosis, however, ileocolic or ileoileal intussusceptions may be reduced using water-soluble contrast material and balloon retention catheters. A further discussion of intussusception is presented in Chapters 17 and 19.

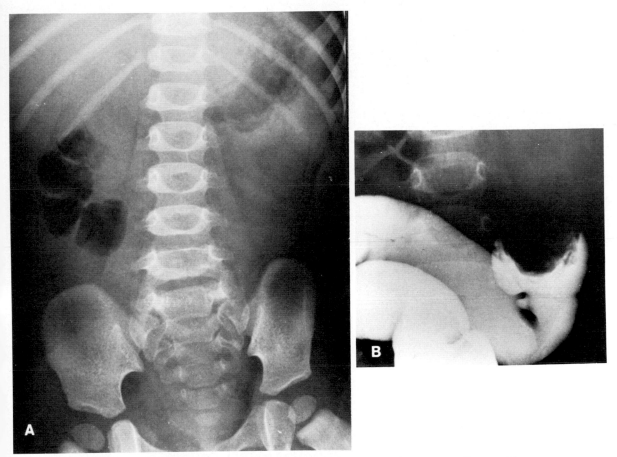

FIG. 5.27. LONG INTUSSUSCEPTION MASQUERADING AS PROXIMAL SMALL BOWEL
OBSTRUCTION

This 13-month-old girl had three bloody stools and persistent bilious vomiting for
12 hr. (**A**) A supine film of the abdomen reveals a little air in the stomach and a few
loops of dilated small bowel. (**B**) The barium enema demonstrates an intussusception
into the sigmoid colon. A long intussusception plus vomiting can produce a near
gasless abdomen.

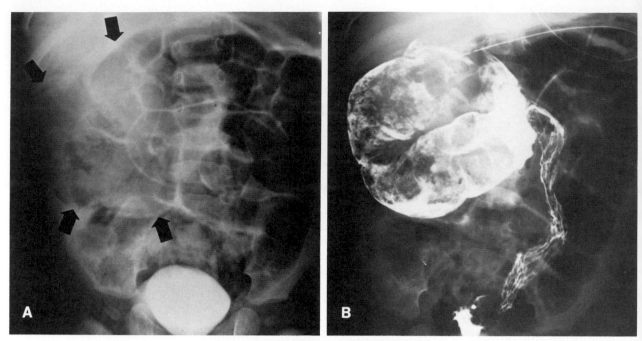

FIG. 5.28. A GANGRENOUS ILEOCOLIC INTUSSUSCEPTION IN AN 8-MONTH-OLD BOY

The child was referred because of a right abdominal mass. (**A**) A partially gas filled, *avascular* mass (arrows) was shown by high dose urography. (**B**) A barium enema could not reduce an intussusception at the hepatic flexure. The intussusception proved to be gangrenous at laparotomy.

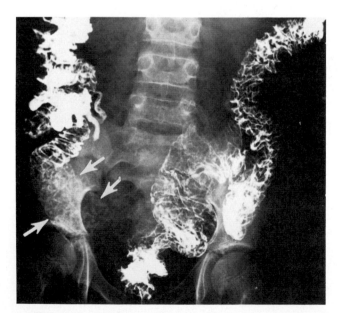

FIG. 5.29. CYSTIC FIBROSIS WITH INSPISSATED STOOL PLUGGING THE TERMINAL ILEUM

This 11-year-old boy had vomited for 12 hr and had not passed stools for 4 days. A barium enema shows hyperplasia of the colonic mucosa and a stool plug (meconium equivalent) in the ileum (arrows).

CYSTIC FIBROSIS

The colon may be involved in children with cystic fibrosis. The mucosa may be hypertrophic throughout the colon from enlargement of mucous glands and hyperplasia of the mucosa (Fig. 5.29). The appearance may resemble diffuse lymphosarcoma, except that nodularity of the wall is absent, or disimpacted psychogenic megacolon except that the colon diameter is normal. Adherent plugs of stool may cause obstruction of the colon or small bowel in patients with cystic fibrosis (meconium equivalent) and require hydrostatic dislodgement using a water-soluble contrast material. Prolapse of the rectum is common in patients with cystic fibrosis, as well as in patients with overwhelming trichuriasis.

BIBLIOGRAPHY

Ament, M. E.: Inflammatory disease of the colon: Ulcerative colitis and Crohn's colitis. J. Pediatr., 86: 322, 1975.

Aziz, E. M.: Neonatal pneumatosis intestinalis associated with milk intolerance. Am. J. Dis. Child., 125: 560, 1973.

Bar-Ziv, J.: Hemolytic uremic syndrome: A case presenting with acute colitis. Pediatr. Radiol., 2: 203, 1974.

Berger, L. A., and Wilkinson, D.: The investigation of colitis in infancy. Pediatr. Radiol., 2: 145, 1974.

Cardoso, J. M., Kimura, K., Stoopen, M., Cervantes, L. F., Elizondo, L., Churchill, R., and Moncada, R.: Radiology of invasive amebiasis of the colon. Am. J. Roentgenol., 128: 935, 1977.

Devroede, G. J., Taylor, W. F., Sauer, W. G., Jackman, R. J., and Stickler, G. B.: Cancer risk and life expectancy of children with ulcerative colitis. N. Engl. J. Med., 285: 17, 1971.

Donaldson, M. H., Taylor, P., Rawitscher, R., and Sewell, J. B.: Colon carcinoma in childhood. Pediatrics, 48: 307, 1971.

Ein, S. H., Lynch, M. J., and Stephens, C. A.: Ulcerative colitis in children under 1 year: A 20 year review. J. Pediatr. Surg., 6: 264, 1971.

Farman, J., Rabinowitz, J. G., and Meyers, M. A.: Roentgenology of infectious colitis. Am. J. Roentgenol., 119: 375, 1973.

Franken, E. A., Jr.: *Gastrointestinal Radiology in Pediatrics,* Chap. 6. Harper & Row, Hagerstown, MD, 1975.

Friedland, G. W., and Filly, R.: Evanescent colitis in a child. Pediatr. Radiol., 2: 73, 1974.

Golden, G. T., Rosenthal, J. D., and Shaw, A.: Carcinoma of the rectum in adolescence. Am. J. Dis. Child., 129: 742, 1975.

Hardy, J. D., Savage, T. R., and Shirodaria, C.: Intestinal perforation following exchange transfusion. Am. J. Dis. Child., 124: 136, 1972.

Holsclaw, D. S., Rocmans, C., and Schwachman, H.: Intussusception in patients with cystic fibrosis. Pediatrics, 48: 51, 1971.

Howell, H. S., Bartizal, J. F., and Freeark, R. J.: Blunt trauma involving the colon and rectum. J. Trauma, 16: 624, 1976.

Jaffe, N., Carlson, D. H., and Vawter, G. F.: Pneumatosis intestinalis cystoides in acute leukemia. Cancer, 30: 239, 1972.

Karjoo, M., and McCarthy, B.: Toxic megacolon of ulcerative colitis in infancy. Pediatrics, 57: 962, 1976.

Korelitz, B. I., Gribetz, D., and Kopel, F. B.: Granulomatous colitis in children: A study of 25 cases and comparison with ulcerative colitis. Pediatrics, 42: 446, 1968.

Kottmeier, P. K., and Clatworthy, H. W., Jr.: Aganglionic and functional megacolon in children— A diagnostic dilemma. Pediatrics, 36: 572, 1965.

Leonidas, J. C., and Hall, R. T.: Neonatal pneumatosis coli: A mild form of neonatal necrotizing enterocolitis. J. Pediatr., 89: 456, 1976.

Pochaczevsky, R., and Kassner, E. G.: Necrotizing enterocolitis of infancy. Am. J. Roentgenol., 113: 283, 1971.

Rabinowtiz, J. G., and Siegle, R. L.: Changing clinical and roentgenologic patterns of necrotizing enterocolitis. Am. J. Roentgenol., 126: 560, 1976.

Roy, C., and Mareschal, J. L.: Pneumoperitoneum of iatrogenic origin: Ten cases of perforation by thermometer in the premature newborn. Ann. Radiol., 16: 149, 1973.

Singleton, E. B., and Johnson, F.: Localized lesions of the colon in infants and children. Semin. Roentgenol., 11: 111, 1976.

Singleton, E. B., Wagner, M. L., and Dutton, R. V.: *Radiology of the Alimentary Tract in Infants and Children,* 2nd ed., Chap. 17. W. B. Saunders, Philadelphia, 1977.

Santulli, T. V., Schullinger, J. N., Heird, W. C., Gongaware, R. D., Wigger, J., Barlow, B., Blanc, W. A., and Berdon, W. E.: Acute necrotizing enterocolitis of infancy: A review of 64 cases. Pediatrics, 55: 376, 1975.

Tumen, H. J., Valdes-Dapena, A., and Haddad, H.: Indications for surgical intervention in ulcerative colitis in children. Am. J. Dis. Child., 116: 641, 1968.

Wagner, M. L., Rosenberg, H. S., Fernbach, D. J., and Singleton, E. B.: Typhlitis: A complication of leukemia in children. Am. J. Roentgenol., 109: 341, 1970.

Wilkinson, R. H., Bartlett, R. H., and Eraklis, A. J.: Diagnosis of appendicitis in infancy. The value of abdominal radiographs. Am. J. Dis. Child., 118: 687, 1969.

Wood, R. E., Herman, C. J., Johnson, K. W. and Di Sant'Agnese, P.: Pneumatosis coli in cystic fibrosis. Am. J. Dis. Child., 129: 246, 1975.

6

Pathology of Diverticular Disease

AUSTIN L. VICKERY, JR., M.D.

INCIDENCE

Diverticulosis is one of the most common abnormalities of the colon. It occurs with greatest frequency in populations of the western world where the incidence increases with age, ranging from very infrequent under age 40 to about one-third of the population aged 60 and over.

PATHOGENESIS

Although several causative factors have been described, the seemingly random and widespread occurrence of diverticular disease in afflicted populations cannot be adequately explained. For many years, diverticular disease was simply equated with "diverticulitis" and the diagnostic criteria of radiologists, surgeons, and pathologists were often different and difficult to correlate. For example, generations of radiologists were taught that a saw-toothed outline of the colon was a diagnostic feature of "chronic diverticulitis." Correlated radiologic and pathologic studies eventually showed that this finding was primarily due to spasm and muscle hypertrophy, inconstantly related to pathologic evidence of inflammation in or around diverticula. Indeed, it could be found in the absence of diverticula. Morson defines diverticular disease as a disorder of muscle function with abnormality of the muscle being the most consistent and striking pathologic feature of sigmoid diverticulosis. The fact that muscle hypertrophy may occasionally be found in colons without diverticula is interesting evidence supporting the importance of this abnormality as a primary rather than secondary feature in the pathogenesis of diverticular disease. Perhaps the most plausible theory is based on a relationship between the so-called "irritable colon syndrome" and subsequent development of diverticular disease. This is supported by findings of increased intraluminal pressures in segments of bowel involved by the irritable colon syndrome and is helpful in explaining many clinical and pathologic features of this common illness.

PATHOLOGY

Diverticula are acquired mucosal defects which may occur anywhere in the colon but are by far more common in the left colon, particularly the sigmoid. They consist of outpouchings of the mucosa and muscularis mucosa through the circular and longitudinal muscular coats of the bowel (Fig. 6.1).

On the mucosal surface, the ostia of the diverticula are usually very small and often difficult to locate; they communicate via narrow necks of the mucosal invaginations with bulbous-like tips which, when fully developed, protrude through the colonic muscular coats, often into the pericolic fatty tissues.

Microscopically, only a very thin layer of muscle fibers is present at the periphery of fully developed flask-shaped diverticula accounting for impairment of their emptying ability and a tendency for chronic impaction of inspissated feces and vulnerability to perforation (Fig. 6.2). These complications fortunately develop in only a small percentage of individuals with diverticulosis.

Thickening of the bowel wall in chronic diverticular disease is an important pathologic feature and is largely due to hypertrophy of the muscular layers which is in keeping with the theory that long standing elevation of intraluminal pressure is a key factor in the pathogenesis of diverticular disease. Although edema and occasionally fibrosis (mainly in the pericolic tissues) may contribute to thickening of the bowel wall in patients with diverticular disease, these are minor features compared to muscle hypertrophy (Fig. 6.3).

In non-inflammatory diverticular disease, the mucosal surface is frequently thrown into exaggerated folds which tend to make even narrower the bowel lumen which is already compromised by muscular thickening (Fig. 6.4). A stenotic bowel segment with an accentuated but intact mucosal pattern are important correlative pathologic aspects for radiographic diagnosis.

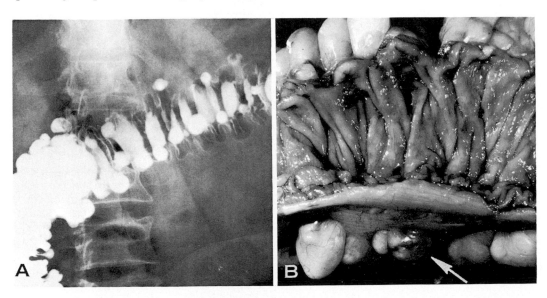

FIG. 6.1. DIVERTICULOSIS
(A) Detail from film of a barium-filled transverse colon. Scattered diverticula are present but with preservation of the normal haustral pattern and luminal diameter. **(B)** An opened segment of colon showing a thin-walled diverticulum (arrow) and numerous appendices epiploica. Although scattered diverticula are present, there is no luminal narrowing or axial shortening.

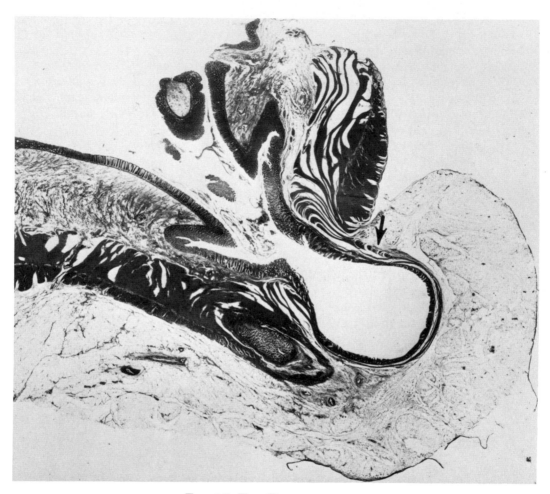

FIG. 6.2. THE DIVERTICULUM

Anatomy of a diverticulum with the flask-shaped diverticulum penetrating into the pericolic fat. Note the very thin layer of muscle at the outer margin of the diverticulum (arrow).

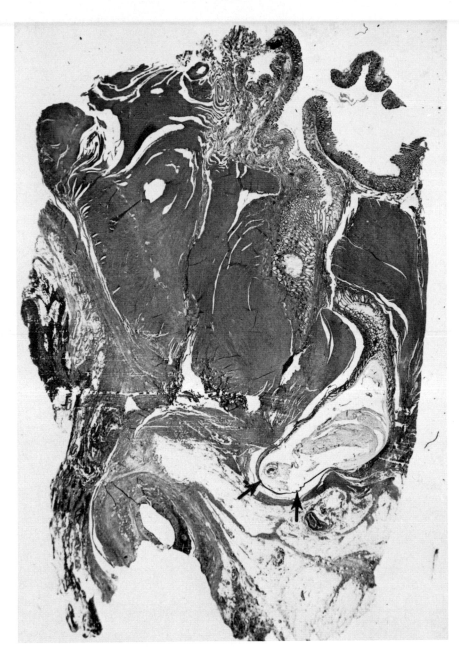

FIG. 6.3. MUSCLE HYPERTROPHY IN DIVERTICULOSIS
Microscopic section of bowel wall with the lumen at the top and a diverticulum with a long neck penetrating into the pericolic fat (arrow). Note the markedly hypertrophied dark staining muscular coat which is 3 or 4 times normal thickness.

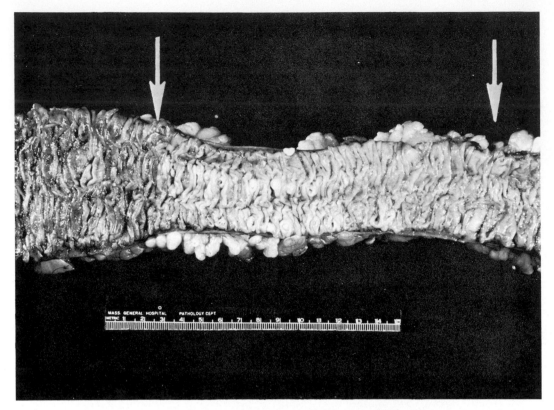

FIG. 6.4. AXIAL SHORTENING AND LUMINAL NARROWING IN DIVERTICULOSIS
Resected sigmoid colon showing marked axial shortening and reduction in size of
the lumen (between arrows). Scattered diverticula are present. The remainder of
the sigmoid, to the left, is normal. Histologic examination showed no evidence of
inflammation.

COMPLICATIONS

It has already been mentioned that the clinical symptoms of diverticular disease
may be present in the absence of any associated inflammation and, indeed, may
actually exist in the absence of diverticula. However, the most serious complication
of this disorder is the vulnerability of the thin-walled sacs to local injury.

Inflammation (Peridiverticulitis)

Joint radiologic and pathologic investigations have indicated that the pathogenesis
of diverticulitis is not analogous to acute appendicitis, as was formerly stated.
Rather than primary inflammation of the wall of a diverticulum, the essential lesion
is microperforation of a diverticulum and inflammation of the peridiverticular tissues
(Fig. 6.5). Thus, the expression "peridiverticulitis" is a more precise description of
the pathologic process. The practice of pathologists gratuitously to diagnose "chronic
diverticulitis" merely on the basis of the presence of diverticula in the absence of
any inflammation tended to perpetuate the misconception about clinical disease
associated with diverticulosis. Indications for surgery have become more precise in
medical centers where there is an awareness that symptomatic diverticulosis need
not be associated with inflammation. It has been estimated that between 10 and
25% of patients with diverticulosis will, however, develop peridiverticulitis at some
time in their life.

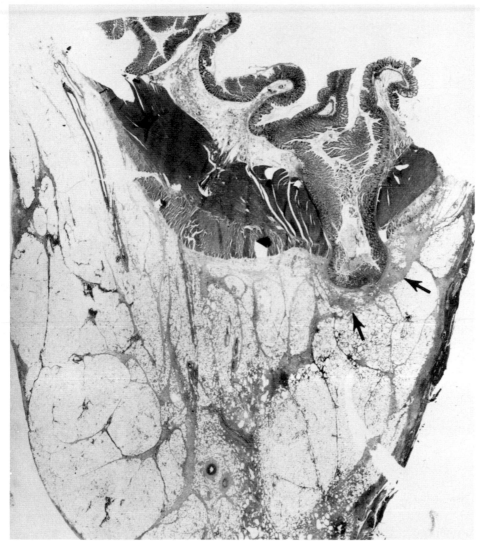

FIG. 6.5. MICROPERFORATION OF A DIVERTICULUM

Photomicrograph of a perforating diverticulum in the colon wall with chronic inflammation surrounding the tip. This appears as the irregular cloudy-gray staining zone (arrows) around the diverticulum in which there is microscopic foreign body giant cell reaction typical of peridiverticulitis.

Even with the complication of severe peridiverticulitis, the ostia of diverticula may appear deceptively normal on the mucosal surface, giving no clue to the inflammatory reaction in the surrounding pericolic tissues. The degree of inflammation in the peridiverticular tissues may range from a small localized process to a diffuse inflammatory reaction with induration and edema of the pericolic tissues and even frank necrosis and abscess formation (Fig. 6.6). Fistulous tracks may develop between the inflammatory focus and adjacent organs, such as the vagina and bladder.

An unusual and unique complication associated with peridiverticulitis is the development of a paracolonic sinus track extrinsic to the muscularis and communicating with one or more ruptured diverticula. Such a longitudinal abscess parallel to the bowel lumen results in the radiographic sign of "double tracking." A similar appearing abscess track may occasionally be seen in Crohn's disease of the colon.

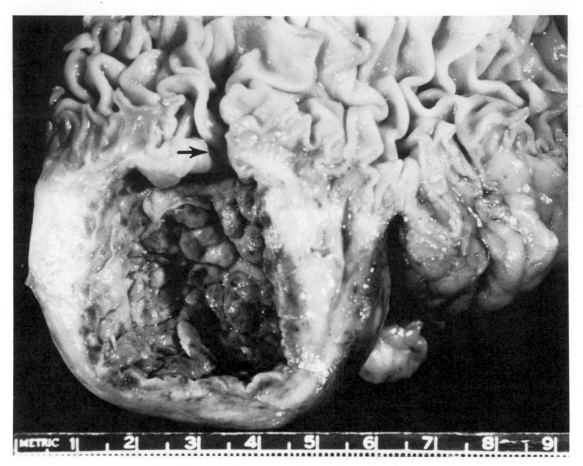

FIG. 6.6. PERICOLIC ABSCESS IN DIVERTICULITIS

Diverticulitis involving the sigmoid with a large chronic abscess in the pericolic fat. Note the cleft-like communication of the abscess with the bowel lumen (arrow) and the exaggerated folds of mucosa.

Hemorrhage

Bleeding from a diverticulum is the most common cause of massive rectal bleeding. A curious feature of this serious complication is that the majority of bleeding diverticula are located in the right colon where the incidence of diverticulosis is much lower than in the left colon. The pathogenesis of the bleeding episode is probably on the basis of erosion of the thin-walled diverticulum into an adjacent blood vessel. The fact that diverticula are thought to develop along the pathway of penetrating nutrient blood vessels seems a valid explanation for this serious complication. Most of the reported cases of massive hemorrhage due to diverticular disease in which the precise bleeding point has been identified by the pathologist have not revealed associated inflammation. Thus, while there is a relationship between diverticulosis and bleeding, no definite correlation has ever been established between diverticulitis and bleeding.

Obstruction

Narrowing of the bowel lumen is a common accompaniment of diverticular disease and is produced by one or a combination of factors including marked muscular thickening, chronic spasm, axial shortening with accordian-like pleating of mucosa and, when associated with inflammation, induration and fibrosis of pericolic tissues.

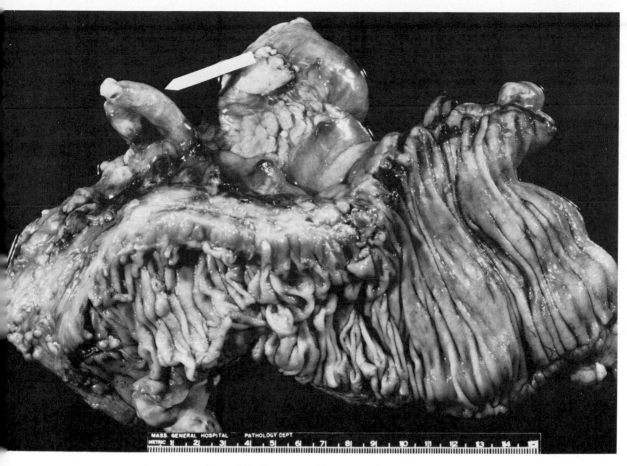

FIG. 6.7. CHRONIC DIVERTICULITIS

Sigmoid segment with chronic peridiverticulitis from a patient with signs of obstruction simulating malignancy. Note the marked thickening of the narrowed segment, the accentuation but preservation of mucosal markings, and the dilated proximal limb with its more normal appearance. The arrow marks the appendix, removed because it was adherent to the inflamed pericolic tissues. (Reprinted by permission from The New England Journal of Medicine, *279:* 597, 1968.)

The degree of chronic or acute bowel obstruction thus produced may be so severe as to simulate malignancy both by radiographic examination and gross inspection at surgery (Fig. 6.7).

BIBLIOGRAPHY

Casarella, W. J., Kanter, I. E., and Seaman, W. B.: Right-sided colonic diverticula as a cause of acute rectal hemorrhage. N. Engl. J. Med., *286:* 450, 1972.

Case Records of the Massachusetts General Hospital, Case 37-1968. N. Engl. J. Med., *279:* 597, 1968.

Ferrucci, J. T., Jr., Ragsdale, B. D., Barrett, P. J., *et al.*: Double tracking in the sigmoid colon. Radiology, *120:* 307, 1976.

Kempczinski, R. F., and Ferrucci, J. T., Jr.: Giant sigmoid diverticula: A review. Ann. Surg., *180:* 864, 1974.

Ming, S-C., and Fleischner, F. G.: Diverticulitis of the sigmoid colon. Reappraisal of the pathology and pathogenesis. Surgery, *58:* 627, 1965.

Morson, B. C.: Pathology of diverticular disease of the colon. Clin. Gastroenterol., *4:* 37, 1975.

Parks, T. G.: Natural history of diverticular disease of the colon. Clin. Gastroenterol., *4:* 53, 1975.

Parsa, F., Gordon, H. E., and Wilson, S. W.: Bleeding diverticulosis of the colon. A review of 83 cases. Dis. Colon Rectum, *18:* 37–41, 1975.

7

Diverticular Disease

JOSEPH T. FERRUCCI, JR., M.D.

BACKGROUND

Diverticular disease of the colon is an acquired disease of adult life occurring principally in highly industrialized western societies. In recent years the natural history of diverticular disease has been greatly clarified by contributions from the fields of pathology, epidemiology, surgery and radiology. At present it is believed that the pathogenesis of colonic diverticular disease is intimately related to a functional overactivity and work hypertrophy of colonic smooth muscle while the remote etiology of the disorder is postulated to be an inadequate intake of vegetable fiber. Indeed, colonic diverticular disease, like scurvy, has been considered a dietary deficiency disorder. As currently conceived, diverticular disease possesses three overlapping stages with differing clinical, radiologic, and pathologic findings. The initial phase or the "prediverticular" stage is characterized by prominent muscular thickening in the wall of the sigmoid colon without frank diverticulum formation. In the second phase, or diverticulosis, pulsion-type mucosal herniations are found passing through the muscular layers of the bowel wall presenting as false diverticula. Diverticulitis, the third phase, represents perforation of a diverticulum with formation of a pericolic abscess and clinical signs of sepsis.

PATHOLOGIC FINDINGS

Evidence from various sources (surgical, radiologic, necropsy) indicates that diverticular disease increases with age, occurring in as many as 50% of patients over the age of 60 years. Of these, 20% will at some time in their lives suffer the complication of acute diverticulitis. On the other hand, pathologic evidence of diverticulitis is occasionally found in autopsy specimens of patients who have been otherwise asymptomatic, while surgical specimens resected for diverticulitis have often shown no evidence of inflammatory reaction. Thus, precise clinical-pathologic correlations have been difficult to establish in diverticular disease and this remains one of the principal problems in understanding the pathogenesis of this disorder. The pathology of diverticular disease is further elaborated in Chapter 6.

The Muscle Abnormality

In 95% of patients with diverticular disease the sigmoid is the principal site of involvement. The striking feature on gross examination of sigmoid segments involved with diverticular disease is the thickened colonic wall composed largely of accentuated circular muscle bundles. Prominent tenia coli are usually found along with thickening of the adjacent mesentery. Numerous interdigitating processes of circular muscle fibers criss-cross the lumen of the bowel giving a corrugated or sacculated appearance. The colonic lumen appears narrowed in caliber while the bowel appears longitudinally shortened as well. Roentgenologically the involved segment does not distend or elongate fully on barium enema examination, and some have applied the term "contracture of the colon" to these features. Fleischner suggested that the overall process reflects work hypertrophy of the colonic circular muscle. Histologically there is evidence of muscular thickening but no clear-cut hyperplasia. It is to be emphasized that this muscular thickening is regularly encountered in the absence of histologic evidence of chronic inflammation, although in the presence of recurrent or chronic diverticulitis, fibrosis of the colonic wall certainly can supervene.

The Diverticulum

Colonic diverticula are pulsion-like protrusions of mucosa and muscularis mucosa between the circular layers of the bowel wall. They are most commonly found in the sigmoid colon and usually appear between the mesenteric and lateral tenia where the longitudinal nutrient arteries penetrate the inner circular muscle layer to form a submucosal capillary plexus.

Diverticula are visible as rounded sac-like or ovoid protrusions ranging between 0.5 and 1.0 cm during colon examinations. Often they are best seen during the early filling phase, becoming relatively obliterated on fully distended overhead radiographs and then reappearing quite prominently when the collapsed colon is demonstrated on postevacuation films. Diverticula are found in all regions of the large bowel with the exception of the rectum but are far more frequently found in the sigmoid where they are usually accompanied by considerable muscle hypertrophy. In a smaller percentage of cases, myriads of diverticula appear throughout the remainder of the colon including the transverse and ascending portions, a condition best described as diffuse diverticulosis. Prominent muscular thickening is not encountered in this variant. Rarely, isolated pericecal diverticula are also observed. These are often larger than sigmoid diverticula and are of uncertain origin.

Colonic diverticula often contain varying degrees of inspissated fecal material on gross examination. However, the radiologic demonstration of fecal residue within colonic diverticula is generally considered to be of no clinical consequence despite the assumption that fecal stasis is the underlying mechanism for the complications of diverticular hemorrhage and peridiverticulitis.

ETIOLOGY AND PATHOGENESIS

Evidence from recent manometric and epidemiologic studies contributes to our understanding of the mechanisms underlying the development of diverticular disease.

Intrasigmoidal pressure determinations performed by Painter and associates have shown that patients with diverticulosis generate higher focal segmental sigmoid pressures in response to food and pharmacologic stimuli than do normal subjects. These exaggerated segmental pressures are readily reversed by the administration of narcotics or anticholinergic drugs. The occurrence of marked muscular thickening and abnormally exaggerated intraluminal pressure responses within the sigmoid colon strongly suggests that the two are related and probably represent a "prediverticular" phase of diverticulosis. Whether the abnormal pressure response or the muscle thickening is the principal factor is unclear. Nevertheless, the net result is predisposition to herniation of mucosal outpouchings at sites of weakness adjacent to penetrating mucosal vessels.

A central question is why the sigmoid colon is so often the site of the pressure, muscular and finally diverticular changes of this disorder. It has been suggested that if the colon behaves as a cylinder, the Law of LaPlace could be invoked. In the distal colon, the fecal stream caliber has been reduced to a minimum by water absorption and thus according to LaPlace's Law, with a given tension (T) the pressure (P) is inversely related to the radius (R) of the cylinder ($P = T/R$). Thus, in a narrow caliber sigmoid, tensions generated by circular muscle bundles will produce higher pressures than in the more proximal portion of the colon where lumen diameter is larger. Thus, mucosal herniations are more likely to occur in the sigmoid colon than more proximally.

Epidemiologic studies indicate that diverticular disease is essentially unheard of in underdeveloped areas of Africa and Asia. It is believed that the rather high dietary fiber content of native diets results in large volume semisolid stools, large caliber colonic lumens and rapid fecal transit times. In contrast, the increasing intake of refined fiber low roughage diets in the United States and Western Europe is believed to cause a dehydrated low residue fecal stream. According to Burkitt this results in excessive segmentation of the sigmoid in order to halt the fecal stream which is associated with a corresponding increase in intraluminal pressure and subsequent "work hypertrophy" of smooth muscle. The protrusions of mucosa through sites of nutrient artery penetration in the colonic wall result in diverticular formation.

Clinical Features

The potential for significant symptom production by uncomplicated diverticular disease (without inflammation) has generally been misunderstood and underestimated. Pain is a predominant feature of diverticular disease, often located in the lower abdominal quadrants, and frequently precipitated by or related to meals and emotional stress. Alternating bouts of diarrhea and constipation are common and a tender, palpable mass is often present in the left lower quadrant. It is likely that this symptom complex actually represents the altered motor activity of the thickened colonic musculature and has nothing to do with inflammation. Indeed, symptoms caused by prediverticular muscle dysfunction only cannot be distinguished from those occurring with frank diverticulum formation. Further, younger patients in the third, fourth, and fifth decade, often exhibit symptoms in the presence of muscle changes only, with no visible diverticula radiographically. Obviously, such complaints are nonspecific and other significant colonic pathology must be excluded. Finally, it should be also emphasized that while rectal bleeding may occur in diverticulosis this is invariably related to the presence of blood vessel erosion at the apex of a diverticulum and will be considered in more detail below.

Relationship to Irritable Colon Syndrome

In recent years the concept of the irritable colon syndrome has been somewhat legitimatized as it has been recognized that the majority of such patients are probably manifesting the prediverticular phase of colonic diverticular disease (Fig. 7.1). In practical terms the clinical hallmarks of intermittent crampy lower abdominal pain and change in bowel habits are essentially indistinguishable from the features of diverticulosis. Further, patients with the irritable colon syndrome also possess similar exaggerated manometric pressure responses within the sigmoid colon although roentgenographic evidence of actual muscular thickening is not often present. As in the case of frank diverticular disease, the diagnosis is one of exclusion and is advanced when radiographic and colonoscopic studies fail to demonstrate other pathology.

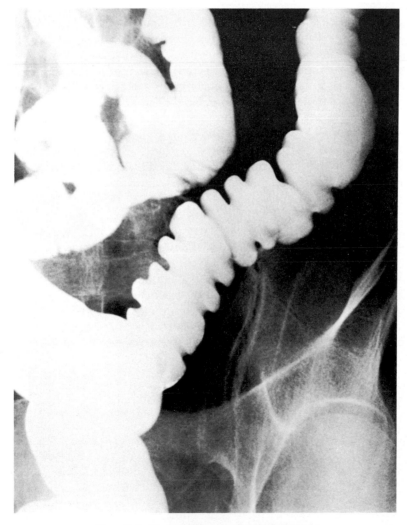

FIG. 7.1. THE MUSCLE ABNORMALITY

Prediverticular disease. The haustral markings in the sigmoid are accentuated in depth, crowded together, and increased in number. The effective lumen is slightly narrowed. Symptoms of irritable colon may accompany this appearance.

While the irritable colon syndrome usually affects younger patients, in the third and fourth decade, it is difficult to document that such patients clearly proceed to the development of true radiographic and pathologic diverticulosis. Similarly, it is difficult to demonstrate that patients with obvious diverticulosis have previously evolved through an irritable colon stage. By the same token, many patients with classic diverticulitis have never experienced any prior colonic symptoms whatsoever. Thus, circumstantial evidence of an association is strong although not conclusive. Proof of the link will require accumulation of longitudinal data on the clinical course of patients with "irritable colon" symptoms (Fig. 7.2).

Roentgen Findings

Colonic diverticula appear as round or oval sac-like outpouchings projecting beyond the confines of the colonic lumen and range in size between 0.5–1.5 cm (Fig. 7.3). Often, a short neck is visible. Typically, the lumen is narrowed by a series of sacculations due to deep criss-crossing ridges of thickened circular muscle (Fig. 7.4). In the sigmoid, individual diverticula often arise from the apex of saw-tooth-like corrugations in the barium column (Fig. 7.5). This configuration is, however, confined to the sigmoid and is not seen in other regions of the colon. Inspissated fecal material is often visible within the apex of the diverticular sacs and is frequently outlined by a surface meniscus of barium. Although diverticula tend to be arranged anatomically along the tenia coli this feature is usually not prominent or significant from the radiologic standpoint. As previously noted, the sigmoid is most commonly affected but scattered diverticula are often evident in other portions of the colon as well. In some patients diffuse diverticulosis occurs (Fig. 7.6).

On fluoroscopic examination, the features of muscular thickening, spasm and consequent luminal narrowing of the sigmoid colon are sometimes more striking than the actual presence of diverticula. Typically, the sigmoid presents a relatively fixed appearance, shortened in its axial dimension with a somewhat serpiginous course through the left hemipelvis. Initial attempts at retrograde filling may meet with severe sigmoid spasm and complete obstruction to retrograde flow, especially if the hydrostatic pressure is excessive or the enema solution too cold. Generally, lowering the hydrostatic pressure (height of the enema bag) and proceeding with small incremental volumes and words of gentle reassurance will overcome the problem. When severe spasm persists, antispasmodic drugs, especially the anticholinergic agents, and more recently glucagon, have been used as adjuncts during fluoroscopic study (Fig. 7.7). In general, the antispasmodic drug is administered whenever significant sigmoid spasm occurs either with pain or transient obstruction to retrograde flow.

FIG. 7.2. DOCUMENTATION OF PROGRESSION FROM "IRRITABLE COLON" TO DIVERTICULAR DISEASE IN 4 YEARS

A 47-year-old male was studied on 3 occasions because of intermittent left lower quadrant pain and constipation. (**A**) On the first barium enema, the haustral markings in the sigmoid colon are accentuated and increased in number and the effective lumen is slightly narrowed. The clinical and radiographic findings are consistent with an irritable colon syndrome. (**B**) Two years later, there is still further accentuation of the haustral pattern, evidence of muscle hypertrophy. (**C**) Four years after the first barium enema, the sigmoid shows evidence of still further muscle hypertrophy and axial shortening, and now, a few diverticula are present.

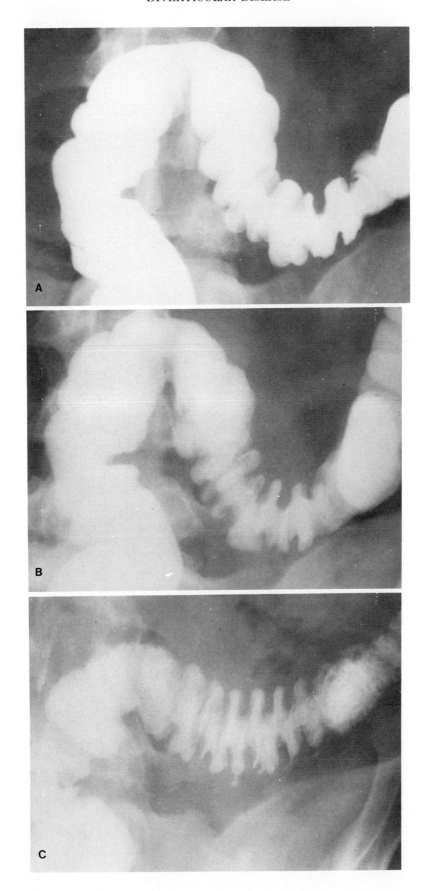

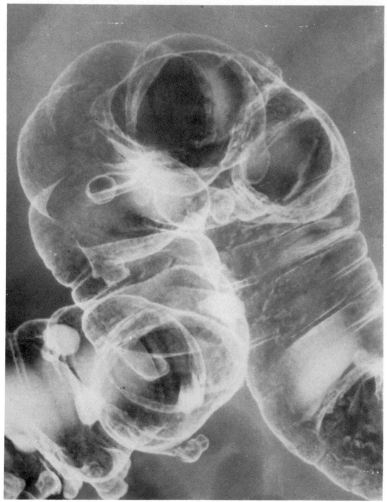

FIG. 7.3. THE DIVERTICULUM
Multiple diverticula ranging from 0.5–1.0 cm in diameter protrude from the colonic lumen. Double-contrast enema, hepatic flexure.

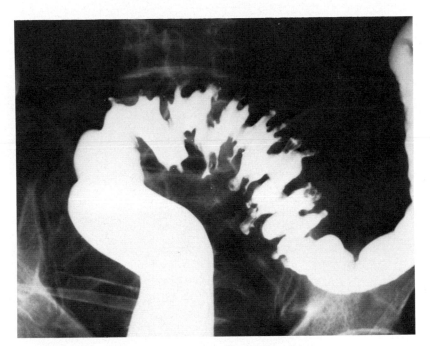

FIG. 7.4. SIGMOID DIVERTICULOSIS

Note the sacculated "saw tooth" appearance with diverticula protruding from each saccule. There is considerable narrowing of the lumen and axial shortening due to deep criss-crossing circular muscle bundles.

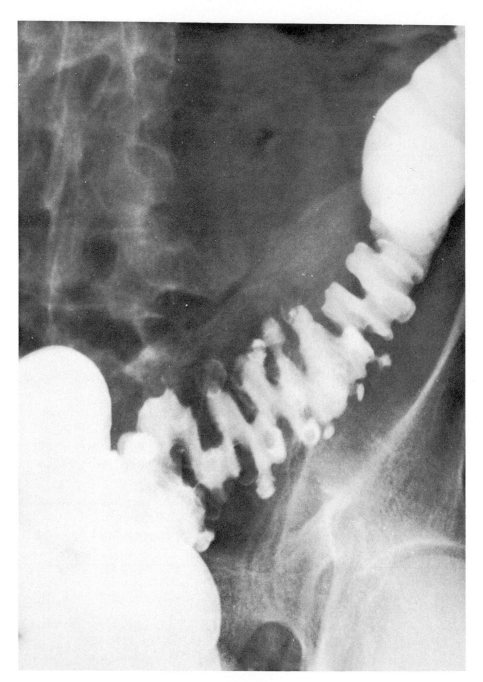

FIG. 7.5. SIGMOID DIVERTICULOSIS

Typical appearance showing thickened interdigitating circular muscle bundles similar to Fig. 7.4. The colon has a sacculated appearance with narrowing of the effective lumen and axial shortening. A few diverticula with inspissated fecal material protrude from the apex of some of the saccules.

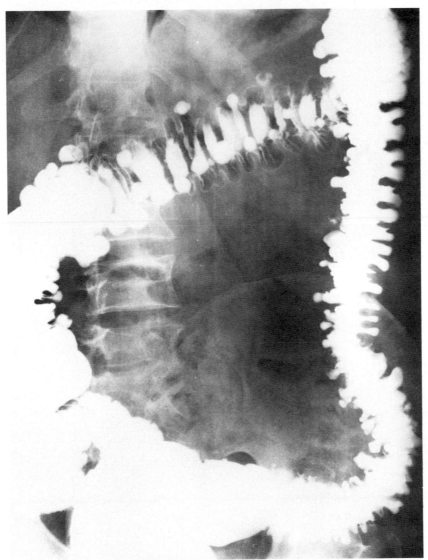

FIG. 7.6. DIFFUSE DIVERTICULOSIS
The colon is studded with innumerable diverticula.

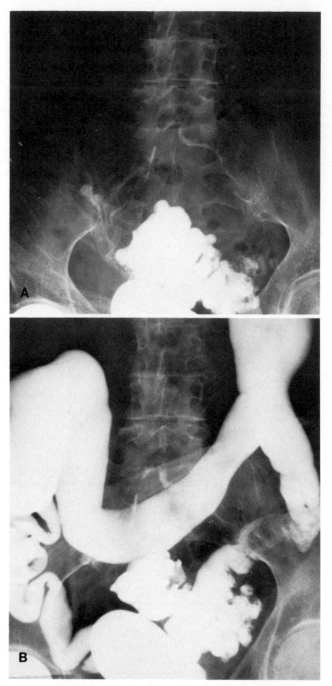

FIG. 7.7. COMPLETE RETROGRADE OBSTRUCTION DUE TO FUNCTIONAL SPASM IN SIGMOID DIVERTICULOSIS OVERCOME BY ADMINISTRATION OF AN ANTISPASMODIC DRUG

(A) Initial filling showing sigmoid diverticulosis with complete obstruction to retrograde flow. (B) After administration of an antispasmodic drug, the lumen fully distends and complete colon filling is achieved. (Reprinted with permission from Ferrucci, J. T., Jr.: Hypotonic barium enema examination. Am. J. Roentgenol., *116*: 304, 1972, American Roentgen Ray Society.)

An additional common and significant concern is the necessity to evaluate a hidden polypoid or constricting carcinoma in the patient with severe sigmoid deformity and associated smooth muscle spasm. In such cases multiple films in both left and right oblique projections, angled views including the Chassard-Lapiné view and the use of antispasmodic drugs and double contrast techniques may all be required. In these cases the maximal skills of the radiologist are surely on trial.

DIVERTICULITIS

Clinical and Pathologic Features

Diverticulitis, the principle complication of colonic diverticular disease, is a clinical-pathologic entity characterized by perforation of a diverticulum and the formation of a peridiverticular abscess. Clinical findings resulting from purulent perisigmoiditis include lower abdominal pain usually associated with fever, mass or tenderness and laboratory evidence of infection.

Since diverticula are mainly extramural structures protruding into the pericolic fat, retained fecal material may become inspissated as a result of the narrow diverticular neck. Inflammation of the mucosal lining ensues which gradually or acutely produces frank diverticular perforation with formation of a peridiverticular abscess. Histologically, evidence of undigested muscle fibers, foreign body giant cell granulomas, pus and necrotic tissue are found in the pericolic fat. In most cases peridiverticular abscesses become walled off by fibrous tissue and are chronic in character although occasionally a free intraperitoneal perforation occurs. Fistulas to adjacent organs are common, especially to the bladder, vagina, small bowel and skin. In some instances dissection of the inflammatory process extends parallel to the bowel lumen in the pericolic fat with perforations or communications into a series of adjacent diverticula forming pericolonic longitudinal sinus tracks. When the inflammatory process is severe, surgical obstruction of the large bowel may occur with typical clinical and radiographic features. Occasionally in such cases, the pericolonic pelvic abscess may cause entrapment of a loop of distal small bowel and produce concomitant signs of mechanical small bowel obstruction. Other organs occasionally encased in the pelvic inflammatory process include the left ureter, pelvic adnexa, and the appendix. On rare occasions extensive dissection of pelvic abscesses along soft tissue planes has resulted in abscesses presenting in the upper thigh, perineum, and anterior abdominal wall.

Roentgen Findings

Plain Film Findings

Plain roentgenographic studies of the abdomen in active diverticulitis may disclose a number of important findings. Large bowel obstruction occurs commonly and is often accompanied by either generalized small bowel ileus or mechanical obstruction of a loop of small bowel adhering to the inflamed sigmoid colon. In such cases, analysis of plain films may be extremely difficult. A gas-containing pelvic abscess is occasionally encountered and rarely pneumoperitoneum is seen when free diverticular perforation is present. In all patients with suspected acute diverticulitis the pelvis and lower abdominal quadrants should be carefully inspected for evidence of a radiopaque foreign body.

Fluoroscopic Technique

Most authorities advise delaying the performance of a retrograde barium enema for several days in the presence of acute diverticulitis, fearing that the increased pressure exerted by the barium column will expel even more luminal contents through the perforated diverticulum. After several days of medical management consisting of bowel rest and antibiotics, the inflammatory reaction has usually subsided enough to permit a safe enema examination. However, when clinical findings suggest the possibility of acute pelvic sepsis, bowel obstruction or free perforation, an immediate colon examination may be performed. A water-soluble contrast agent is preferred if perforation is suspected. Otherwise, conventional barium preparations are used because of the superior radiographic detail they afford. Obviously, gentle technique with incremental filling and use of antispasmodic drugs contributes to a successful examination (Fig. 7.8).

Contrast Extravasation

Extraluminal barium or water-soluble contrast material extravasating from the tip of a diverticulum as a micro- or macroperforation is the most specific, although not the most frequent, evidence of acute diverticulitis. The extravasated contrast material may occur as a tiny microprojection from the tip of the diverticulum or as a free-flowing perforation from the mesocolic or antimesocolic margin of the sigmoid (Figs. 7.9 and 7.10). When it perforates, a diverticulum may no longer be identifiable as a discrete structure—only the extravasation may be seen. Often, even the presence of extravasation is not suspected during fluoroscopic filling or on the filled overhead radiographs, but becomes visible on postevacuation films as the increased pressure generated by evacuation expels the contrast material into the abscess. Occasionally, gas-containing abscesses do not communicate with the colonic lumen, and these can be easily misinterpreted on colon radiographs as pockets of gas within adjacent intestinal loops.

Pericolic Abscess

A slightly less specific although probably more common finding is a pericolic soft tissue mass due to a localized abscess (Fig. 7.11). Characteristic signs of an extraluminal mass include eccentric narrowing and displacement of the bowel lumen. The mucosal folds may be edematous but are almost always preserved. A diverticulum may or may not be seen in the immediate area of the abscess. A pericolic mass is a relatively nonspecific sign, however, and the differential diagnosis includes entities such as metastatic serosal implant and endometriosis.

Nonspecific Stenosis

In some instances, a nonspecific narrowing of the sigmoid lumen occurs as a result of varying degrees of spasm and mural inflammatory induration (Fig. 7.12). Typically, both proximal and distal margins of the stenotic segment have a gradual tapered symmetrical configuration in contradistinction to the eccentric shelf-like appearance in primary carcinoma. The mucosal folds through the stenotic region are usually thickened and edematous, and may appear smudged or indistinct due to poor barium coating. In carcinoma, the mucosa presents a bland appearance due to ulcerative mucosal destruction. However, in a small percentage of cases, the features do not permit an x-ray diagnosis or even a morphologic diagnosis at the time of surgery. Other entities in the differential diagnosis include segmental ischemic colitis, segmental involvement by Crohn's colitis, and other infectious colitides.

Fistula Formation

Colo-vesical, colo-vaginal, colo-enteric, and colo-cutaneous fistulas are distinctive

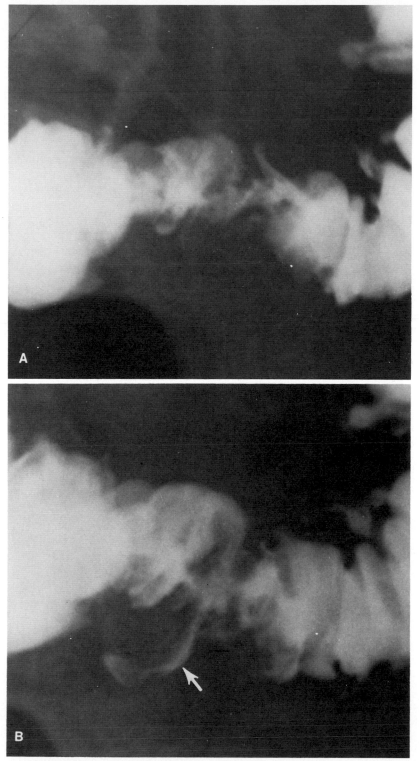

FIG. 7.8. ACUTE DIVERTICULITIS WITH ABSCESS FORMATION—SHOWN AFTER A
HYPOTONIC ENEMA

(A) Initial filling shows nonspecific stenosis with suggestion of an extrinsic mass
against the underside of the sigmoid. (B) Immediately following administration of
an antispasmotic drug, there is relaxation of the narrowed area and filling of the
abscess cavity (arrow).

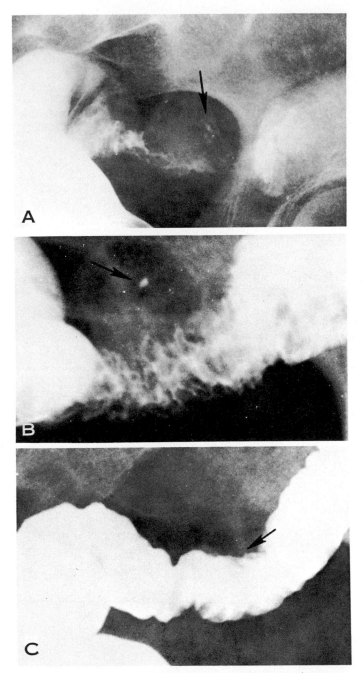

FIG. 7.9. ACUTE DIVERTICULITIS WITH MICROPERFORATION
(A) Barium enema performed on admission shows a microperforation (arrow) of
the sigmoid colon with partial obstruction. The tapered margins and the preservation
of mucosa through the narrowed segment are in favor of diverticulitis rather than
carcinoma. (B) After 4 days of conservative treatment, there is less spasm and an
intramural mass surrounds the microperforation (arrow) and indents the bowel
lumen. (C) One month later the sigmoid colon has a normal appearance except for
a minimal residual intramural mass (arrow). The extravasated particle of barium is
now covered by distended colon.

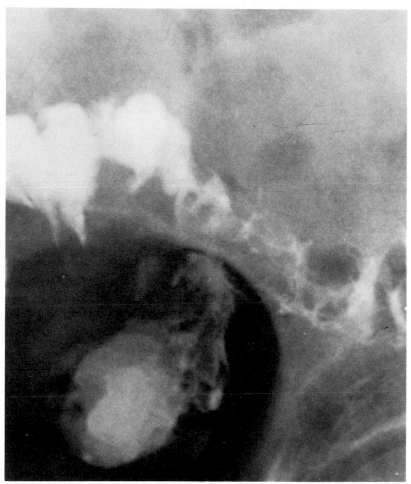

FIG. 7.10. ACUTE DIVERTICULITIS WITH MACROPERFORATION
The midsigmoid is irregularly narrowed with preserved but swollen mucosa.
Barium from a perforated diverticulum fills a 4 × 6 cm left pelvic abscess.

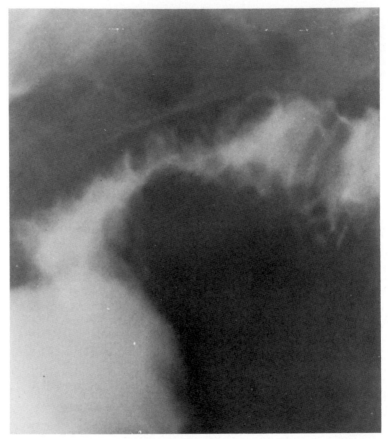

FIG. 7.11. EXTRAMURAL PERISIGMOIDAL MASS DUE TO ACUTE DIVERTICULITIS WITH
ABSCESS FORMATION

Note the characteristic signs of an extramucosal mass including eccentric narrowing and displacement of the bowel lumen. No extravasation is seen nor is the
offending diverticulum evident. This pattern is not specific but is strongly suggestive
of diverticulitis given the proper clinical setting.

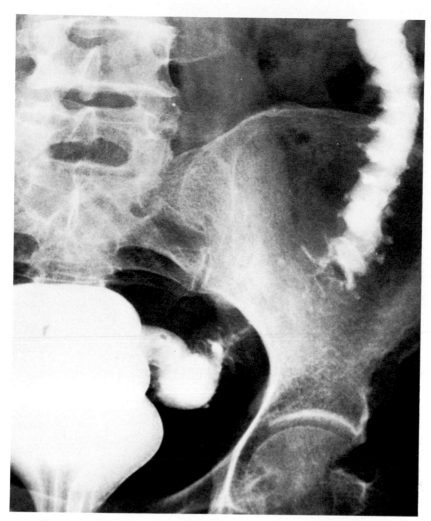

FIG. 7.12. SIGMOID DIVERTICULITIS WITH INTENSE SPASM

There is a segment of narrowing in the distal descending colon. Diverticula are present proximally. The length of the segment, the preservation of some mucosal pattern, and the absence of tumor shelf at each end are all in favor of diverticulitis rather than carcinoma.

albeit unusual complications of acute and chronic diverticulitis. Fistulas to the bladder and vagina occur most commonly and result in the passage of air and feces per urethra and vagina. While barium studies may show the fistulous communication, often clinical inspection by cystoscopy or vaginal speculum examination is necessary to confirm the diagnosis. The differential diagnosis of colonic fistula formation includes Crohn's ileo-colitis and primary rectosigmoid carcinoma.

Paracolonic Tracking

Longitudinal paracolonic sinus tracks are manifestations of an unusual variety of dissecting peridiverticulitis. These are readily demonstrated on barium enema examinations and are somewhat more frequently detected if careful pathologic examination of the pericolic fat envelope is conducted on resected surgical specimens. These tracks are rather short, measuring 3–5 cm in length and may show multiple communications to the bowel lumen via additional serially involved adjacent diverticula (Fig. 7.13). Their exact pathogenesis is unclear. While coincidental peridiverticular perforations could account for the involvement of multiple succes- sive diverticula to form these sinus tracks, it is more likely that a paracolic abscess arising from a single diverticulum dissects longitudinally involving several diverticula in sequence (Fig. 7.14). However, paracolonic sinus tracking is not specific for diverticulitis and indeed rather long tracks occur in Crohn's colitis with or without the presence of underlying diverticular disease. (Fig. 7.15). In addition, primary carcinoma of the colon may cause a short paracolonic track indistinguishable from diverticulitis, and thus colonic malignancies should always be excluded when a paracolonic fistulous track is encountered.

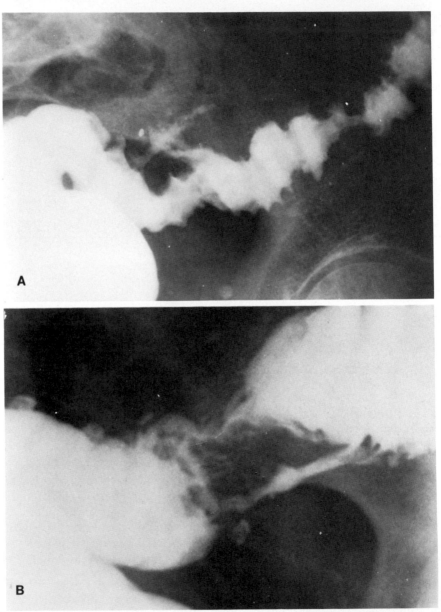

FIG. 7.13. PARACOLONIC SINUS TRACKS IN DISSECTING PERIDIVERTICULITIS OF THE SIGMOID

Tracks may involve the mesocolic (**A**) or antimesocolic (**B**) borders of the sigmoid. Such tracks usually extend for 3–5 cm longitudinally paralleling the colonic lumen and may end blindly (**A**) or re-enter the lumen (**B**) at one or more points.

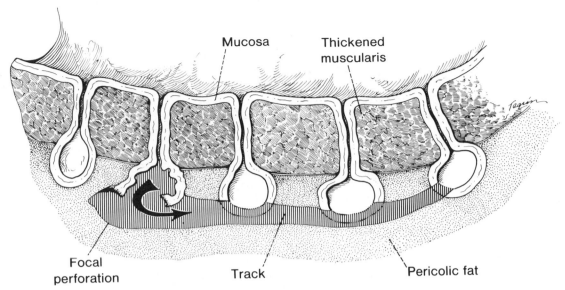

Mucosa　　　Thickened muscularis

Focal perforation　　　Track　　　Pericolic fat

FIG. 7.14. POSTULATED MECHANISM OF PARACOLONIC LONGITUDINAL SINUS TRACKS IN DISSECTING PERIDIVERTICULITIS

Following perforation of a single diverticulum into the pericolic fat, the abscess extends along the axis of the colon to involve adjacent diverticular sacs sequentially. Multiple sites of communication with the colonic lumen may be evident. (Reprinted with permission from Ferrucci, J. T., Jr., Ragsdale, B. D., Barratt, P. J., *et al.*: Double tracking of the sigmoid colon. Radiology, *120:* 307, 1976.)

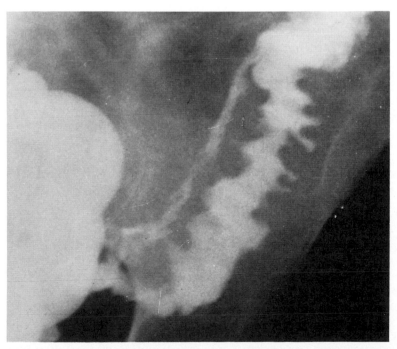

FIG. 7.15. A 10 CM PARACOLONIC SINUS TRACK IN DISSECTING PERIDIVERTICULITIS
Long tracks in the sigmoid may also be encountered in Crohn's colitis.

SPECIAL FEATURES

Diverticular Hemorrhage

Painless, bright red rectal bleeding in an elderly patient without shock followed by gradual spontaneous cessation is often due to a bleeding diverticulum. In recent years, the mechanism of bleeding from colonic diverticula has been elucidated by angiographic techniques which have stimulated a more detailed analysis of the microvascular anatomy of colonic segments involved by diverticular disease. It is presently believed that submucosal branches of the penetrating arteries are stretched over the apex of the diverticulum as it bulges beyond the colonic wall into the pericolic fat (Fig. 7.16). Focal inflammation of diverticular mucosa due to fecal inspissation subsequently leads to erosion of arterial walls and brisk hemorrhage. Usually the size of the artery is such that frank clinical shock does not supervene. As the artery gradually contracts, thrombosis occurs and bleeding ceases.

Selective mesenteric angiographic examinations performed during the phase of active bleeding may show frank contrast extravasation within the lumen of the diverticulum or within the adjacent colonic lumen providing bleeding occurs at a rate of 0.5 ml/min or greater (Fig. 7.17). This subject is covered in detail in Chapter 13. Several investigators have provided angiographic documentation that bleeding is twice as frequent from right-sided colonic diverticula as from diverticula in the descending and sigmoid colon even though diverticula are far more common in the

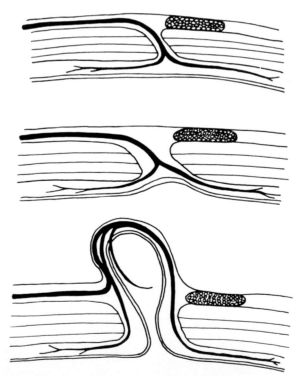

FIG. 7.16. SCHEMATIC REPRESENTATION OF MICROVASCULAR ANATOMY
UNDERLYING COLONIC DIVERTICULAR HEMORRHAGE

A penetrating branch of vasa recta is displaced over the dome of a protruding diverticular sac. Erosion of the arterial wall results in massive painless colonic bleeding. (Reprinted with permission from Meyers, M. A., Volberg, F., Katzen, B., et al.: The angio-architecture of colonic diverticula. Radiology, 108: 249, 1973.)

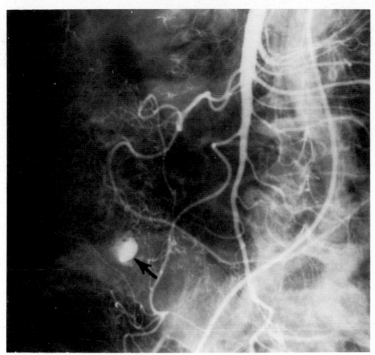

FIG. 7.17. ANGIOGRAPHIC DEMONSTRATION OF DIVERTICULAR HEMORRHAGE
Note the pooled collection of extravasated contrast in the lumen of the cecum (arrow). Right sided colonic diverticula are especially susceptible to bleeding, but the rate of blood loss must exceed 0.5 ml/min before angiographic detection of contrast extravasation is possible. Bleeding can sometimes be controlled by intra-arterial infusion of vasoconstrictor substances.

latter locations. The explanation for this phenomenon is not yet apparent. When hemorrhage is severe, administration of intra-arterial vasoconstrictor substances selectively injected into the area of the bleeding diverticulum may control hemorrhage nonoperatively although rebleeding is not uncommon.

Giant Diverticula

Rarely, a so-called giant diverticulum may be encountered as a discrete gas-containing structure on a plain abdominal film or by communication with the colonic lumen on barium enema examination (Fig. 7.18). Such diverticula are most commonly found in the sigmoid colon and may reach rather enormous dimensions, as much as 25 cm in diameter. Presentation as a tympanitic abdominal mass has been recorded although they may be only intermittently palpable due to episodic inflation and deflation. Volvulus of a giant diverticulum has also occurred. Pathologic examination discloses a fibrous wall usually lined with a granulating mucosal surface but sometimes the lining is composed of low cuboidal epithelium. Many authorities consider giant sigmoid diverticula to be manifestations of a chronic healed peridiverticular abscess with subsequent gradual air distention by a check-valve phenomenon. Surgical resection is usually indicated.

Cecal Diverticula

Individual or multiple diverticula are occasionally found in the cecal area. They are often larger than the usual sigmoid diverticula measuring as much as 2–3 cm in size and otherwise appear unassociated with any local muscular abnormality in the

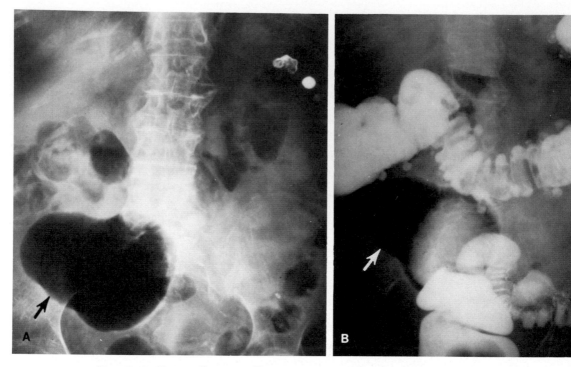

FIG. 7.18. GIANT SIGMOID DIVERTICULUM (GIANT GAS CYST OF THE SIGMOID)
Note the large gas-containing structure (arrow) on plain roentgenogram (**A**) and
with partial filling following barium enema (**B**).

cecal wall. Often they occur in association with diverticular disease of the sigmoid.
Clinically, the majority of cecal diverticula are asymptomatic, but perforation with
pericecal diverticulitis may occur and simulate appendicitis. The origin of cecal
diverticula is uncertain.

DIFFERENTIAL DIAGNOSIS AND ASSOCIATED DISEASES

In view of the prevalence of diverticular disease in the adult and aged population,
coincidental occurrence of other disorders must be constantly born in mind. Coexisting carcinoma of the sigmoid may be notoriously elusive within the spastic and
compartmentalized sigmoid of severe diverticular disease. In addition, a sigmoid
carcinoma (even in the absence of diverticulitis) may be associated with mural
penetration and an inflammatory reaction indistinguishable from diverticulitis.
Similarly, in the aged patient ischemic colitis may occur segmentally and simulate
acute diverticulitis with spasm and mucosal edema. Pain and occasional bleeding
may occur in both disorders although the bloody diarrhea of ischemic colitis is
generally more severe. Sigmoidoscopic findings are frequently helpful in differential
diagnosis. Both ulcerative and Crohn's colitis can also be engrafted upon diverticular
disease. Important differential points include the typical mucosal edema and ulcerations on barium studies and sigmoidoscopy. Paracolonic sinus tracks occurring in
Crohn's disease may be initiated by pre-existing diverticula. Long paracolonic tracks
in excess of 10 cm are more compatible with Crohn's colitis whereas shorter tracks
between 3–5 cm are more consistent with diverticular disease. Often radiographic
evidence of inflammatory bowel disease elsewhere in the colon will settle the
differential diagnosis. If inflammatory changes are not present elsewhere in the
colon, diverticulitis and primary carcinoma are both considerations and thus surgical
resection should be considered.

BIBLIOGRAPHY

Arfwidsson, S., Knock, N. G., Lehmann, L., *et al.*: Pathogenesis of multiple diverticula of the sigmoid colon in diverticular disease. Acta Chir. Scand., Suppl. 342, 1964.

Burkitt, D. P., Walker, A. R. P., and Painter, N. S.: Effect of dietary fibre on stools and transit-time, and its role in the causation of disease. Lancet, *2:* 408, 1972.

Cassarella, W. J., Kanter, I. E., and Seaman, W. B.: Right-sided colonic diverticula as a cause of acute rectal hemorrhage. N. Engl. J. Med., *286:* 450, 1972.

Ferrucci, J. T., Jr.: Hypotonic barium enema examination. Am. J. Roentgenol., *116:* 304, 1972.

Ferrucci, J. T., Jr., Jaffer, F., and Seidler, R.: Muscle spasm in sigmoid diverticulosis: Evaluation of retrograde colon obstruction by hypotonic barium enema. J. Can. Assoc. Radiologists *25:* 269, 1974.

Ferrucci, J. T., Jr., Ragsdale, B. D., Barrett, P. J., *et al.*: Double tracking of the sigmoid colon. Radiology *120:* 307, 1976.

Fleischner, F. G.: Diverticular disease of the colon. New observations and revised concepts. Gastroenterology, *60:* 316, 1971.

Fleischner, F. G., and Ming, S. C.: Revised concepts on diverticular disease of the colon. II. So-called diverticulitis; diverticular sigmoiditis and peridiverticulitis; diverticular abscess, fistula, and frank peritonitis. Radiology *84:* 599, 1965.

Fleischner, F. G., Ming, S. C., and Henken, E. M.: Revised concepts on diverticular disease of the colon. I. Diverticulosis; emphasis on tissue derangement and its relation to the irritable colon syndrome. Radiology *83:* 859, 1964.

Horner, J. L.: Natural history of diverticulosis of the colon. Am. J. Dig. Dis. *3:* 343, 1958.

Hughes, L. E.: Postmortem survey of diverticular disease of the colon. I. Diverticulosis and diverticulitis. Gut *10:* 336, 1969.

Kempczinski, R. F., and Ferrucci, J. T., Jr.: Giant sigmoid diverticula: A review. Ann. Surg. *180:* 864, 1974.

Marshak, R. H., Janowitz, H. D., and Present, D. H.: Granulomatous colitis in association with diverticula. N. Engl. J. Med., *283:* 1080, 1970.

Marshak, R. H., Lindner, A. E., Pochaczevsky, R., *et al.*: Longitudinal sinus tracts in granulomatous colitis and diverticulitis. Semin. Roentgenol. *11:* 101, 1976.

Meyers, M. A., Alonso, D. R., and Baer, J. W.: Pathogenesis of massively bleeding colonic diverticulosis: New observations. Am. J. Roentgenol. *127:* 901, 1976.

Meyers, M. A., Volberg, F., Katzen, B., *et al.*: The angioarchitecture of colonic diverticula. Radiology, *108:* 249, 1973.

Ming, S. C., and Fleischner, F. G.: Diverticulitis of the sigmoid colon: Reappraisal of the pathology and pathogenesis. Surgery, *58:* 627, 1965.

Morson, B. C.: The muscle abnormality in diverticular disease of the sigmoid colon. Br. J. Radiol., *36:* 385, 1963.

Painter, N. S., and Burkitt, D. P.: Diverticular disease of the colon: A deficiency disease of western civilization. Br. Med. J., *2:* 450, 1971.

Painter, N. S., and Truelove, S. C.: The intraluminal pressure patterns in diverticulosis of the colon. Gut, *5:* 201, 1964.

Parks, T. G.: National history of diverticular disease of the colon: A review of 521 cases. Br. Med. J., *4:* 639, 1969.

Schatzki, R.: The roentgenologic differential diagnosis between cancer and diverticulitis of the colon. Radiology, *34:* 657, 1940.

Slack, W. W.: Diverticula of the colon and their relation to the muscle layers and blood vessels. Gastroenterology, *39:* 708, 1960.

Slack, W. W.: The anatomy, pathology and some clinical features of diverticulitis of the colon. Br. J. Surg., *50:* 185, 1962.

Sleisenger, M. H., and Fordtran, J. S.: *Gastrointestinal Disease,* pp. 1353–1354. W. B. Saunders, Philadelphia, 1973.

Tagliacozzo, S., and Virno, F.: The vascularization of the colon wall; morphological study. Ann. Ital. Chir., *38:* 301, 1961.

Tagliacozzo, S., and Virno, F.: Vascular relationships of diverticula of the colon; morphological study. Ann. Ital. Chir., *38:* 420, 1961.

Welch, C. E., Allen, A. W., and Donaldson, G. A.: An appraisal of resection of the colon for diverticulitis of the sigmoid. Ann. Surg., *138:* 332, 1953.

Williams, I.: Diverticular disease of the colon without diverticula. Radiology, *89:* 401, 1967.

Williams, I., and Fleischner, F. G.: Diverticular disease of the colon. In *Alimentary Tract Roentgenology,* 2nd ed., edited by A. R. Margulis and H. J. Burhenne, pp. 1014–1036. C. V. Mosby, St. Louis, 1973.

Wolf, B. S., Khilnani, M., and Marshak, R. H.: Diverticulosis and diverticulitis; roentgen findings and their interpretation. Am. J. Roentgenol. *77:* 726, 1957.

8

Pathology of Ulcerative Colitis and Crohn's Colitis

AUSTIN L. VICKERY, JR., M.D.

INTRODUCTION

Ulcerative colitis and Crohn's disease of the colon (granulomatous colitis) are the most common nonspecific inflammatory diseases of the large intestine with ulcerative colitis being much more frequent. Since these entities share many clinical, radiologic and pathologic characteristics, it is not surprising that distinctions between them are often difficult and controversial.

Since we do not know the cause of either illness, the definition of each is based on a group of clinical, radiologic and pathologic features which best seem to represent the common denominators between the two. Thus, these illnesses might better be termed clinicopathologic entities rather than specific diseases. Some observers have suggested that, instead of a rigid separation, it is better to consider ulcerative colitis and Crohn's colitis as a single disease with each at opposite ends of a spectrum of clinical and pathologic manifestations. Although there is little argument over the diagnostic criteria for so-called "classic" examples of either ulcerative colitis or Crohn's colitis, there is a group of cases in an intermediate "gray" zone of uncertainty where the diseases tend to merge. The differential diagnosis of these debatable cases is dependent on subjective bias and different emphases on arbitrary criteria, which is reflected in the wide variation in the reported incidences of these two diseases from different institutions.

An indefinite designation of "inflammatory bowel disease, unclassified" is the

TABLE 8.1
PATHOLOGIC CLASSIFICATION OF INFLAMMATORY BOWEL DISEASE*

Idiopathic
  Ulcerative colitis and proctitis
  Crohn's disease of the colon
Bacterial
  Dysenteric (Shigella, Salmonella, pathologic *Escherichia coli*, etc.)
  Gonococcal proctitis
  Tuberculous
  Whipple's disease
Parasitic
  Amebiasis
  Balantidiasis
  Schistosomiasis
  Cryptosporidiosis
Viral
  Lymphogranuloma venereum
  Cytomegalovirus
Fungal
  Histoplasmosis
Drug, chemical and foodstuff-related
  Antibiotic-related
  Cytotoxic drugs (5-fluorouracil)-related
  Heavy metal-related
  Milk protein allergy
Irradiation-induced
  Acute irradiation colitis
  Postirradiation colitis
Of intrinsic origin
  Ischemic colitis
  Solitary ulcer syndrome
  Diverticulitis
  Obstruction-related
Pseudomembranous Enterocolitis

* Adapted from Yardley, J. H., and Donowitz, M.: Colo-rectal biopsy in inflammatory bowel disease. In *The Gastrointestinal Tract*, edited by J. H. Yardley, B. C. Morson, and M. R. Abell, Chap. 5, p. 68. Williams & Wilkins, Baltimore, 1977.

diagnostic option preferred by some pathologists and clinicians for the minority of cases which do not fit their criteria for either ulcerative colitis or Crohn's disease. The experience of St. Mark's Hospital in London is that about 10% of colectomy specimens with nonspecific inflammatory bowel disease are diagnosed as "unclassified colitis," and some other institutions report higher percentages. Although the idiopathic types of inflammatory bowel disease, ulcerative colitis, and Crohn's colitis comprise the large proportion of all cases, it is important to exclude entities of known cause in the differential diagnosis (Table 8.1).

ULCERATIVE COLITIS

Definition

Ulcerative colitis is an idiopathic acute or chronic inflammatory and ulcerative disease of the large intestine. The main symptoms are diarrhea, abdominal pain, rectal bleeding, weight loss and anorexia.

Disease Course

The disease tends to be chronic and persistent for years with alternate periods of remission and exacerbation a common characteristic. However, about 10% of patients die within a year of the initial attack.

Incidence and Constitutional Factors

Like Crohn's disease, ulcerative colitis may afflict all ages but it is primarily a disease of young adults with large series of reported cases showing 75% between ages of 15 and 49 years with a peak incidence of about 20 and 40 years. However, occasionally ulcerative colitis is seen in older age groups with a second peak incidence about the age of 60. There is a slightly greater incidence in females and, as with regional enteritis, a higher frequency among Hebrews. Although ulcerative colitis has a worldwide distribution, it has a greater prevalence in more complicated, "civilized" societies.

Etiology and Pathogenesis

The etiology of ulcerative colitis remains a mystery although a large number of theories have been investigated including infection, destructive enzymes and surface irritants, hypersensitivity and autoimmune mechanisms, exogenous antigens (e.g., food allergies), psychosomatic or emotional factors and a basic mucosal cell defect.

Still another possibility is that ulcerative colitis may represent the combined effect of several etiologic factors and therefore that the disease may not be a single entity but rather a syndrome with several causes.

Of the above possible specific etiologic factors, the hypersensitivity and autoimmune mechanisms have received most attention in recent years. Observations favoring these theories include the following:

1. The association of ulcerative colitis with some collagen diseases such as rheumatoid arthritis, rheumatic fever and lupus erythematosus.
2. An increased serum γ-globulin in some cases of ulcerative colitis.
3. The response of the rabbit colon to the arthus test and Shwartzman phenomenon and the production of experimental colitis in animals sensitized to egg albumin.
4. The response of ulcerative colitis to steroid and immunosuppressive drugs.
5. The presence of circulating antibodies to colon extract in patients with ulcerative colitis; however, there is no conclusive evidence of anti-colon antibodies. These findings may represent secondary immune responses to other injury.

Pathology

Gross Pathology of Acute and Chronic Phases

There is a strong predilection for ulcerative colitis to begin in the rectosigmoid with over 90% of cases starting in this location and with a tendency for gradual retrograde extension to the ileocecal valve (Fig. 8.1). In from 10–25% of cases, the disease extends for a short distance into the terminal ileum ("back-wash ileitis") which must be distinguished from the ileocolitis of Crohn's disease. After many years of disease, the colon may become narrowed due to submucosal scarring and the mucosal surface atrophic and flattened with perhaps irregular chronic ulcerations (Fig. 8.2).

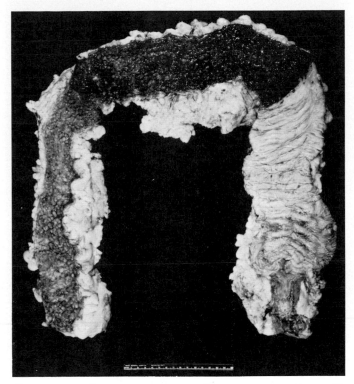

FIG. 8.1. COLECTOMY SPECIMEN FROM A PATIENT WITH LONG-STANDING
ULCERATIVE COLITIS

The bowel is reversed with the ileo-cecal area at the lower right. Note the irregular
and very inflamed mucosal surface of the involved left and transverse colon segments
and the abrupt cessation of the process in the ascending colon.

External Appearance of Bowel

The serosa shows remarkably little considering the severe mucosal damage. In
addition, the wall is characteristically not thickened as in Crohn's colitis and indeed,
may be thin and friable in fulminant cases, "toxic megacolon."

Mucosal Changes

The opened bowel presents a dramatic picture with severely congested, angry red
purple mucosa overlayed with blood and mucus (Fig. 8.3). Ulcerations are variable
in size but tend to be shallow and coalescent along the long axis. With alternate
periods of activation and remission, the mucosa tends to assume a geographic
topography representing various stages of tissue repair, regeneration, and scarring.

Pseudopolyposis is a nonspecific term used to describe the effect produced by
islands of inflamed, uninvolved, or regenerative mucosa which are surrounded by
zones of ulceration and thus tend to protrude into the lumen as polypoid lesions
(Fig. 8.4). The term pseudopolyposis is grammatically incorrect for, as stated on the
section on polypoid tumors, a "polyp" may be *any* process which protrudes into the
bowel lumen, neoplastic or inflammatory. Nonetheless, "pseudopolyposis," by common usage, has become an established term meaning simulation of a benign
neoplastic polyp.

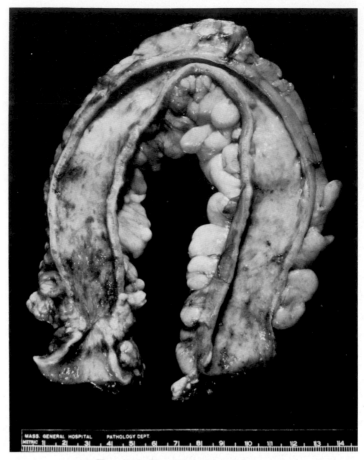

FIG. 8.2. ULCERATIVE COLITIS

"Burnt out" ulcerative colitis showing smooth atrophy of mucosa.

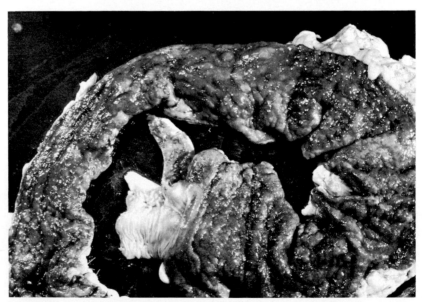

FIG. 8.3. MODERATE ULCERATIVE COLITIS

Detail of resected colon showing obliteration of normal mucosal detail and inflammatory reaction. Also note sudden termination of the disease at the ileocecal valve (center of picture).

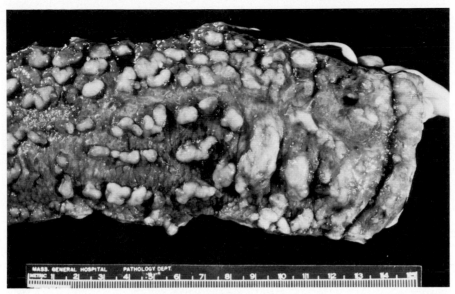

FIG. 8.4. ULCERATIVE COLITIS

Pseudopolyposis in ulcerative colitis, produced by islands of mucosa surrounded by areas of ulceration.

Pseudopolyposis, although more commonly present in ulcerative colitis, may also be seen in Crohn's colitis and therefore is not a reliable discriminating finding. Occasionally, the process may be so extensive in inflammatory bowel disease, particularly ulcerative colitis, that it may be difficult to distinguish from familial adenomatous colonic polyposis.

Microscopic Pathology

In the acute stage, ulcers show a heavy infiltration of chronic inflammatory cells (lymphocytes, plasma cells, eosinophils, and macrophages) associated with congested granulation tissue. The ulcers are characteristically superficial, confined to the mucosa and submucosa.

The tendency for these superficial ulcers to undermine the adjoining mucosa can produce defects which resemble "collar buttons" when seen on radiographic examination (Fig. 8.5) The confinement of the ulcerative inflammatory reaction to the mucosa and submucosa is perhaps the single most distinctive pathologic feature in ulcerative colitis and constitutes the major difference from Crohn's colitis. It is, indeed, remarkable to observe the abrupt cessation of an extensive ulcerative process at the submucosal-muscularis junction (Fig. 8.6) in a patient with known ulcerative colitis of many years duration. Micro-abscesses of the crypts are typical. Granulomas characteristic of Crohn's disease are absent. None of these changes are specific and no common denominator of morphologic change has been recognized. Therefore, it is important to rule out all possible other known causes of colon inflammatory lesions with ulcers such as amebiasis and ischemic colitis before a diagnosis of idiopathic ulcerative colitis is made.

Complications

The most serious aspect of ulcerative colitis is the multiplicity of its complications which include in order of frequency: severe hemorrhage, perforation with peritonitis, intestinal obstruction due to strictures, and carcinoma.

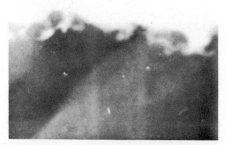

FIG. 8.5. COLLAR BUTTON ULCERS

Detail film demonstrating submucosal burrowing of deep ulcers along the inferior margin of the transverse colon.

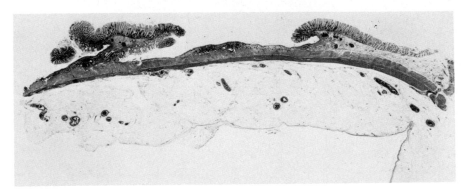

FIG. 8.6. ULCERATIVE COLITIS

Microscopic section through an ulcer in ulcerative colitis showing undermining of the adjacent mucosa with overhanging margins. Also evident is the characteristic confinement of the lesion to the mucosa and submucosa. Note the absence of thickening of the wall.

Carcinoma

The incidence of carcinoma developing in patients with ulcerative colitis is about 10 times that of the normal population and is highest in those patients who have had the illness for 10 years or more. Since ulcerative colitis is mainly a disease of young people, it would be reasonable to predict that cancer, if related, would appear in younger age groups than does colon carcinoma in the general population and this proves to be true. The average age for the development of cancer is about 35 years in patients with ulcerative colitis compared to about 60 years in the normal population. The neoplastic change is probably associated with a long period of intermittent destruction and regeneration of mucosa. These cancers are located most often in the distal colon but are more widely distributed elsewhere in the colon than in non-colitis carcinomas. Their gross appearance is often atypical for colonic cancer with a flattened and less discrete outline (Fig. 8.7). Histologically, carcinomas associated with ulcerative colitis tend to be less differentiated than the usual colon cancer and they have a poor prognosis. This may also be related to delayed diagnosis due to the masking of clinical and radiographic signs of malignancy by the basic inflammatory disease.

Although ulcerative colitis is associated with a relatively high incidence of colon cancer, the great majority of patients do not develop carcinoma. This has stimulated search for criteria to assist in the identification of that group of patients with the highest cancer risk. Various observers have noted that the risk of the development of cancer in ulcerative colitis is principally in those patients with extensive involvement of the colon for many years, while disease confined to the distal colon is associated with little cancer risk. Investigators at St. Mark's Hospital in London have performed rectal and colonic biopsies in ulcerative colitis patients with extensive disease to detect early or premalignant mucosal changes. It has been demonstrated that such atypical or dysplastic mucosal changes may be present in biopsies distant from an actual carcinoma so that a rectal biopsy with a "premalignant" histologic appearance may be associated with a cancer in the transverse colon.

Despite the proven ability of this diagnostic technique to help identify the high cancer risk patient, the method is associated with various limitations, including:

1. *A low yield of biopsies suggestive of cancer.* In the St. Mark's Hospital study on 229 patients with extensive ulcerative colitis, 1,570 biopsies were performed of which only 32 from 13 patients showed severe dysplasia. Seven of these 13 had colectomies and 4 cancers were detected.

2. *Difficulty in pathologic interpretation of the biopsy.* Regenerative mucosa associated with active inflammatory disease may simulate precancerous changes. Experience is a prerequisite for the pathologist.

3. *Severe dysplasia may not be a reliable guide to the presence of cancer.* This change may be present in the absence of carcinoma. In a review of published cases of rectal biopsies on ulcerative colitis patients with a duration of over 10 years, Dobbins noted that, although 19% showed precancerous changes, only one-third of these patients had colonic cancer.

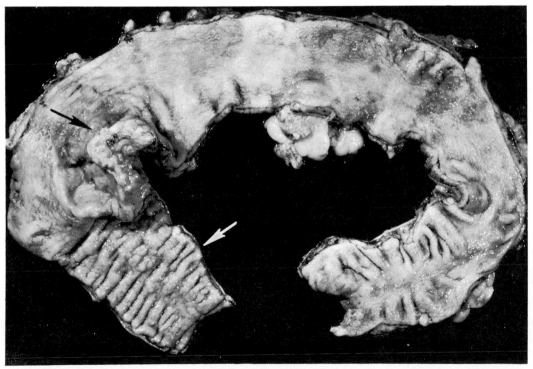

FIG. 8.7. ADENOCARCINOMA ASSOCIATED WITH CHRONIC ULCERATIVE COLITIS
Resected right colon. The normal mucosal pattern has been totally effaced. There is marked atrophy and an adenocarcinoma (black arrow) is present just distal to the ileo-cecal valve. The terminal ileum (white arrow) shows inflammatory changes.

There seems to be general agreement that rectal and colonic biopsy may be useful in discovering the ulcerative colitis patient with a higher cancer risk but that this evidence alone is an insufficient indication for colectomy and should be combined with other clinical and radiographic factors in the ultimate decision regarding surgery.

Extracolonic or Systemic Manifestations

Other diseases which may be associated with and possibly related to ulcerative colitis include uveitis, arthritis, bile duct sclerosis, and cirrhosis.

Treatment and Prognosis

Conservative medical management is the treatment of choice with steroid therapy often being beneficial. Colectomy, however, is occasionally necessitated usually due to complications. About 10% of the patients eventually have radical surgery after their initial attack because of medical management failure and in one large reported series of patients who have been followed many years, 27% eventually had some form of radical surgery.

CROHN'S COLITIS

Introduction

Although it had been recognized for many years that regional enteritis involving the terminal ileum occasionally extended a short distance beyond the ileocecal valve, acceptance of the concept that Crohn's disease might primarily involve the colon did not occur until three decades after the original paper on regional ileitis in 1932. The major reason for this delay was difficulty in distinguishing "Crohn's colitis" from other bowel lesions associated with inflammation, *e.g.*, ischemic colitis, diverticulitis and especially, ulcerative colitis. This long lag period in the recognition that Crohn's disease could be localized to the colon is sufficient evidence in itself to indicate that the diagnostic criteria are nonspecific and that the diagnosis often depends on the correct interpretation of a combination of clinical, radiologic, and pathologic features.

Terminology

Crohn's disease of the colon or Crohn's colitis is a more accurate designation of this lesion than "granulomatous colitis," a term which adds some confusion for it suggests that the disease involving the colon is different from regional enteritis or Crohn's disease of the small intestine. We no longer refer to Crohn's disease of the small bowel as "granulomatous enteritis" and it seems illogical to call its disease counterpart in the colon by a different name. Furthermore, the term "granulomatous" is imprecise for about half of the cases of Crohn's disease of the intestines are not associated with the formation of granulomas.

Clinical Features

As with Crohn's disease of the small intestine, involvement of the colon is also an illness of young adults with a peak age incidence between 10 and 20 years with a slight female predominence and a higher incidence among Hebrews. The most common symptoms of both ilecolitis and colitis are diarrhea, abdominal pain, weight loss, toxemia, fever, and perianal disease.

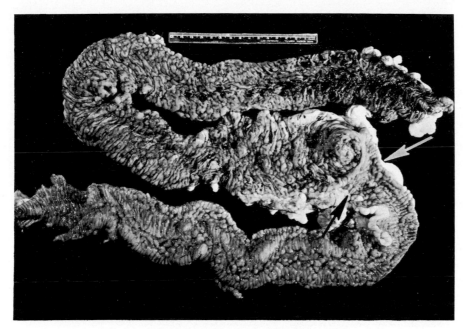

FIG. 8.8. CROHN'S COLITIS

Diffuse "cobblestone" mucosal pattern of the transverse and right colon and of the ileum which is at the bottom of the photograph. The ileo-cecal valve is marked by arrows.

Distribution of Lesions

Most cases (50–80%) of Crohn's colitis are associated with disease of the terminal ileum, usually continuous (Fig. 8.8) and occasionally with a second distal segment ("skip lesion") of colon involvement. A minority of cases (20–50%) consist of colon involvement alone. Although the right colon is the most common site of disease, the incidence of rectal involvement is relatively high in all cases, being present in one-third of patients reported from Mount Sinai Hospital of New York and in about one-half of patients with disease localized to the colon. Perianal lesions are common in both ileocolitis and colitis, being found in over 50% of the Mount Sinai cases.

Pathology

The pathology of Crohn's disease of the colon is basically that seen in regional enteritis with the main gross features including: penetrating ulcers or fissures, confluent linear ulcers, a discontinuous (segmental) pattern and a thickened bowel wall (Figs. 8.9 and 8.10). The major microscopic findings are: penetrating ulcers or fissures, transmural inflammatory reaction including proliferation of lymphoid tissue, submucosal fibrosis, and granulomas.

The major differences in the gross pathology of Crohn's colitis and ulcerative colitis have been compared by Morson and these may be so distinctive as to be strongly suggestive of the diagnosis (Table 8.2). However, it is important to bear in mind that despite a so-called "classic" gross pathologic picture, the microscopic criteria are the most reliable and, in the great majority of cases, must be present to make the diagnosis.

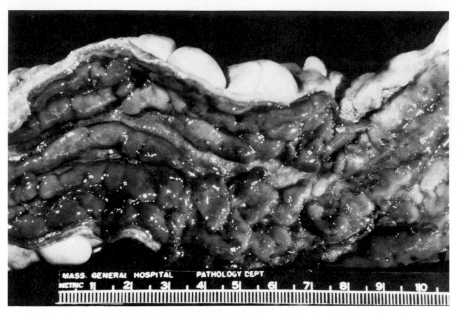

FIG. 8.9. CROHN'S COLITIS
Linear ulcerations are responsible for the edematous islands of inflamed colonic
mucosa. The ileum was also involved in this 16-year-old girl with anal fissures.

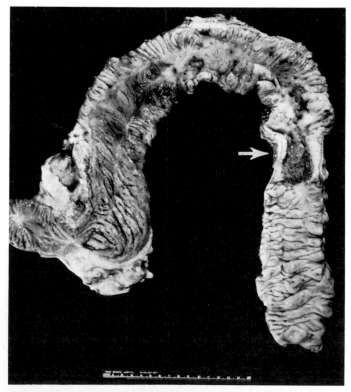

FIG. 8.10. CROHN'S COLITIS WITH EXTENSIVE INVOLVEMENT OF TRANSVERSE AND
PROXIMAL DESCENDING COLON
Note the segmental narrowing at the distal point of disease with striking fibrous
thickening of the wall and severe ulceration of the mucosa (arrow).

Cobblestoning

The deep, irregular mucosal ulcerations (fissures) of Crohn's colitis may separate intervening edematous but nonulcerated islands of mucosa resulting in a cobblestone pattern (Fig. 8.11). Although this observation may be very suggestive of Crohn's disease, as with other gross pathologic features, this is not a specific finding and "cobblestoning" may also be seen in ulcerative colitis.

Microscopically, submucosal edema and fibrosis largely account for the narrowed lumen while the irregular mucosal ulceration pattern is associated with an infiltrate of chronic inflammatory cells. As with regional enteritis, lymphoid hyperplasia is present both within the bowel wall and regional lymph nodes (Fig. 8.12).

Although there is general agreement among pathologists that microscopic evidence of penetrating ulcers, transmural inflammation, and granulomas strongly favor a diagnosis of Crohn's colitis, none of these findings is specific. Although

TABLE 8.2

GROSS DIFFERENCES IN THE PATHOLOGY OF ULCERATIVE COLITIS AND CROHN'S DISEASE OF THE COLON*

Ulcerative Colitis	Crohn's Disease
1. Disease in continuity	1. Disease discontinuous
2. Rectum almost always involved	2. Rectum normal in 50%
3. Terminal ileum involved in 10–25%	3. Terminal ileum involved in 50–80%
4. Granular and ulcerated mucosa; no fissuring	4. Discretely ulcerated mucosa; cobblestone appearance; fissuring
5. Often intensely vascular	5. Vascularity seldom pronounced
6. Normal serosa (except in acute fulminating colitis)	6. Serositis common
7. Muscular shortening of colon; fibrous strictures very rare	7. Shortening due to fibrosis; fibrous strictures common
8. Never spontaneous fistulas	8. Enterocutaneous or intestinal fistula in 10%
9. Inflammatory polyposis common and extensive	9. Inflammatory polyposis less prominent and less extensive
10. Malignant change—well recognized	10. Malignant change—probable increased incidence
11. Anal lesions in less than 25%; acute fissures, excoriation and rectovaginal fistula	11. Anal lesions in 75%; anal fistulas (often multiple); anal ulceration or chronic fissure; edematous anal tags

* Adapted from Morson, B. C., and Dawson, I. M. P.: *Gastrointestinal Pathology*, p. 477. Blackwell Scientific Publications, Oxford, 1972.

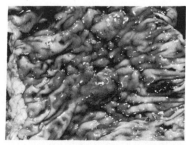

FIG. 8.11. COBBLESTONE MUCOSAL PATTERN IN CROHN'S COLITIS
Detail of a segment of resected colon.

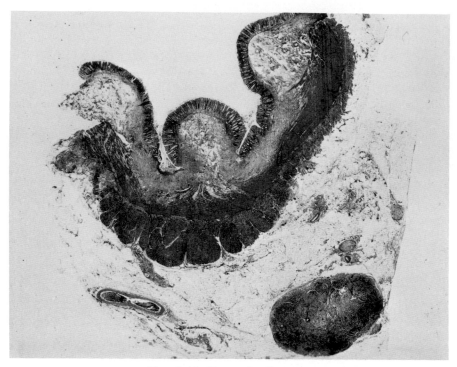

FIG. 8.12. CROHN'S COLITIS
Photomicrograph of Crohn's colitis showing narrow, cleft-like ulcerations on either side of a central mucosal island. Note the severe submucosal edema and thickened wall involved with transmural inflammation and granulomas. There is an enlarged lymph node in the mesenteric fat, also with granulomas.

Glotzer *et al.* from the Beth Israel Hospital in Boston found that the presence of microscopic sinuses and/or granulomas correlated significantly with clinical features of Crohn's colitis and their absence with clinical features of ulcerative colitis, there was still an overlap in about 25% of the cases.

Noncaseous granulomas are found in about 50% of Crohn's colitis cases and are the nearest to a specific histopathologic feature. They are not seen in ulcerative colitis and must not be confused with the foreign body granulomas incidental to secondary inflammatory reactions to perforations and chronic abscesses in that disease. Granulomas may be seen anywhere in the bowel wall in Crohn's colitis and also in lymph nodes. McGovern and Goulston regard granulomas as a reaction to the disease rather than related to its cause, and feel that their inconstant presence in Crohn's disease indicates that they are not an essential part of the process.

Aphthoid Ulcers

Morson has referred to "aphthoid" ulcers as possibly the earliest macroscopic lesion of Crohn's colitis. These lesions are tiny, shallow ulcers situated distant to obviously diseased bowel. (The term "aphthoid" is derived from the Greek meaning "thrushlike," referring to the small ulcers with a white base seen in candidiasis or thrush infections of the oral mucosa.) Some pathologists (McGovern and Goulston) believe that such ulcer formation is preceded by infiltrations of lymphocytic aggregations which may have initiated the process. Since so-called "aphthoid" ulcers are basically small lesions which may vary in size from pinpoint to a few millimeters,

Morson states these may easily be overlooked by the pathologist examining the specimen, and he suggests that these early lesions may take many years to give rise to detectable clinical or radiologic signs. It would therefore seem difficult for a radiologist to identify lesions which are aphthoid ulcers in a true pathologic sense.

Complications

Complications, as with Crohn's disease of the small intestine, are directly related to the nature and chronicity of the pathologic changes.

Internal and External Fistulas

These include perianal disease (abscess and fistula) and are due to the penetrating ulcers and involvement of all bowel layers in the inflammatory process.

Intestinal Obstruction

Although less common than in a small intestinal involvement, obstruction may occur due to lumen stenosis and/or adhesions secondary to serositis.

Hemorrhage

Hemorrhage is an infrequent complication but is considerably more common than in regional enteritis.

Recurrent Disease

As with regional enteritis of the ileum, segmental resection and anastomosis in Crohn's disease of the colon are associated with a high (50% or more) rate of recurrent disease. Although opinions vary on the actual incidence of recurrent ileal disease after colectomy with ileostomy procedures in Crohn's disease of the colon, there is general agreement that such recurrences are more common than after similar operations for ulcerative colitis.

Extraintestinal Complications

The New York Mount Sinai Hospital has reported that skin, joint, eye, mouth, and hepatic diseases are significantly higher in patients with Crohn's colitis than in enteritis confined to the small bowel.

Malignancy

Although about 40 cases of carcinoma associated with Crohn's disease of the small intestine have been reported, the issue is still controversial. Favoring a relationship is the fact that most of these occurred in the distal rather than proximal small bowel, a reversal of the usual distribution of small intestinal cancer. Nonetheless, the normal incidence of small bowel carcinoma is so low that more data are needed to demonstrate that this association has statistical relevance. On the other hand, in the colon, the evidence seems more convincing of a relationship between Crohn's disease and cancer, although there are conflicting opinions with some believing the association is coincidental. A study from the Mayo Clinic of 356 patients who were 21 years of age or younger at the time of the original diagnosis of Crohn's disease of the colon showed the incidence of colorectal carcinoma was 20 times that expected in a control population. As with cancer appearing in ulcerative colitis, patients with Crohn's disease of the colon who developed carcinoma in this Mayo series were relatively young (average age 34).

BIBIOGRAPHY

Dobbins, W. O.: Current status of the precancer lesion in ulcerative colitis. Gastroenterology, *73:* 1431, 1977.

Edwards, F. C. and Truelove, S. C.: The course and prognosis of ulcerative colitis. Gut, *4:* 299, 1962 (A follow up study of 624 patients).

Glotzer, D. J., Gardner, R. C., Goldman, H., *et al.*: Comparative features and course of ulcerative and granulomatous colitis. N. Engl. J. Med., *282:* 582, 1970.

Greenstein, A. J., Geller, S. A., Dreiling, D. A., *et al.*: Crohn's disease of the colon. Am. J. Gastroenterol. *64:* 191, 1975.

Korelitz, B. I., Present, D. H., Alpert, L. I., *et al.*: Recurrent regional ileitis after ileostomy and colectomy for granulomatous colitis. N. Engl. J. Med., *287:* 110, 1972.

Kraft, S. C., and Kirsner, J. B.: Immunological apparatus of the gut and inflammatory bowel disease. Prog. Gastroenterol., *60:* 922, 1971.

Leonard-Jones, J. E., Morson, B. C., Ritchie, D. M., *et al.*: Cancer in colitis: Assessment of the individual risk by clinical and histological criteria. Gastroenterology, *73:* 1280, 1977.

Lightdale, C. J., Sternberg, S. S., Posner, G., *et al.*: Carcinoma complicating Crohn's disease. Report of seven cases and review of the literature. Am. J. Med., *59:* 262, 1975.

Lockhart-Mummery, H. E., and Morson, B. C.: Crohn's disease (regional enteritis) of the large intestine and its distinction from ulcerative colitis. Gut, *1:* 87, 1960.

McGovern, V. J., and Goulston, S. J. M.: Crohn's disease of the colon. Gut, *9:* 164, 1968.

Michener, W. M., Gage, R. P., Sauer, W. G., *et al.*: The prognosis of chronic ulcerative colitis in children. N. Engl. J. Med. *265:* 1075, 1961.

Morson, B. C.: The early histological lesion of Crohn's disease. Proc. R. Soc. Med. *65:* 71, 1972.

Morson, B. C., and Dawson, I. M. P.: *Gastrointestinal Pathology.* Blackwell Scientific Publications, Oxford, 1972.

Mottet, N. K.: *Histopathologic Spectrum of Regional Enteritis and Ulcerative Colitis.* W. B. Saunders, Philadelphia, 1971.

Price, A. B., and Morson, B. C.: Inflammatory bowel disease. The surgical pathology of Crohn's disease and ulcerative colitis. Hum. Pathol. *6:* 7, 1975.

Weedon, D. D., Shorter, R. G., Ilstrup, D. M., *et al.*: Crohn's disease and cancer. N. Engl. J. Med., *289:* 1099, 1973.

Wright, R.: Ulcerative colitis progress review. Gastroenterology, *58:* 875, 1970.

Yardley, J. H., and Donowitz, M.: Colo-rectal biopsy in inflammatory bowel disease. In *The Gastrointestinal Tract*, edited by J. H. Yardley, B. C. Morson and M. R. Abell, Chap. 5, p. 68. Williams & Wilkins, Baltimore, 1977.

9

Ulcerative Colitis

MURRAY L. JANOWER, M.D.

BACKGROUND

Nonspecific or idiopathic ulcerative colitis is an inflammatory disease of the large bowel, the cause of which has yet to be found. Many theories have been advanced to explain the onset and unpredictable course of this debilitating disease, such as bacterial or viral infection, immunologic reactions, allergy and hypersensitivity, the destructive effect of enzymes, and emotional disorder. None of these theories has been proved, nor is it conceded that any of them may even play a significant role in the etiology of ulcerative colitis. The total lack of progress in establishing an etiology for this entity is frustrating, and simply points out our ignorance in many other areas of the disease. The failure of improved prognosis in these patients over the last 25 years is undoubtedly related.

There is no reliable estimate of the incidence of ulcerative colitis. Statistics include only the more florid cases—frequently only those patients seen in a hospital or similar setting. The indolent and subacute forms of the disease, including the majority of patients who are seen only in a private office setting are usually not included in statistical summaries. Ulcerative colitis is a much more frequent disease than the statistics would suggest.

Females are involved slightly more often than males. About one-half of the cases begin between the ages of 20 and 40, about one-quarter between the ages of 40 and 60, with the remainder about equally divided before age 20 or after age 60. Ulcerative colitis seems to be more common in patients who are Hebrew, caucasian, unmarried, and college graduates. There is no proven familial incidence.

CLINICAL FEATURES

Although ulcerative lesions may be seen in a wide variety of colonic diseases, there is a characteristic appearance and clinical course of ulcerative colitis that marks it as a discrete entity.

The onset of symptoms in ulcerative colitis may be insidious or fulminating. The *usual* course is one of gradual development of lower abdominal cramps, tenesmus, increasing frequency of bowel movements proceeding to watery or bloody diarrhea with mucus, together with anorexia, malaise, and occasional fever. One of the characteristic features of ulcerative colitis is a tendency to alternating periods of remission and exacerbation. While it might be expected that patients with more extensive involvement or with more severe *initial* attacks might have a more guarded long-term prognosis in terms of remission, medical failure or mortality, this is not necessarily correct. There does appear to be a closer correlation between the severity of *subsequent* attacks with eventual outcome, however. In other words, prognostication based upon the initial presentation of the patient is fraught with error, while prognosis may be related to subsequent presentations. As the attacks become more severe and the disease spreads to involve the entire colon, the prognosis becomes more guarded. While the likelihood of developing a recurrence during a given year is about 50% regardless of severity of disease, those patients with total colonic involvement have a much higher incidence of recurrences. Furthermore, in one series of patients with total colon involvement, there was a mortality rate of about 50% after 25 years of follow-up. In this group, about 50% of the patients died of unrelated causes; of the remaining deaths related to ulcerative colitis, many patients died in the immediate postoperative period and a few died from cancer.

A decidedly *unusual* presentation is one of an explosive onset with severe abdominal pain, toxemia, high fever, and a violent, frequent, foul, watery diarrhea that often contains pus and gross blood.

The initial diagnosis is usually established by proctosigmoidoscopic or colonoscopic examination. In early and mild cases, typical findings reveal swelling and hyperemia of the mucosa, an excess of mucus, and easy bleeding after swabbing. As the disease progresses, the mucosa becomes red, granular, ulcerated, and islands of hyperplastic mucosa may predominate. Oozing of blood is almost always noted as well as a covering of mucopurulent exudate.

Extracolonic manifestations include hepatic involvement, arthritis, uveitis, erythema nodosum, and pyoderma gangrenosum. The incidence of one or another of these associations has been reported to be as high as 20%; however, clinical experience suggests that these associated conditions are unusual.

Complications include severe hemorrhage, toxic megacolon with perforation, and carcinoma. Of these, considerable attention has been paid to the subsequent development of carcinoma which is said to be considerably more virulent than the usual carcinoma. It has been estimated that the chances of developing carcinoma in patients who have had ulcerative colitis for at least 10 years is 20% per decade thereafter. The overall incidence of cancer in this population is between 2–4%, which is about 6 times higher than in the general population. Further extrapolation of these figures would suggest that as many as 1 patient in 6 might be expected to develop carcinoma if a colectomy had not been performed for some other reason. These statistics must be viewed warily since, again, they are based primarily on only those patients seen in the hospital or similar settings. The incidence may be even lower as the population at risk is diminished in view of the recent tendency to perform earlier colectomies.

There has been recent interest in attempting to relate an increased incidence of developing carcinoma to the histologic findings of severe, consistent, epithelial dysplasia found in rectal biopsies. Such changes have been reported in about 20% of patients who have had ulcerative colitis for at least 10 years, and it has been postulated that these patients represent the high-risk group in which carcinoma will develop. This is an interesting concept, but one which requires further follow-up before a definite conclusion can be reached.

ROENTGEN EXAMINATION

Plain Abdominal Film

The x-ray examination of the patient with ulcerative colitis must include a preliminary film of the abdomen. In extremely ill patients, the signs of obstruction, toxic dilatation, or perforation must be ruled out before a barium enema is performed. Even if these ominous signs are not present, much information can be gained from the plain film about the probable location and severity of the disease (Fig. 9.1). For example, it is rare to find normal-appearing haustra outlined by gas in areas of marked colitis. Similarly, narrowed gas-filled segments of the colon frequently can be seen in areas which, when later filled with barium, will show advanced mucosal changes. It may also be possible to define the soft tissue outline of an apparently thickened descending colon or sigmoid, especially where these portions of the bowel are seen against the relatively homogeneous density of the left iliac bone.

The plain film x-ray signs of toxic dilatation, which may occur in either fulminating or chronic ulcerative colitis, are dilatation of the colon, large nodular protrusions of hyperplastic mucosa, and deep ulcers which may be seen outlined by intraluminal air (Figs. 9.2 and 9.3). Because of its anterior position when the patient is supine, the transverse colon usually shows the most striking air distention. These findings may confirm the clinical impression and obviate a barium enema (Fig. 9.4), which is contraindicated in toxic megacolon because of the danger of perforating the bowel.

Barium Enema

While a great deal has been written about the roentgen appearance of the colon in ulcerative colitis, very little has appeared pertaining to the role of this vital examination in the management of the patient or about the preparation and actual performance of the examination. In discussing this subject, one must differentiate between the examination performed on a new patient, one with an exacerbation of symptoms, or one having a routine follow-up study.

There are few, if any, indications for the performance of a barium enema on a patient who is having frequent, violent, bloody bowel movements. Usually, the diagnosis has been established previously by clinical and sigmoidoscopic findings. It is very uncomfortable for the patient to have an examination performed at this time, and the films will be frequently less than ideal, although there is no evidence that such an enema will cause an exacerbation of symptoms. A retrospective review of 507 patients with ulcerative colitis was conducted at the Massachusetts General Hospital. No deterioration in clinical condition could be documented in the 403 patients who had undergone at least one barium enema.

It is true that an occasional patient may experience an increase in bowel movements following a barium enema, but many more patients have exacerbation without having undergone a barium enema. There is plenty of time to do a proper barium enema after the patient's symptoms have subsided. These statements should not be interpreted as suggesting that the barium enema has no role in the management of the patient with acute ulcerative colitis. It is simply that the timing of the examination should be correct.

The purpose of the barium enema in a fresh case of ulcerative colitis is to confirm the diagnosis and to establish the severity and extent of disease. In a follow-up examination, any change in status is documented, and complications, such as carcinoma, are identified.

Assuming that a barium enema is to be perfomed, all patients *must* be prepared. This is a point which is often frequently misunderstood by both the clinician and

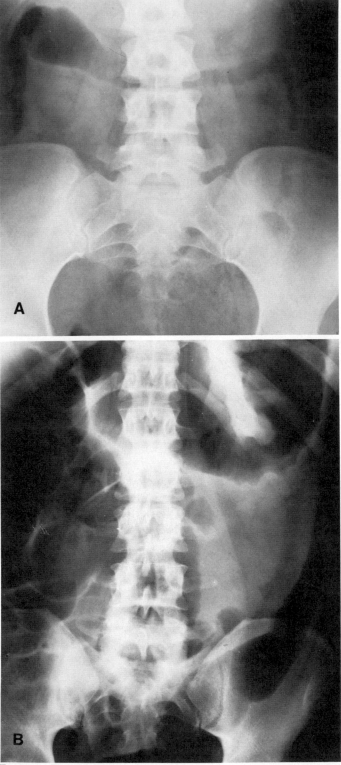

FIG. 9.1. PLAIN ABDOMINAL FILMS IN ULCERATIVE COLITIS
(**A**) The transverse and proximal descending colon are narrow and tubular in appearance. (**B**) The proximal splenic flexure is narrow and edematous and the descending colon is narrowed. (**C**) The walls of the distal descending colon are irregular and the lumen is narrowed. (**D**) The entire descending colon is shortened and markedly narrowed.

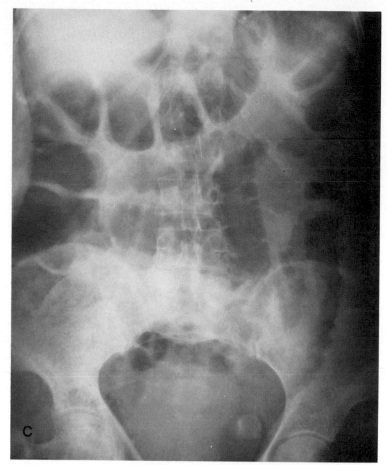

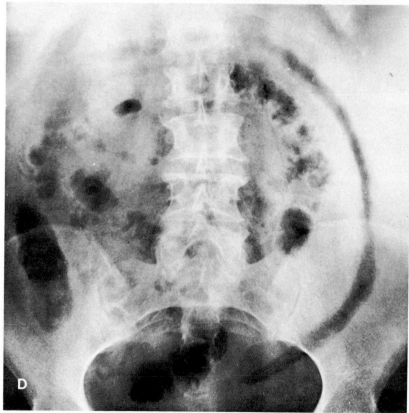

FIG. 9.1. (C) AND (D)

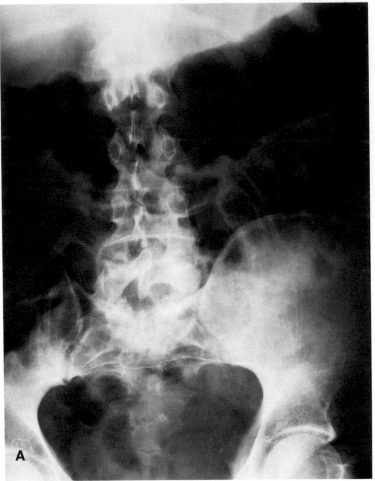

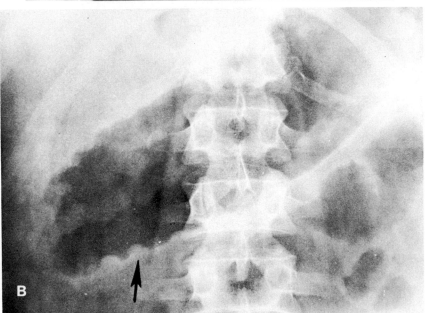

FIG. 9.2. TOXIC DILATATION IN ULCERATIVE COLITIS
(A) The transverse colon is markedly dilated. Its walls, particularly on the inferior surface, appear nodular. (B) Detail film (from another patient) well demonstrates the nodules of hyperplastic mucosa (arrow) indenting the dilated air column of the transverse colon.

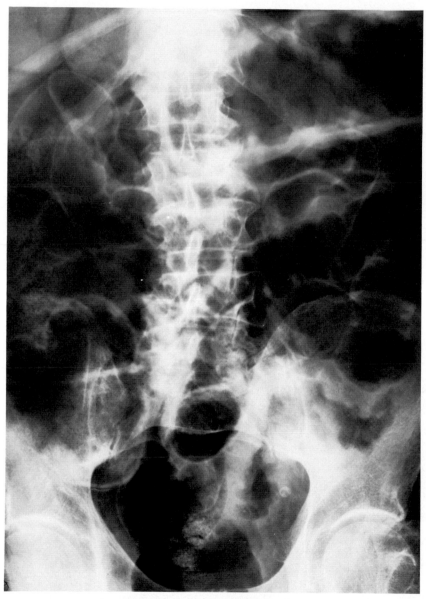

FIG. 9.3. TOXIC DILATATION WITH PERFORATION

Flat film of the abdomen demonstrating dilatation of the transverse colon and much of the remainder of the large bowel and the small bowel. The white line around many of the bowel loops represents the bowel wall outlined by intraluminal gas on one side and free peritoneal air on the other.

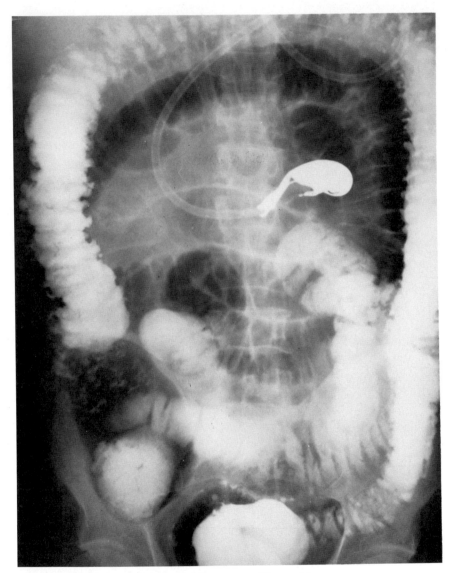

FIG. 9.4. BARIUM ENEMA IN TOXIC DILATATION

The barium outlines multiple deep ulcers in a dilated colon. A barium enema is definitely contraindicated in this type of case.

the radiologist. The problem is one of understanding the necessity of increasing the number of bowel movements in a patient whose prime complaint centers on too many movements. The very fact that the patient is having diarrhea means he must have a colon full of liquid stool. Furthermore, if the patient's clinical condition is such that he cannot tolerate proper preparation, he is too ill to undergo a barium enema examination. It is frequently impossible to distinguish watery stool from tiny ulcerations, and it is impossible to assess the integrity of the mucosa in the presence of stool. Since only patients who are having relatively few movements are candidates for a barium enema, either preparation suggested in Chapter 3 may be used. In selected cases, some minor modifications may be implemented, but the preparatory process should not be so diluted that it becomes a sham. This type of patient is also the ideal one to receive a 2000 cc tap-water enema; in fact, this may be the best way to wash liquid stool from the colon in most patients.

Two additional points should be made about the preparation and performance of the examination. The use of a rectal balloon in patients with ulcerative colitis is contraindicated; the risk of perforating an ulcerated segment of the rectum is too great. Tannic acid has also been said to be contraindicated in these patients because of the presence of ulcerated mucosa and the greater possibility of systemic absorption. This theoretical contraindication was not borne out in the study cited in Chapter 3, but the point is moot under the present FDA ban of tannic acid.

A current controversy exists over the type of barium enema which should be performed, i.e., a single-contrast barium enema or a primary double-contrast study; each group believes their technique to be superior. On the one hand, many of the single-contrast advocates have little experience with the primary double-contrast air examination, but experience with their own technique has been extensive. The proponents of the primary double-contrast enema feel that they have the ability to be far more accurate in the establishment of a diagnosis and assessment of the extent of the disease. However, they have been accused of a few intellectual sins and, perhaps, as in any relatively new technique, this is to be expected. For example, claims have been made that it is possible to be 100% accurate (obviously wrong, since no examination is 100% accurate—see Chapter 10 on Crohn's disease of the colon). The primary double-contrast group has also been guilty of comparing the accuracy of their examination performed after meticulous cleansing of the colon with results of older studies using the single-contrast barium technique, in which preparation was often minimal at best. It is likely that either technique will be acceptable and comparable if the colon has been properly cleansed. Preparation is the absolute prerequisite to a satisfactory colon examination of any type.

Single-Contrast Enema

The roentgen findings in the single-column technique will be described first. The earliest radiographic signs of ulcerative colitis are so little beyond the range of normal that they must be looked for carefully; they are real and can be seen on both the full and evacuation films. The colon may show no change in caliber or haustral markings, but in areas of involvement, the margin of the barium-filled colon may be "fuzzy," as if it were out of focus. In addition to this sign of edema, there may be tiny hairline spiculations that represent pinpoint ulcerations (Fig. 9.5). Since identical findings can be caused by fecal sludge (Figs. 9.6–9.8) or the innominate grooves (Figs 9.9 and 9.10) (see Chapter 2 on Anatomy), these minimal abnormal findings must be carefully looked for on fluoroscopic compression spot films and on good evacuation mucosal films. Additional evidence for ulcerative colitis is a slight coarsening of the mucosal folds, some of which tend to run in the axis of the bowel rather than having the more normal rosette or crenated appearance. The folds may

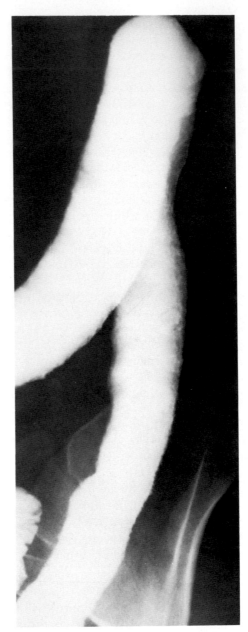

FIG. 9.5. EARLY ULCERATIVE COLITIS

The margins of the barium column appear hazy and indistinct. Careful inspection
reveals multiple tiny ulcerations. The haustral pattern has been lost in this case.

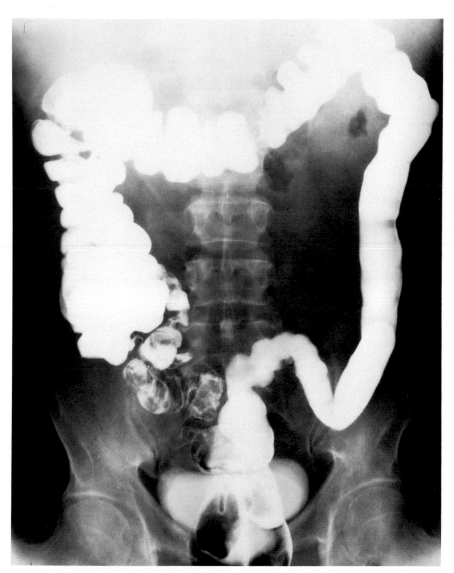

FIG. 9.6. FECAL SLUDGE MIMICKING ULCERATIVE COLITIS
The left colon appears ahaustral and its walls appear minimally indistinct. In this patient with symptoms suggestive of ulcerative colitis, colonoscopy revealed only liquid stool.

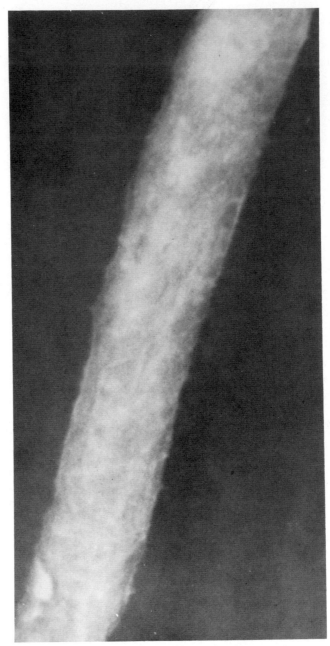

FIG. 9.7. FECES SIMULATING ULCERATIVE COLITIS
Detail film of the descending colon. The margin of the bowel appears spiculated
and the mucosa appears indistinct. Colonoscopy—normal.

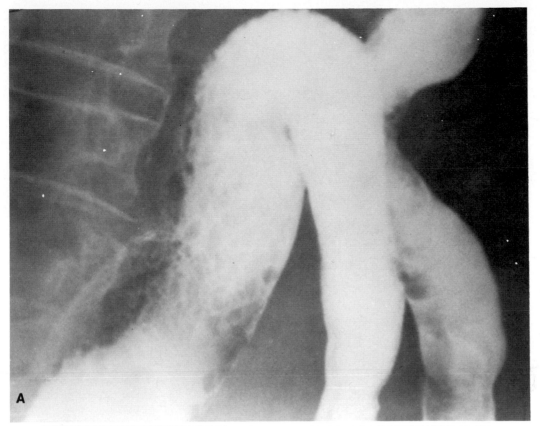

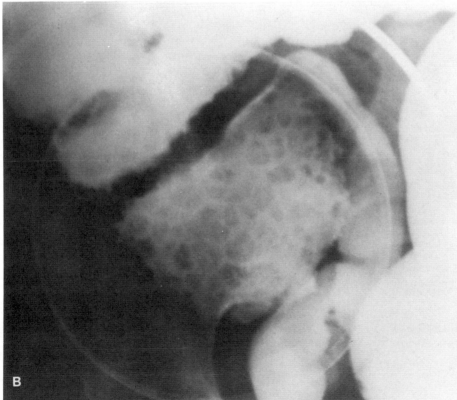

FIG. 9.8. FECAL MATERIAL SIMULATING ULCERATIVE COLITIS
Detail films of the transverse colon (**A**) and cecum (**B**). The large irregular nodules represent adherent feces.

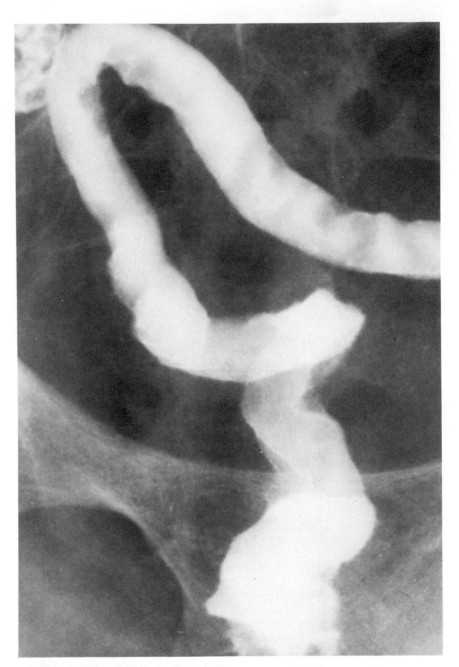

FIG. 9.9. INNOMINATE LINES SIMULATING ULCERATIVE COLITIS
Detail film of the sigmoid colon. The margins of the bowel appear smudged and
multiple spiculations are seen. Colonoscopy was entirely normal.

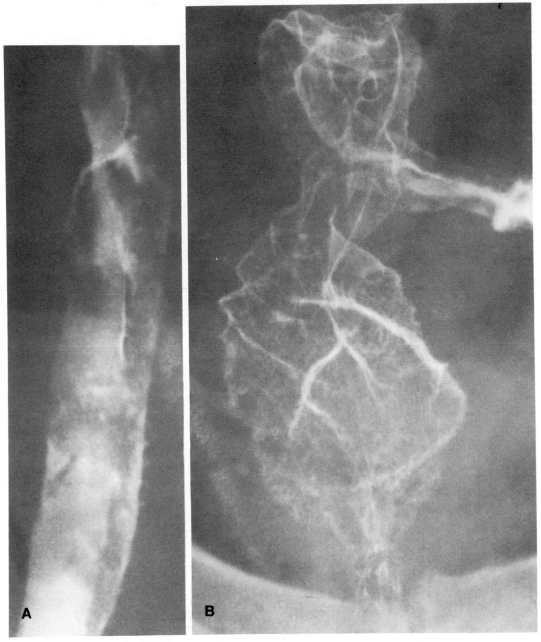

FIG. 9.10. INNOMINATE LINES SIMULATING ULCERATIVE COLITIS
(**A**) Detail film of the descending colon. Multiple spiculations are evident, particularly laterally. Colonoscopy—normal. (**B**) (Different patient.) Postevacuation detail film of the rectum. Multiple pinpoint collections of barium are evident when seen *en face* while the margins of the bowel wall show multiple spiculations. Colonoscopy—negative.

also appear smudged or slightly indistinct (Fig. 9.11). These areas of minimal change may be seen along the entire length of the colon, but they are usually present first in the left colon. Where possible to define it, the bowel wall may appear slightly thicker than normal in areas that also show mucosal involvement.

Ulcerative colitis usually begins in the rectum and early cases may involve only the rectum, sigmoid, or descending colon. It should be noted, however, that in about 15% of cases, the rectum is spared. The disease frequently spreads to involve the whole colon. This spread is usually gradual, but it may occur very rapidly (Fig. 9.12). In general, ulcerative colitis is a disease of the left or entire colon (Fig. 9.13). Isolated involvement of the right colon or short involved segments with normal intervening bowel does not occur.

With progression of the disease, the haustral markings decrease in number and depth and ulcerations can be defined along the edge of the bowel. The ulcers vary greatly in size and shape (Figs. 9.14 and 9.15), and they cannot be easily categorized. As previously stated, the early ulcers appear as tiny projections, so-called spiculations. At the opposite end of the spectrum are the "collar button" ulcers (Fig. 9.16) which are formed as the ulcers burrow through the bowel wall to terminate at the submucosal-muscularis junction; on occasion, these ulcers may become confluent (Fig. 9.17). Although ulcerative colitis is considered a "mucosal" disease, the ulcers penetrate into the submucosa in almost 50% of cases, and "collar button" ulcers reach all the way to the muscular layer. In spite of this penetration, the bowel wall remains relatively thin and fistula formation is very uncommon. Although the ulcers can assume a wide range of sizes and shapes, they are usually monotonous in appearance and are *symmetrically* distributed around the circumference of the bowel wall. Furthermore, the intervening mucosa is abnormal in that there are thickened mucosal folds or pseudopolyps.

Pseudopolyps are islands of hyperplastic, inflamed mucosa that remain between ulcers (Fig. 9.18). They will vary in size, shape, and pattern reflecting the degree and variability of the ulceration and inflammatory response in the bowel. At times, the pseudopolyps may appear as smaller, regular nodules resembling a "cobblestone" road (Figs. 9.19 and 9.20). Although this term has been used more often as an identifying feature of the longitudinal ulceration with cross-fissuring sometimes seen in Crohn's colitis, it should be appreciated that "cobblestones" can also be seen in ulcerative colitis where they are usually more uniform in size and appearance than in Crohn's colitis. Recent terms such as "filariform polyposis," "mucosal bridging," etc. only denote several other appearances of the remaining mucosa. On rare occasions, these islands of mucosa can undergo such extreme hyperplasia that they may appear as large masses which cannot be distinguished from polypoid tumors (Figs. 9.21–9.23).

With still further progression, the colon may appear markedly narrowed and foreshortened and take on a tubular appearance (Fig. 9.24). The haustral pattern is absent and all signs of mucosal detail may be lost or there may only be a few thickened mucosal ridges running in the long axis of the colon. While this appearance may be secondary to fibrosis, it may equally well be secondary to muscular spasm. Accordingly, one may see a narrow, short colon return to a colon of almost normal caliber and length on a follow-up study (Fig. 9.25). This return of the colon to a near-normal appearance is not a well-appreciated condition.

When colitis involves the ascending colon and cecum, the terminal ileum may be involved and show changes ranging from shaggy mucosa to narrowing and rigidity of the lumen. The changes of this "backwash ileitis" may be identical to those seen in regional ileitis; however, only the last few centimeters of terminal ileum are involved as contrasted to the greater length of involvement in regional enteritis (Fig. 9.26).

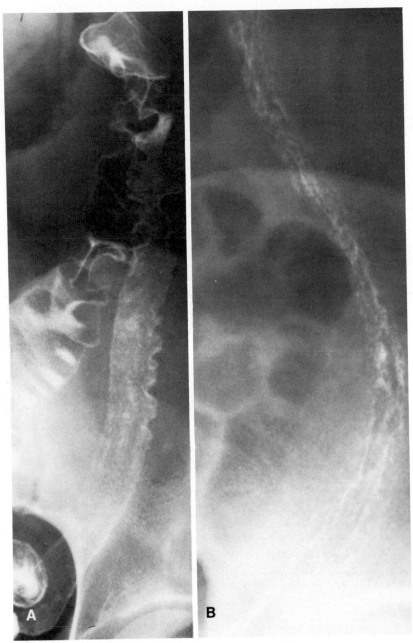

Fig. 9.11. Early Ulcerative Colitis

Detail postevacuation films of two different patients. In (**A**), all mucosal detail is lost and multiple pinhead collections of barium are present. In (**B**), the mucosal folds appear smudged and edematous.

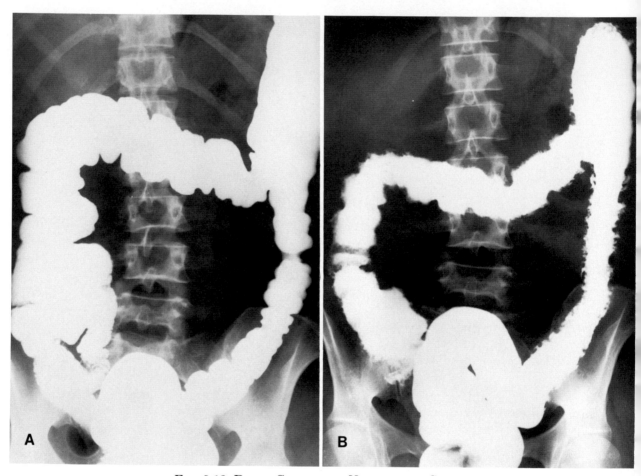

FIG. 9.12. RAPID SPREAD OF ULCERATIVE COLITIS
The initial examination (**A**) was interpreted as normal. Three weeks later (**B**), the entire colon is involved by a diffuse, deeply ulcerating process.

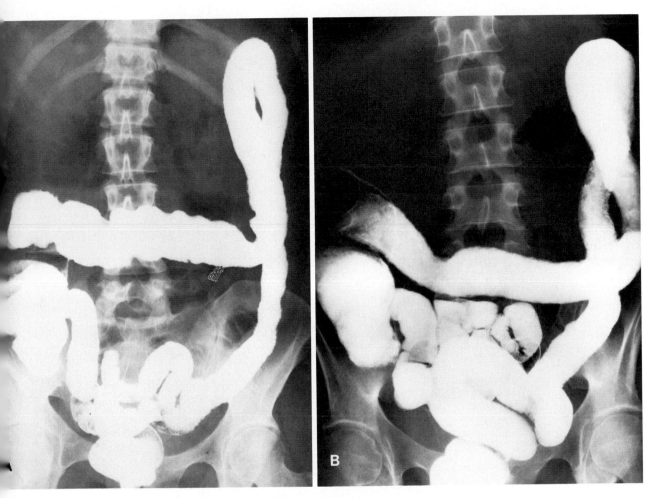

FIG. 9.13. ULCERATIVE COLITIS INVOLVING THE ENTIRE COLON
Two different patients (**A** and **B**) showing total colon involvement.

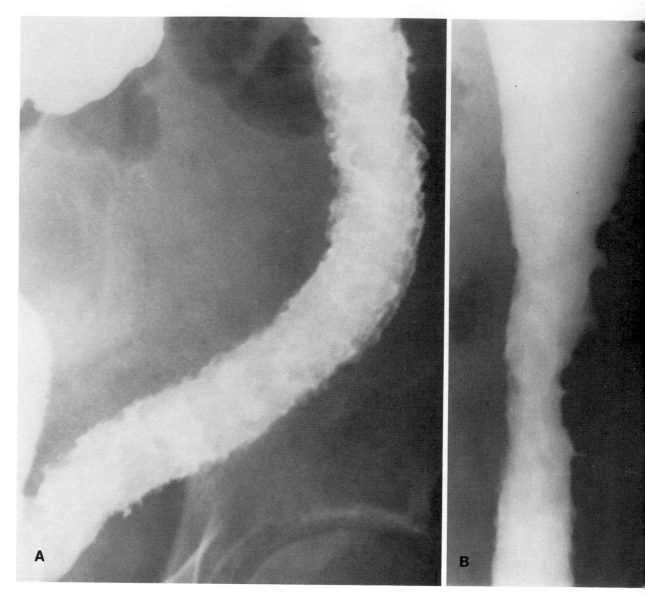

**FIG. 9.14. VARYING APPEARANCES OF ULCERS IN MODERATE ULCERATIVE
COLITIS**
In (**A**), the ulcers are uniform in size and symmetrically distributed around the
circumference of the bowel wall of the sigmoid colon. In (**B**), the ulcers appear
nonuniform, relatively deep, and involve the lateral aspect of the wall of the
descending colon to a greater extent than the medial wall.

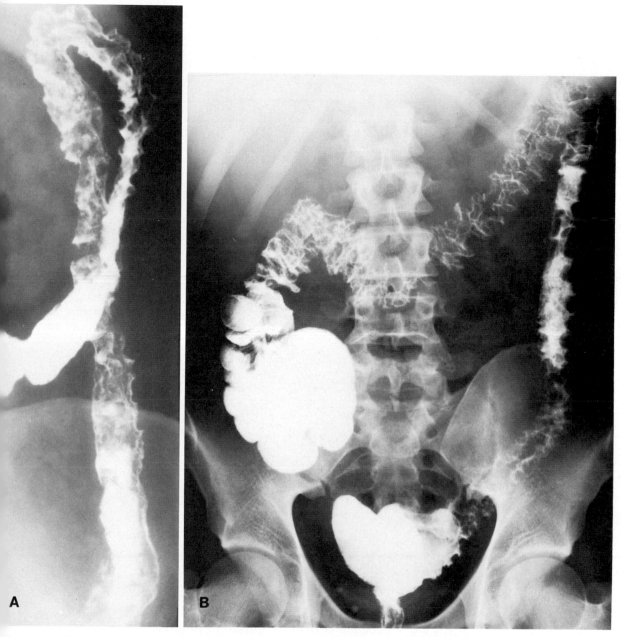

Fig. 9.15. Varying Appearance of Ulcers in Moderate Ulcerative Colitis
Postevacuation films from two different patients (**A** and **B**) demonstrating ulceration and mucosal edema.

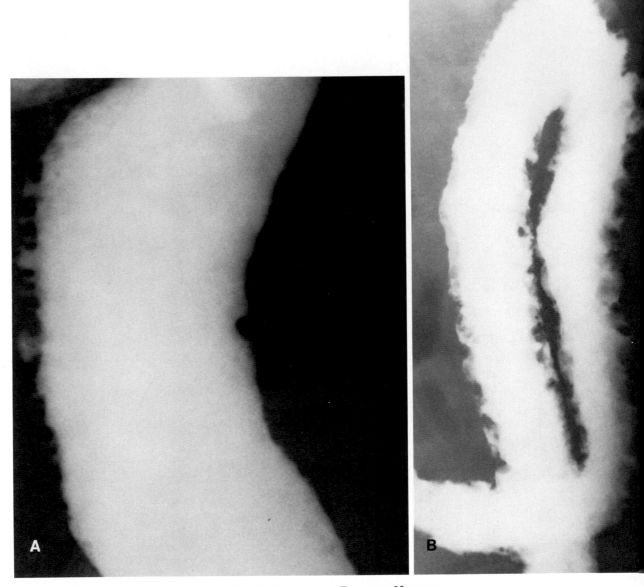

FIG. 9.16. COLLAR BUTTON ULCERS
Detail films of the descending colon (**A**) and splenic flexure (**B**) demonstrating
deep penetration of multiple ulcers, into the bowel wall.

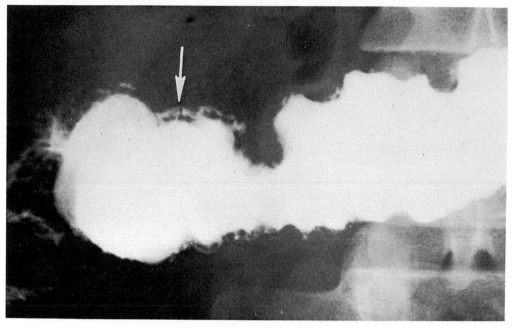

FIG. 9.17. CONFLUENT ULCERS

Numerous deep ulcers are present in the transverse colon, some of which have become confluent (arrow).

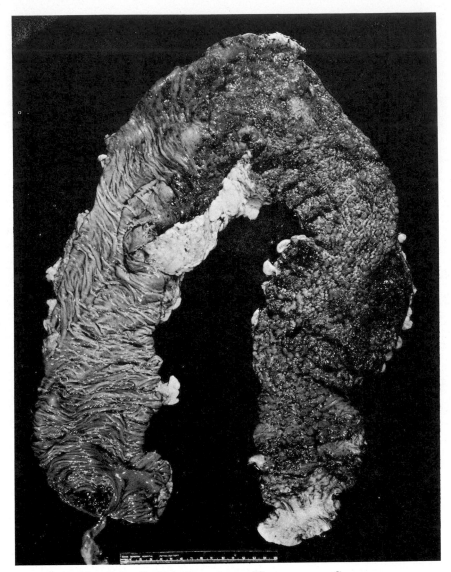

FIG. 9.18. PSEUDOPOLYPS IN ULCERATIVE COLITIS

The cecum is at the lower left and the rectum at the lower right of this resected colon. The ascending and proximal transverse segments appear normal, but the remainder of the bowel is involved by ulcerative colitis with innumerable islands of hyperplastic mucosa (pseudopolyps) studding the luminal surface.

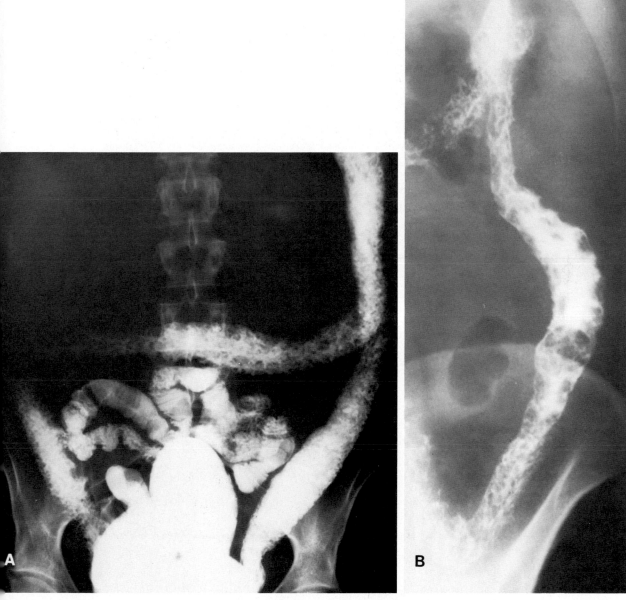

FIG. 9.19. PSEUDOPOLYPS

In (**A**), the mucosal nodules are much more regular, resembling cobblestones, than in (**B**). (Two different patients.)

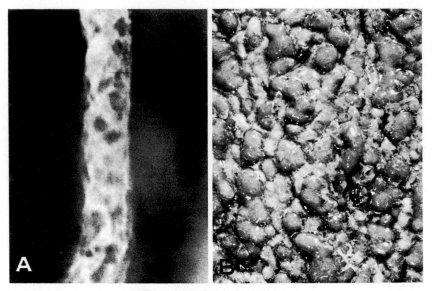

FIG. 9.20. PSEUDOPOLYPS

(**A**) Islands of hyperplastic mucosa are outlined by a criss-crossing pattern of barium-filled mucosal ulcerations. (**B**) Detail of resected colon showing a blanket of pseudopolyps outlined by a thick exudate. A similar "cobblestone" pattern may be seen in Crohn's colitis (see Fig. 10.9).

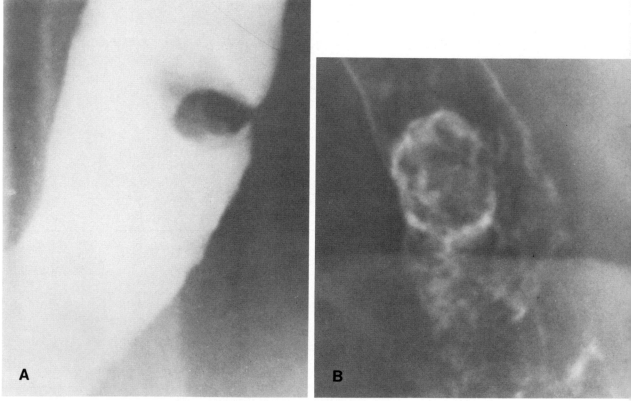

FIG. 9.21. PSEUDOPOLYPS IN ULCERATIVE COLITIS

Detail films with barium (**A**) and following evacuation (**B**) revealing a 2-cm polypoid mass which was proven to be an isolated pseudopolyp. The exact histology of a mass of this type can only be determined by biopsy.

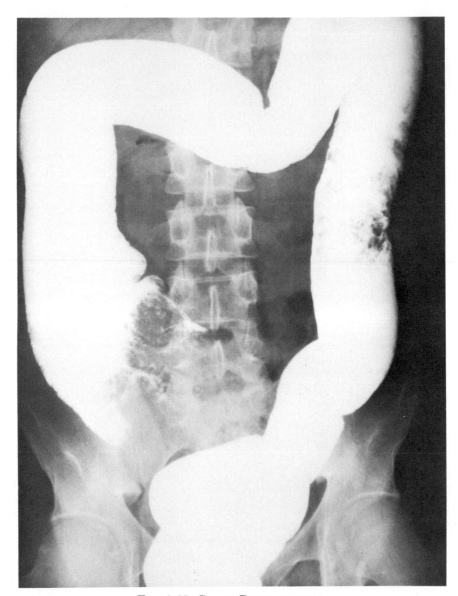

FIG. 9.22. GIANT PSEUDOPOLYPS

The mottled area of increased density in the proximal descending colon was thought to represent feces, while the obstructing lesion at the cecum was thought to be a fungating carcinoma. Both lesions were proven to be massive benign hyperplasia of the mucosa—pseudopolyps.

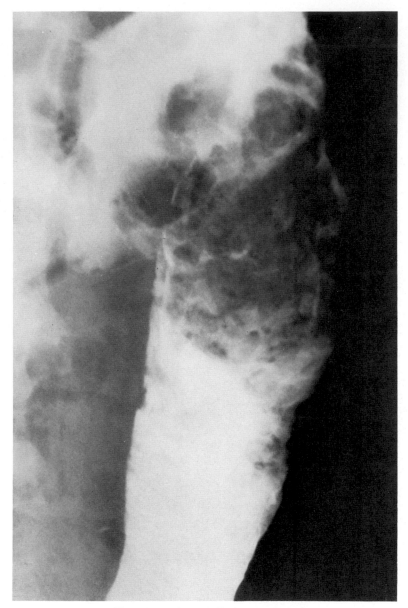

FIG. 9.23. GIANT PSEUDOPOLYP

Detail film of the upper descending colon demonstrating a large fungating mass subsequently shown to be a benign pseudopolyp.

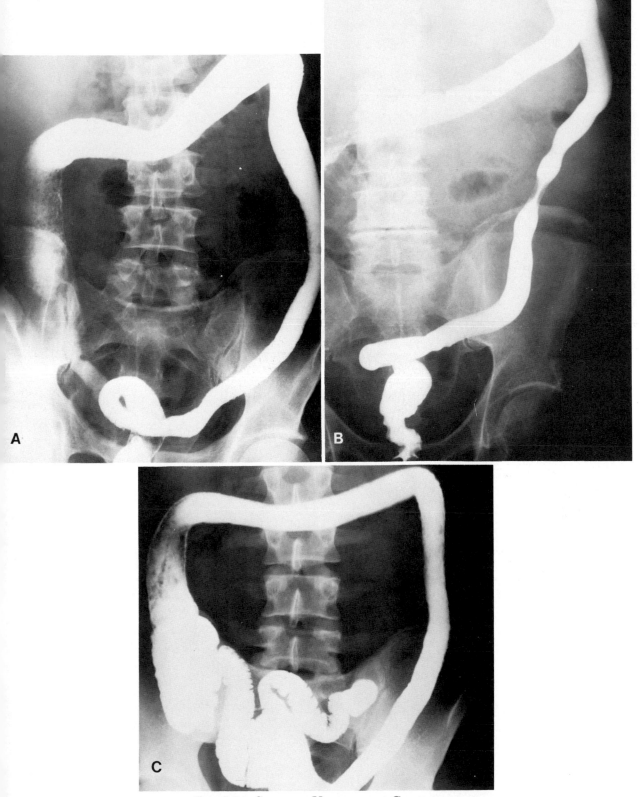

FIG. 9.24. CHRONIC ULCERATIVE COLITIS
The barium-filled colons in three different patients (**A**, **B**, and **C**) appear narrow,
tubular, foreshortened, and ahaustral.

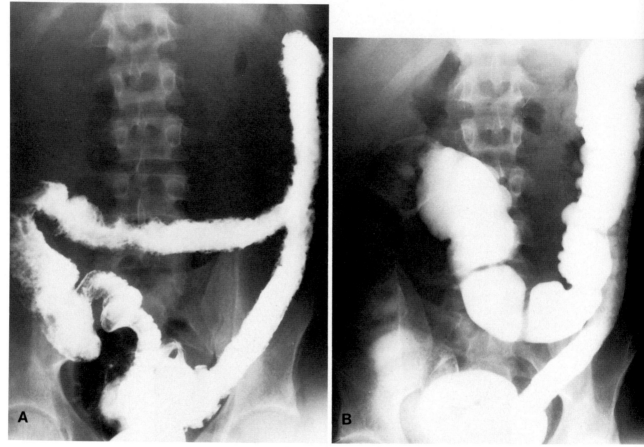

FIG. 9.25. MARKED REGRESSION IN ULCERATIVE COLITIS
The examination in (**A**) was performed 9 months before (**B**). The ulcerations have regressed dramatically, the transverse colon appears much longer and more redundant than previously, and its diameter has doubled.

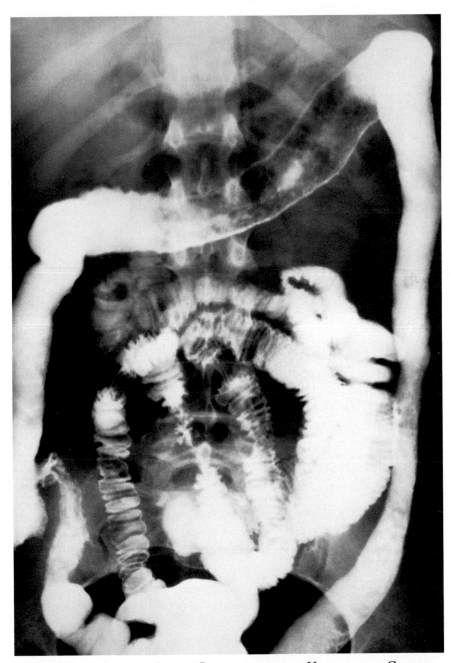

FIG. 9.26. TERMINAL ILEUM INVOLVEMENT IN ULCERATIVE COLITIS
Changes are evident in the entire colon and the last few centimeters of terminal ileum.

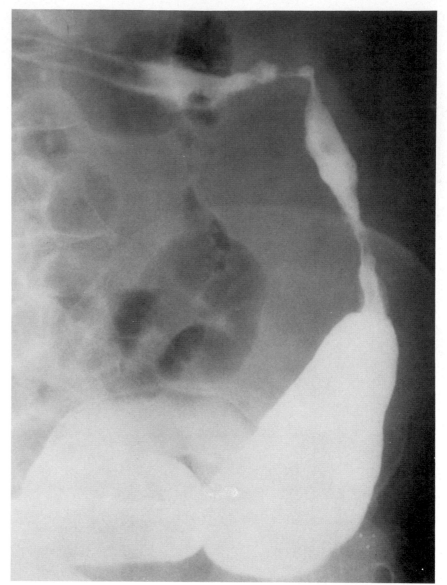

FIG. 9.27. BENIGN STRICTURE IN ULCERATIVE COLITIS
A long area of narrowing involves the entire proximal descending colon.

Benign areas of narrowing may occur in chronic ulcerative colitis, but they are very rare. These benign strictures tend to be concentric and smoothly tapered. They may be secondary to actual fibrosis (Fig. 9.27), or they may simply represent an area of localized spasm and may, therefore, not be constant on the same or a subsequent examination (Figs. 9.28–9.30).

If an area of narrowing is seen, the possibility of a "linitis plastica" type of carcinoma must be considered. Sometimes this type of carcinoma may have abrupt margins (Fig. 9.31), but more often such a carcinoma may mimic identically a benign stricture and may only be excluded by colonoscopy or surgery. A somewhat less common form of carcinoma may also occur—a polypoid, fungating lesion. The appearance is similar to a polypoid carcinoma seen in otherwise normal colons.

In summary, the appearance of ulcerative colitis may vary from minimal, tiny ulceration of some of the left colon to universal involvement of the entire large

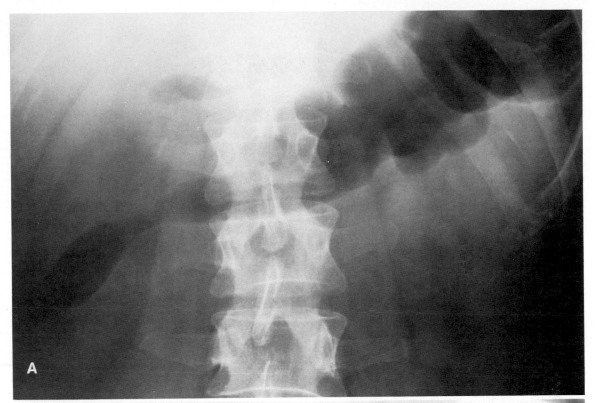

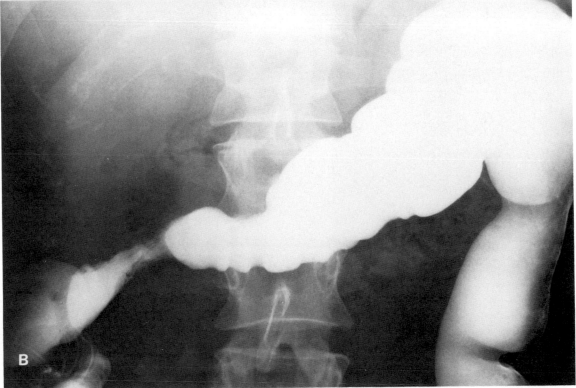

FIG. 9.28. SPASM MASQUERADING AS A STRICTURE

The plain film (**A**) and barium enema (**B**) reveal an identical area of narrowing in the proximal transverse colon. A colectomy was performed on the following day. It was not possible to identify an area of narrowing by examination of the gross specimen. Microscopic sections through the area of interest showed similar histology to the remainder of the colon in this patient with chronic ulcerative colitis.

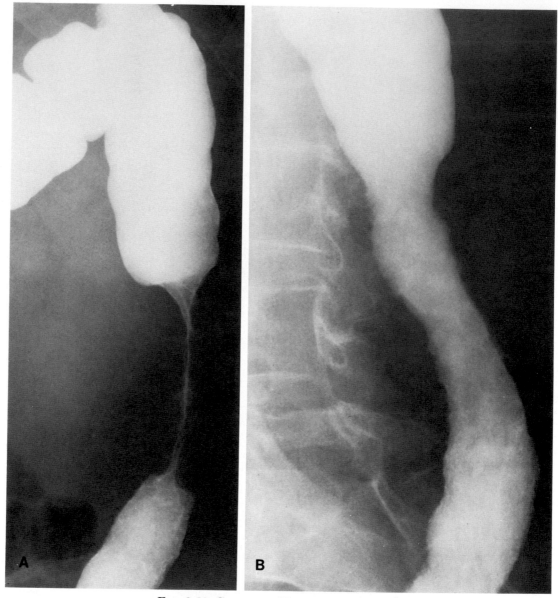

FIG. 9.29. SPASM IN ULCERATIVE COLITIS
The detail film of the proximal descending colon in (A) was obtained approximately 5 min before the film in (B).

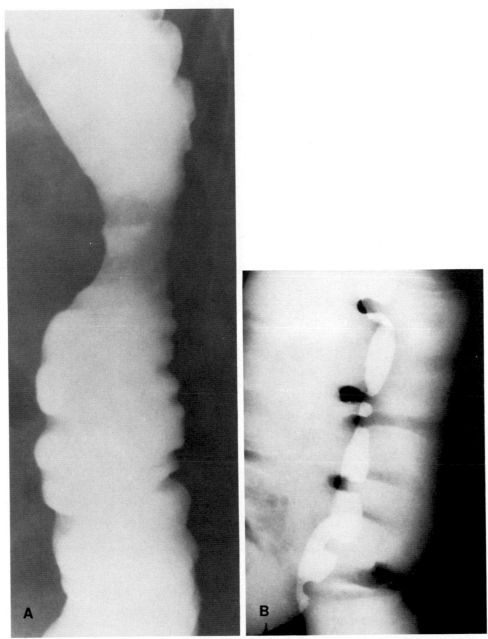

FIG. 9.30. SPASM IN ULCERATIVE COLITIS

One representative film (**A**) from a barium enema shows a constant well-defined area of narrowing. A repeat examination on the following day (**B**) revealed a descending colon of normal caliber.

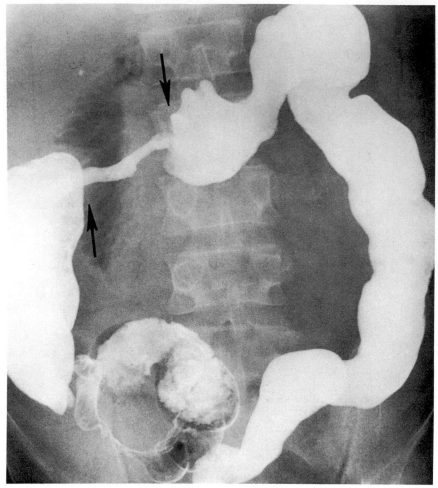

FIG. 9.31. CARCINOMA IN ULCERATIVE COLITIS
The sharp, proximal margins (arrows) of the area of narrowing differentiate this cancer from the smooth tapering of a benign stricture.

intestine. Regardless of the stage of the disease, the hallmarks are uniformity, continuity, and symmetry. These changes are frequently best seen on the postevacuation film and the importance of this film cannot be overemphasized.

Primary Double-Contrast Enema

The appearance of the colon on primary double-contrast enemas varies considerably from that seen on the standard single-contrast barium examination. The earliest finding is a fine granular appearance of the mucosa which reflects the edema present (Fig. 9.32). Granularity precedes ulceration, and the proponents of this technique claim that such a change cannot be appreciated on the standard barium examination. Although the change can be mimicked by adherent fecal material (Fig. 9.33), one school of examiners believes that it is not necessary to prepare the colon before a primary air-contrast study; most adherents of primary air enemas, however, go out of their way to cleanse the colon thoroughly.

Superficial ulcers are seen in the next stage of the disease. The barium adheres to the pit of each ulcer, giving an overall "stippled" appearance to the mucosa. It must be emphasized that normal mucosa is not present between the tiny ulcers and that the "stippling" pattern is uniform and diffuse throughout the length of the involved colon (Fig. 9.34).

The larger ulcers in the next stage of the disease are readily identifiable as large, uniform collections of barium on a background mucosal pattern which appears coarsely granular (Fig. 9.35). These changes may be best appreciated by viewing the ulcers *en face* within the circumference of the lumen rather than by seeing them tangentially along the margins of the bowel. At times, the ulcers can be quite deep (Fig. 9.36). Pseudopolyps (Fig. 9.37) and carcinoma (Fig. 9.38) are also well demonstrated while the shortening of the bowel and loss of haustral pattern are less well-appreciated because of the overdistention inherent in the insufflation of an adequate amount of air. The terminal ileum is also less well-demonstrated by this technique.

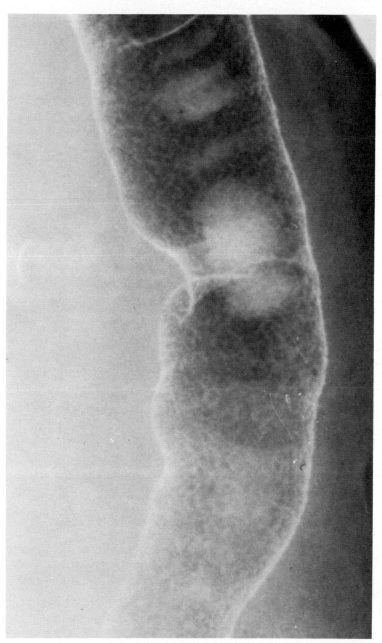

FIG. 9.32. EARLY CHANGES OF ULCERATIVE COLITIS—PRIMARY DOUBLE-CONTRAST ENEMA

Detail film of the descending colon revealing a uniform "granular" appearance of the mucosa. (Reprinted with permission from CRC Critical Reviews in Diagnostic Imaging, *9:* 421, Copyright © 1977, The Chemical Rubber Co., CRC Press, Inc.)

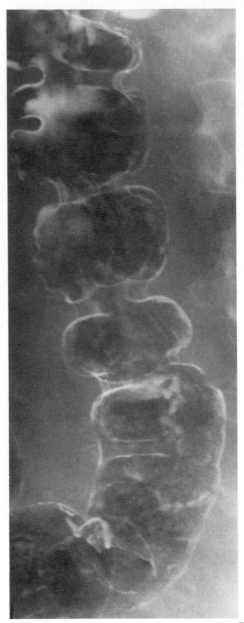

FIG. 9.33. FECES SIMULATING ULCERATIVE COLITIS ON A PRIMARY DOUBLE-
CONTRAST EXAMINATION

The irregularity of the mucosa secondary to fecal debris simulates the true
"granularity" of ulcerative colitis.

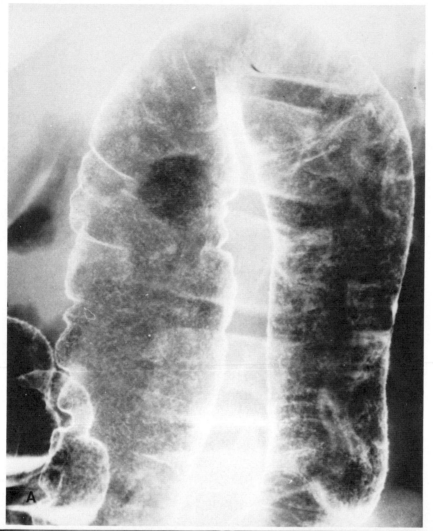

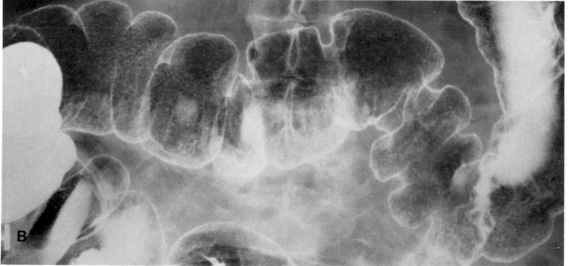

FIG. 9.34. EARLY ULCERATION IN ULCERATIVE COLITIS—PRIMARY DOUBLE-
CONTRAST TECHNIQUE

Detail films of the splenic flexure (**A**) and transverse colon (**B**) reveal the universal
distribution of pinpoint collections of barium (stippling) which is characteristic of
superficial ulceration. [(**A**) Courtesy of I. Laufer, Philadelphia, Pa.; (**B**) Courtesy of
Ervin Philipps, Boston, Mass.]

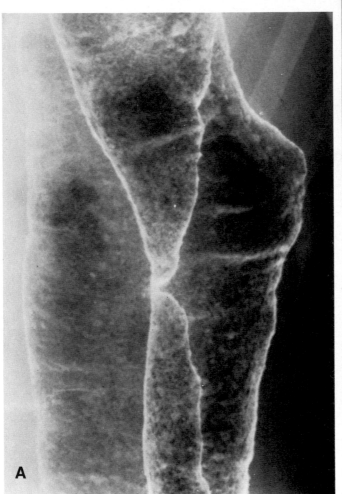
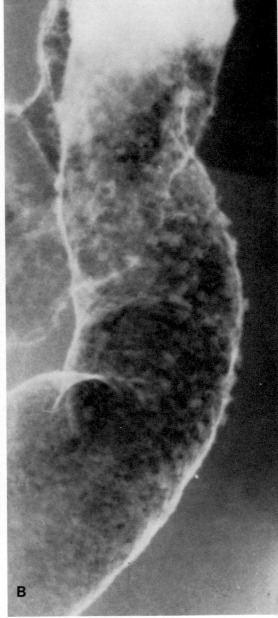

FIG. 9.35. ADVANCED ULCERATIVE COLITIS—PRIMARY DOUBLE-CONTRAST
EXAMINATION
The large ulcers can easily be identified *en face* (**A**) as a myriad of discrete
collections of barium. The background mucosa has a diffuse granular appearance.
The profiles of some of the ulcers can be seen along the lateral wall of the colon (**B**).
(Reproduced by permission from Laufer, I.: *Double Contrast Gastrointestinal
Radiology.* W. B. Saunders, Philadelphia, 1979.)

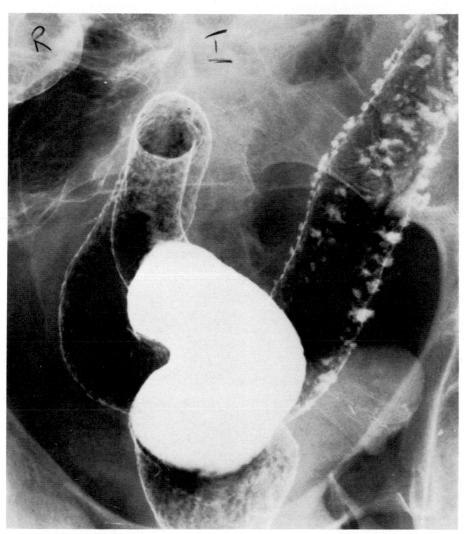

FIG. 9.36. DEEP ULCERS IN ULCERATIVE COLITIS—PRIMARY AIR ENEMA
Detail film of the sigmoid colon revealing multiple deep penetrating ulcers.
(Reproduced by permission from Journal of Canadian Association of Radiologists
26: 116, 1975.)

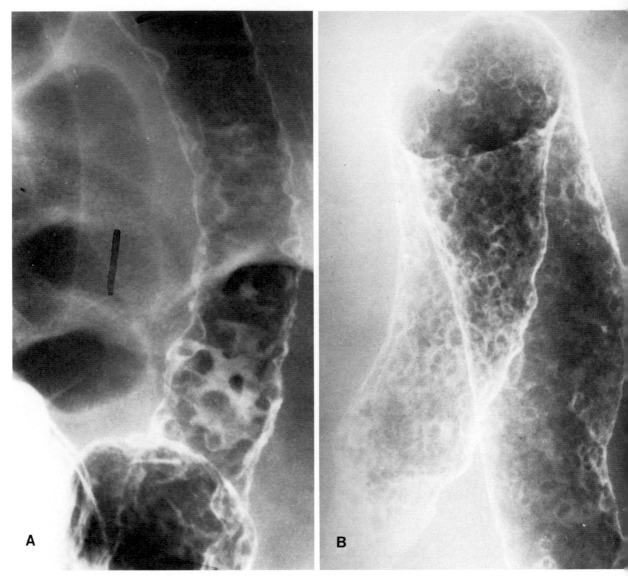

Fig. 9.37. Pseudopolyps in Ulcerative Colitis—Primary Air Enema
In (**A**), the pseudopolyps are larger and more irregular than in (**B**). [(**A**) Courtesy of I. Laufer, Philadelphia, Pa.; (**B**) Reprinted with permission from CRC Critical Reviews in Diagnosic Imaging, *9:* 421, © 1977 The Chemical Rubber Co., CRC Press, Inc.]

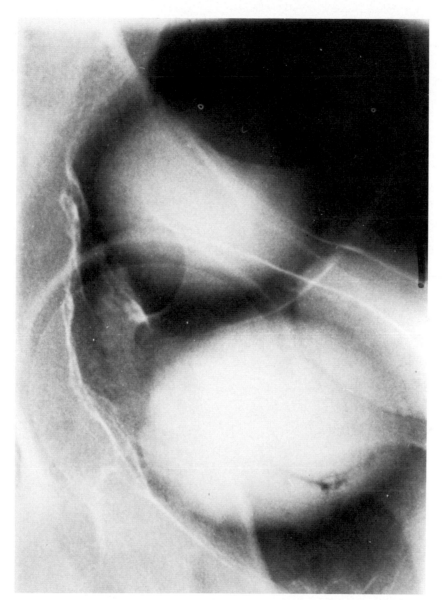

FIG. 9.38. CARCINOMA IN ULCERATIVE COLITIS—PRIMARY AIR ENEMA
Lateral detail film of the rectum demonstrating a long plaque-like carcinoma of
the posterior rectal wall. (Reproduced by permission from Laufer, I.: *Double Contrast Gastrointestinal Radiology.* W. B. Saunders, Philadelphia, 1979.)

BIBLIOGRAPHY

Devroede, G. J., Taylor, W. F., Sauer, W. G., *et al.*: Cancer risk and life expectancy of children with ulcerative colitis. N. Engl. J. Med., *285:* 17, 1971.

Dobbins, W. O.: Current status of the precancer lesion in ulcerative colitis. Gastroenterology, *73:* 1431, 1977.

Glotzer, D. J., Gardner, R. C., Goldman, H., *et al.*: Comparative features and course of ulcerative and granulomatous colitis. N. Engl. J. Med., *282:* 582, 1970.

Gloulston, S. J., and McGovern, V. J.: The nature of the benign strictures in ulcerative colitis. N. Engl. J. Med., *281:* 290, 1969.

James, E. M., and Carlson, H.: Chronic ulcerative colitis and colon cancer: Can radiographic appearance predict survival patterns? Am. J. Roentgenol., *130:* 825, 1978.

Janower, M. L., Robbins, L. L., and Wenlund, D. E.: A review of the use of tannic acid in patients with ulcerative colitis. Radiology, *89:* 42, 1967.

Joffee, N.: Localized giant pseudopolyposis secondary to ulcerative or granulomatous colitis. Clin. Radiol., *28:* 609, 1977.

Kalil, T. H., and Robbins, L. L.: Early roentgenologic changes in idiopathic ulcerative colitis. Radiology, *53:* 1, 1949.

Kelvin, F. M., Oddson, T. A., Rice, R. P., *et al.*: Double contrast barium enema in Crohn's disease and ulcerative colitis. Am. J. Roentgenol., *131:* 207, 1978.

Laufer, I.: *Double Contrast Gastrointestinal Radiology with Endoscopic Correlation.* W. B. Saunders, Philadelphia, 1979.

Laufer, I., Mullens, J. E., and Hamilton, J.: Correlation of endoscopy and double-contrast radiography in the early stages of ulcerative and granulomatous colitis. Radiology, *118:* 1, 1976.

Lennard Jones, J. E., Morson, B. C., Ritchie, J. K., *et al.*: Cancer in colitis: Assessment of the individual risk by clinical and histological criteria. Gastroenterology, *73:* 1280, 1977.

McConnell, F., Hanelin, J., and Robbins, L. L.: Plain film diagnosis of fulminating ulcerative colitis. Radiology, *71:* 674, 1958.

Matsuura, K., Nakata, H., Tahedo, N., *et al.*: Innominate lines of the colon. Radiology, *123:* 581, 1977.

Watts, J. M., deDombal, F. T., Watkinson, G., *et al.*: Long-term prognosis of ulcerative colitis. Br. Med. J., *1:* 1447, 1966.

Welch, C. E., and Hedberg, S. E.: Colonic cancer in ulcerative colitis and idiopathic colonic cancer. J.A.M.A., *191:* 815, 1965.

10

Crohn's Colitis

MURRAY L. JANOWER, M.D.

BACKGROUND

Crohn's disease of the colon is an inflammatory disease with radiographic and histologic features identical to those first described in 1932 in patients with regional enteritis. This entity has been called by many names including granulomatous colitis; since granulomas are found in only about one-half of the cases, and since granulomas may be found in other inflammatory bowel diseases, Crohn's disease is considered to be a more specific name. Most observers believe that Crohn's disease is an entity separable from idiopathic ulcerative colitis because of differences in appearance and behavior; it should be emphasized that the previous statement is unproven and may be incorrect.

CLINICAL FEATURES

Crohn's disease of the colon is a disease of young adult life, with no sex predilection and of unknown etiology. Usually both the small bowel and colon are involved, but in up to 25% of patients, only the colon may show changes. The symptoms include fever, abdominal pain, diarrhea, and malaise. Gross rectal bleeding is very uncommon in contrast to ulcerative colitis.

When the colon alone is involved, the patients may do well following subtotal colectomy in contrast to patients with ulcerative colitis where total colectomy is curative. If both the small and large bowel are involved, there is a high rate of recurrence at the anastomotic site. It should be noted that Crohn's disease of the colon may worsen locally under medical management, but rarely is there axial spread of the disease. Spread along the longitudinal axis is most likely to occur following surgical intervention.

The pathology of Crohn's disease of the colon has been described in Chapter 8 and should be reviewed at this time.

ROENTGEN EXAMINATION

Single-Contrast Barium Enema

A preliminary plain film of the abdomen should always be obtained before a barium examination. The indications and contraindications for a barium enema are similar to those given for ulcerative colitis. The plain film roentgen findings, including the presence of toxic megacolon, are also similar.

The earliest radiographic changes of Crohn's disease of the colon are slight luminal narrowing, nodular indentations of the bowel wall, and small ulcers (Figs. 10.1 and 10.2). The nodularity, often detected first along the inferior surface of the transverse colon, is due to submucosal inflammation and mucosal edema. These scattered irregular areas of nodularity (Fig. 10.3) may progress rapidly to stricture formation, one of the hallmarks of Crohn's disease of the colon.

As the disease progresses, the ulcers become deeper and more irregular and there is great variation in their size, shape, and overall appearance (Fig. 10.4). In contrast to ulcerative colitis, the distribution of the ulcers around the circumference of the bowel and along its length is not uniform and monotonous, and there is frequently more nodularity between them (Fig. 10.5). Sometimes, the edema and ulceration is so severe that all detail is lost (Fig. 10.6).

As in ulcerative colitis, the remaining mucosa between the ulcers is inflamed and edematous. These nodules of hyperplastic mucosa are similar to the "pseudopolyps" of ulcerative colitis, but are frequently more irregular (Figs. 10.7 and 10.8). Occasionally, the ulcers coalesce to form long tracks parallel to the longitudinal axis of the bowel; perpendicular transverse ulcers may also develop. The appearance of the longitudinal and transverse ulcers with edematous tags of remaining mucosa between them has been likened to a "cobblestone road" (Figs. 10.9 and 10.10). As stated previously, too much emphasis has been placed on "cobblestoning"; it can be seen in both ulcerative and Crohn's colitis.

A related feature is the presence of skip lesions or areas of involvement interspersed between areas of normal-appearing colon (Fig. 10.11); this *segmental* involvement is never seen in ulcerative colitis. Classically, Crohn's disease of the colon has been said to be a disease of the terminal ileum, right colon, *i.e.*, the cecum, ascending and transverse colon segments (Fig. 10.12). However, the entire colon may be involved or there may be simply one or many segments involved (Fig. 10.13). The rectum is involved in about 25% of the cases.

The ulcers penetrate deep into the layers of the bowel wall, and transmural involvement is the rule. Perforations are not infrequent and when they occur in the sigmoid colon, the appearance is not unlike diverticulitis (Figs. 10.14 and 10.15). Very rarely, the ulcers may coalesce in the subserosa causing longitudinal tracks; it should be emphasized that the visualization of the long intramural tracks in the sigmoid colon, with the remainder of the colon being normal, *is* almost always diverticulitis.

The deep penetration of the ulcers into the bowel wall is frequently associated with an inflammatory reaction that may progress to fibrotic stricture formation (Figs. 10.16 and 10.17). Sinus tracks and fistulas are also not uncommon (Figs. 10.18–10.20). There is an increased incidence of carcinoma in Crohn's disease of the colon, but it is considerably less than in ulcerative colitis. The cancers are usually fungating rather than "linitis plastica" in type.

Primary Double-Contrast Enema

The earliest findings are those of isolated tiny discrete ulcers on a background of normal mucosa (Fig. 10.21). The ulcers appear as punctate collections of barium

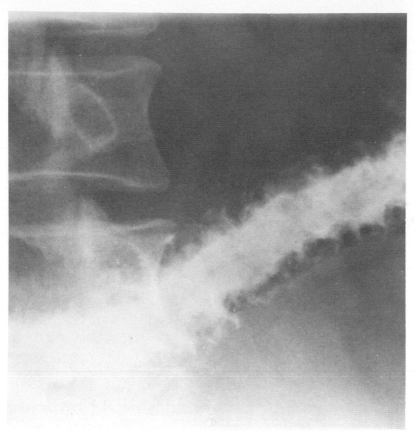

FIG. 10.1. EARLY CROHN'S COLITIS

Detail film of the transverse colon demonstrating nodularity along the margins of the bowel wall with irregular ulcerations.

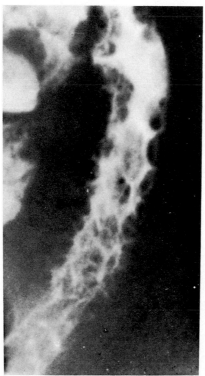

FIG. 10.2. CROHN'S COLITIS

A segment of descending colon showing slight narrowing, nodular indentation of the wall, and numerous transverse ulcers.

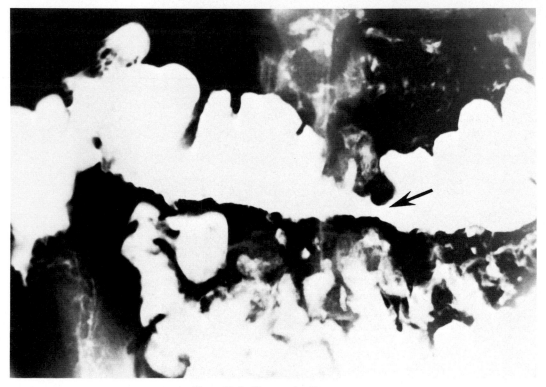

FIG. 10.3. CROHN'S COLITIS

The transverse colon shows extensive ulceration along the inferior margin. An area of nodularity is progressing to stricture formation (arrow).

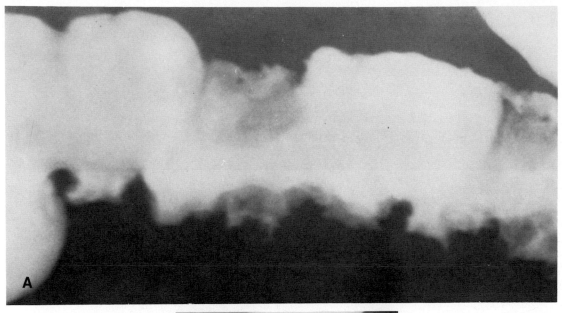

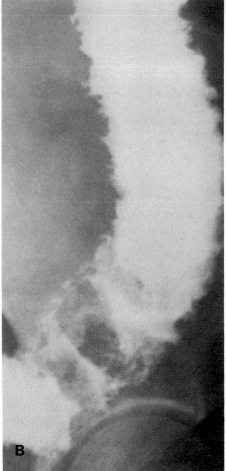

FIG. 10.4. CROHN'S COLITIS

Detail films of the transverse (**A**) and descending (**B**) colons showing ulcers of variable size, shape, and depth.

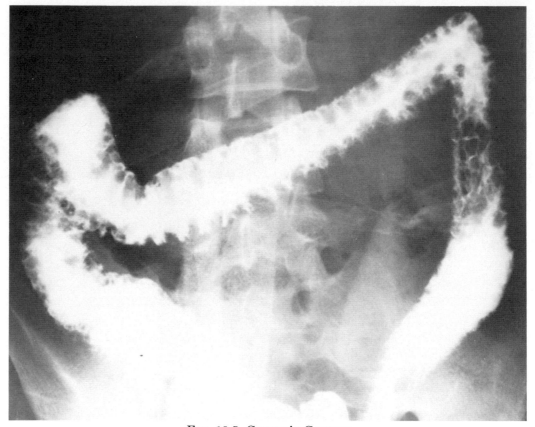

FIG. 10.5. CROHN'S COLITIS

Considerable nodularity is present between the irregular ulcers. There is more involvement of the inferior than the superior margin of the transverse colon, both of which have a different appearance than the descending colon.

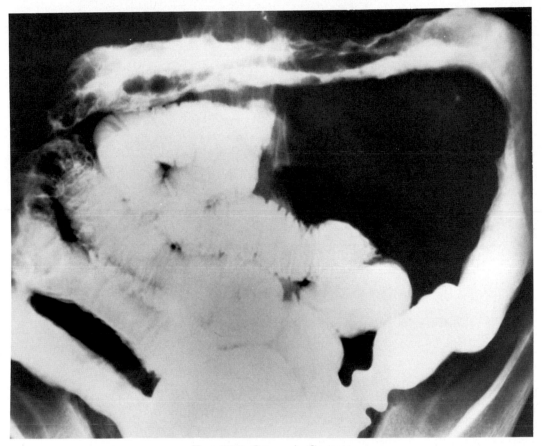

FIG. 10.6. CROHN'S COLITIS
The transverse colon demonstrates extremely wide longitudinal ulcers with thick ridges of inflamed mucosa between them. The patient had undergone a previous right hemi-colectomy.

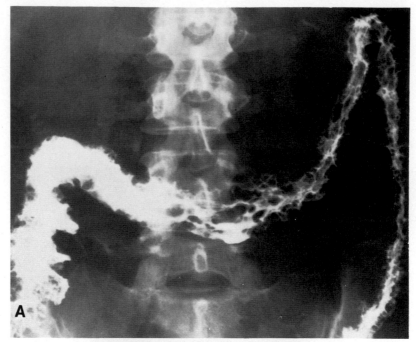

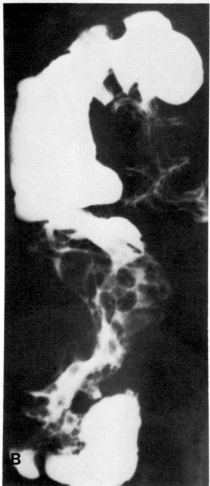

FIG. 10.7. PSEUDOPOLYPS IN CROHN'S COLITIS
Large irregular nodules of hyperplastic mucosa are evident in the transverse (**A**) and ascending (**B**) colons.

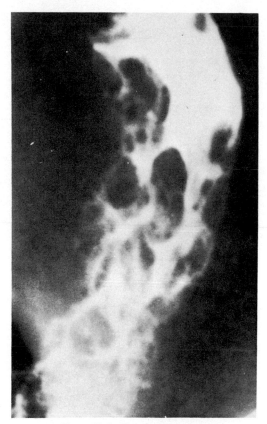

FIG. 10.8. PSEUDOPOLYPS

Detail film of the descending colon showing irregular islands of hyperplastic mucosa between large ulcers.

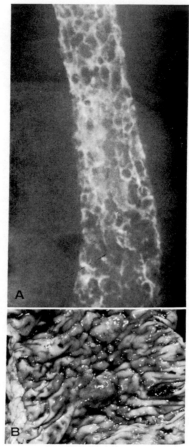

FIG. 10.9. COBBLESTONE MUCOSAL PATTERN IN CROHN'S COLITIS
(A) Detail of evacuation film from barium enema. (B) Detail of a segment of the resected colon. A similar "cobblestone" pattern may be seen in ulcerative colitis (see Fig. 9.20).

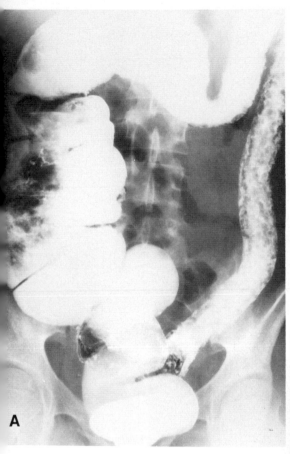

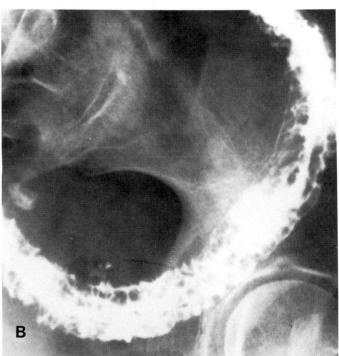

FIG. 10.10. COBBLESTONE MUCOSAL PATTERN IN CROHN'S COLITIS
The relative uniformity of the remaining nodules of mucosa in the descending (**A**)
and sigmoid (**B**) colons has been likened to a cobblestone pavement.

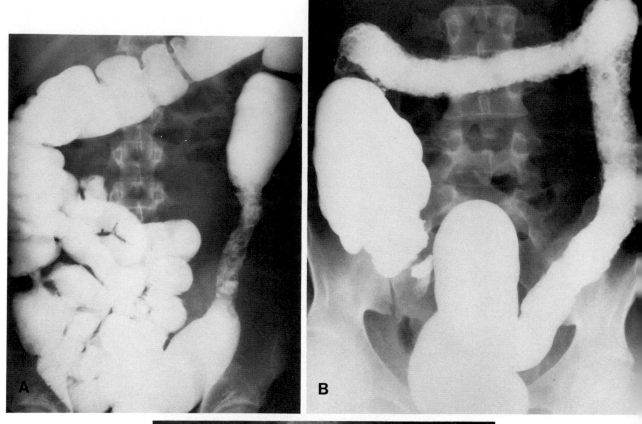

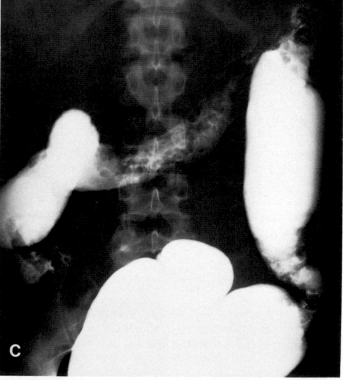

FIG. 10.11. SKIP LESIONS IN CROHN'S COLITIS

(A) An isolated segment in the descending colon. (B) The disease begins in the distal ascending colon and extends to the proximal sigmoid. (C) Areas of disease are present in the cecum and transverse colon including the splenic flexure. A short segment of disease is also present at the junction of the descending and sigmoid colons.

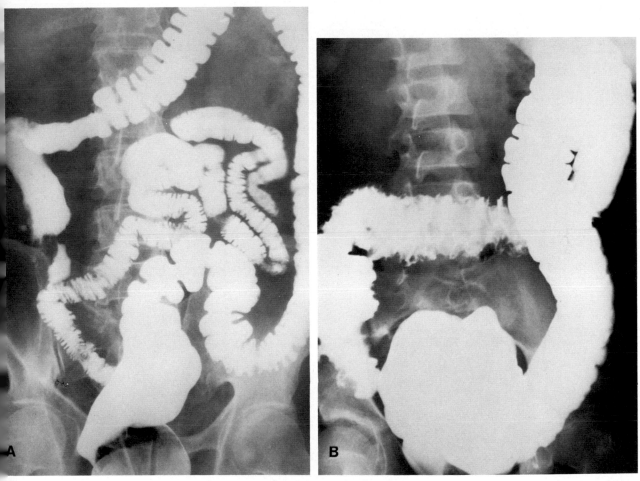

FIG. 10.12. CROHN'S COLITIS
(A) and (B) The ileum, cecum, and ascending colon are narrowed.

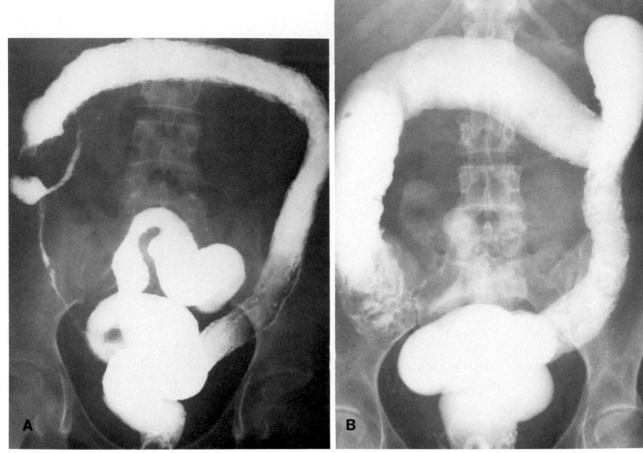

FIG. 10.13. CROHN'S COLITIS

(A), (B), and (C) Varying degrees of ileal and colonic involvement with relative sparing of the sigmoid and rectum.

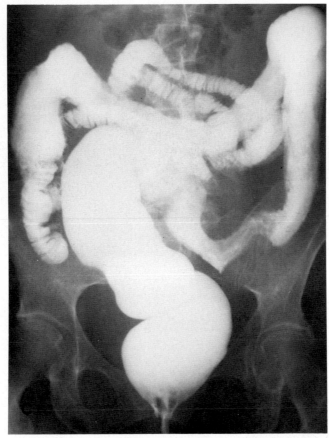

FIG. 10.13. (C)

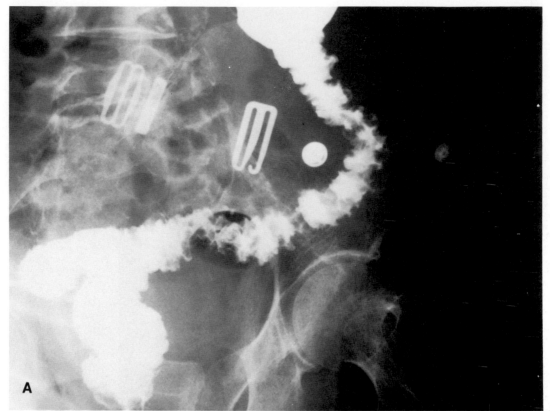

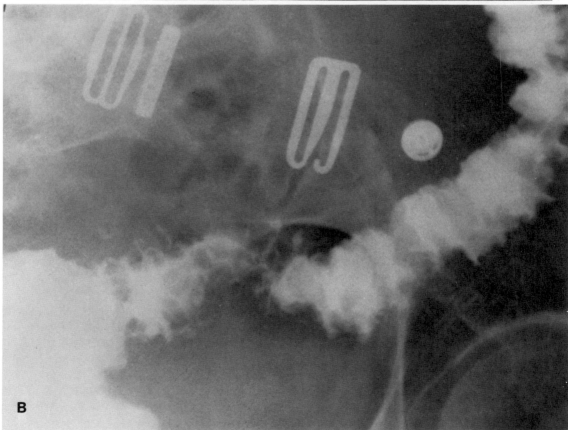

Fig. 10.14. Crohn's Colitis Simulating Perforated Diverticulitis with
Paracolonic Abscess
(A) Full and (B) detail views of the sigmoid colon.

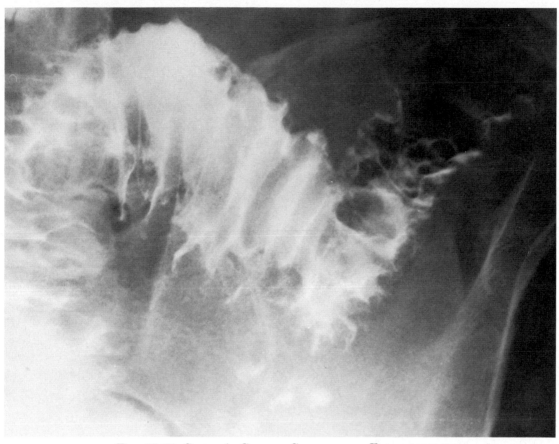

FIG. 10.15. CROHN'S COLITIS SIMULATING DIVERTICULITIS
Detail film of the sigmoid colon revealing markedly edematous mucosa with deep
penetrating ulcers. A perforation is present inferiorly.

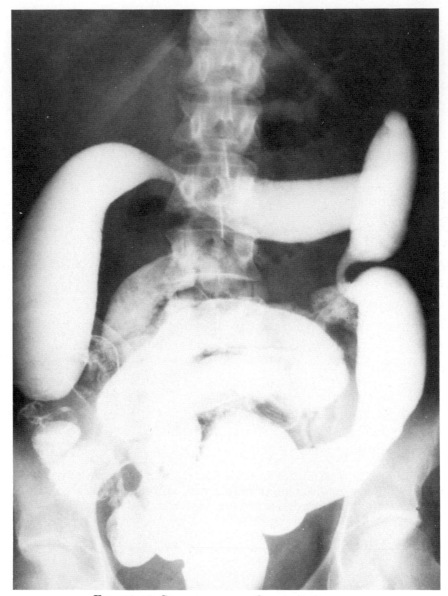

FIG. 10.16. STRICTURES IN CROHN'S COLITIS
Although most of the colon appears tubular and narrow, more marked areas of narrowing are present in the proximal transverse and proximal descending colons.

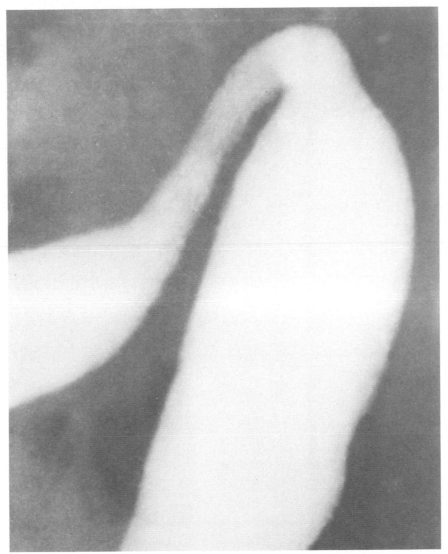

FIG. 10.17. STRICTURE FORMATION IN CROHN'S COLITIS
Detail film of the splenic flexure revealing an area of narrowing with smooth, tapered ends.

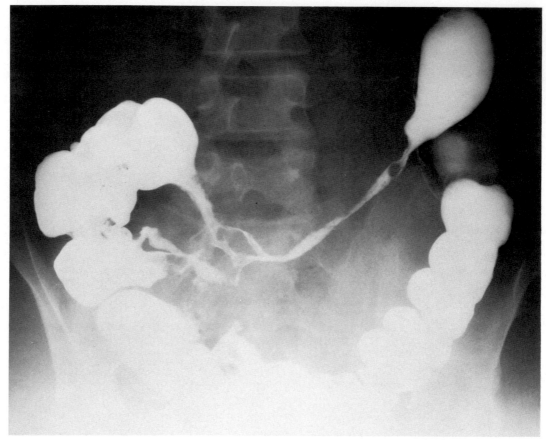

FIG. 10.18. STRICTURE FORMATION AND FISTULA FORMATION
The transverse colon is markedly narrowed. Multiple fistulous tracks are evident on the right.

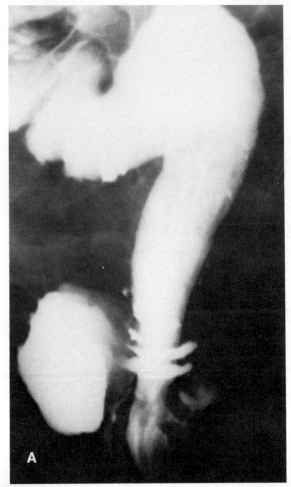

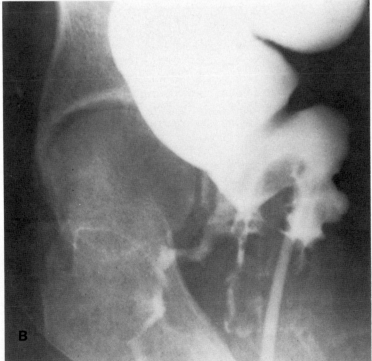

FIG. 10.19. SINUS TRACKS
(A) There are multiple perforations of the rectum, several of which communicate with a large abscess cavity. (B) Several long, narrow sinus tracks originate from the right posterior rectal wall.

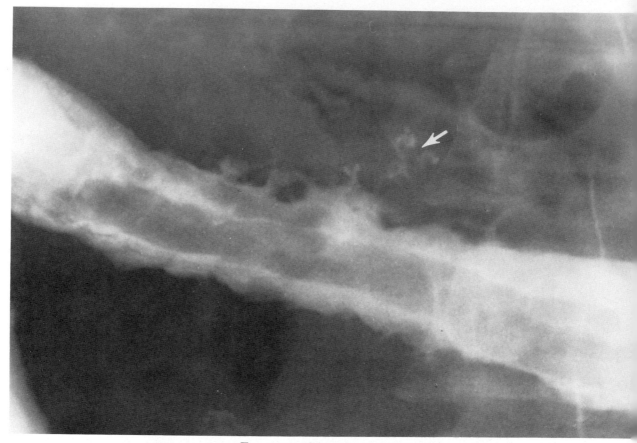

FIG. 10.20. CROHN'S COLITIS

Detail film of the transverse colon showing multiple features of Crohn's colitis. Marked nodularity and pseudopolyp formation with asymmetrical ulceration is present. Several of the ulcers along the superior margin of the bowel wall have begun to coalesce in the subserosa and there has been an early perforation with the formation of an abscess (arrow).

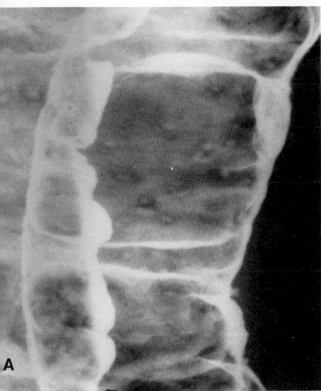

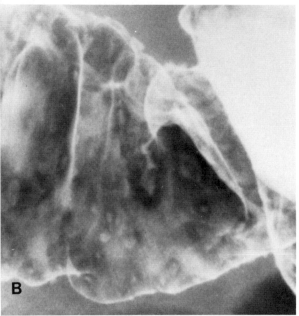

FIG. 10.21. EARLY ULCERATION IN CROHN'S COLITIS—PRIMARY AIR TECHNIQUE
Detail films of the splenic flexure (**A**) and transverse colon (**B**) demonstrating multiple discrete collections of barium. The background mucosa has a normal appearance. (Reproduced by permission from Laufer, I.: *Double Contrast Gastrointestinal Radiology.* W. B. Saunders, Philadelphia, 1979.)

with a thin halo of edema around them. The proponents of this technique believe that these discrete tiny collections correspond to the "aphthoid ulcers" described by some pathologists. It is also their belief that these tiny ulcerations develop in the center of a ring of lymphocytic hyperplasia, which explains the "dot-halo" appearance. It has been claimed that these ulcers can be seen only with the double-contrast technique and that they represent the earliest lesions of Crohn's disease of the colon.

It should be noted that "aphthoid" ulcers are a debatable subject among pathologists (see Chapter 8). Not only is the entity of "aphthoid ulcers" unsettled, but their significance is also unknown. Are they specific for Crohn's colitis? Can they come and go or do they herald future disease in that segment? The answer to these questions is—probably *no.* In view of the secretions which are present within the bowel lumen, can these tiny lesions be visualized roentgenographically?

The ulcers in the later stages of Crohn's colitis appear quite discrete; the background mucosa may appear normal and the ulcers may have a patchy distribution (Figs. 10.22 and 10.23). In general, the ulcers show a greater degree of variability than those in ulcerative colitis. Pseudopolyps are also well demonstrated (Figs. 10.24 and 10.25). The other late changes, such as stricture and fistula formation, are also well shown by the double-contrast technique; the distal ileum is usually less well seen.

In summary, Crohn's disease of the colon is frequently associated with regional

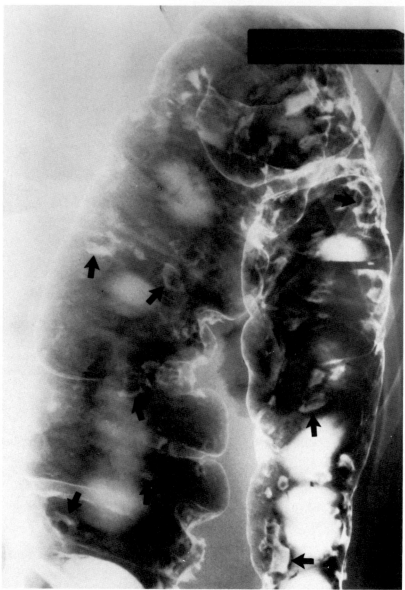

FIG. 10.22. DISCRETE ULCERS IN CROHN'S COLITIS—PRIMARY AIR ENEMA
Detail film of the splenic flexure demonstrates multiple discrete ulcers (arrows)
on a background of normal mucosa. Some of the ulcers are filled with barium, while
others demonstrate barium only in the periphery (ring sign). (Reproduced by
permission from Laufer, I.: *Double Contrast Gastrointestinal Radiology*. W. B.
Saunders, Philadelphia, 1979.)

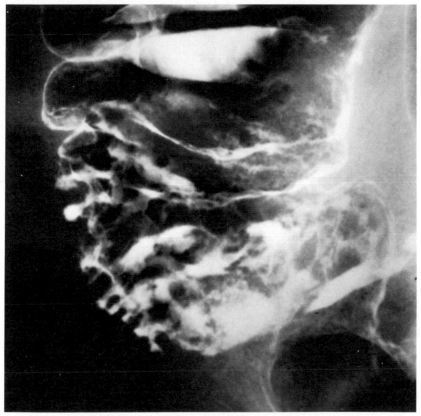

FIG. 10.23. DEEP ULCERS IN CROHN'S COLITIS—PRIMARY AIR TECHNIQUE
Detail film of the cecum demonstrating multiple deep ulcers, with interspersed nodularity between them, arising from the lateral wall of the cecum. (Courtesy of I. Laufer, Philadelphia, Pa.)

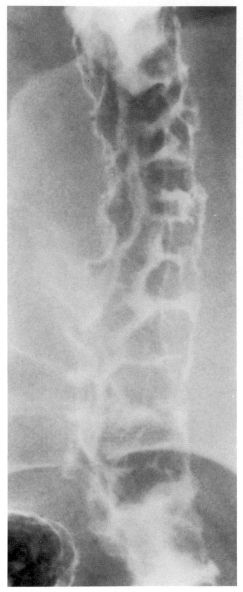

FIG. 10.24. ULCERATION IN CROHN'S COLITIS—PRIMARY AIR ENEMA
Detail film of the descending colon demonstrating longitudinal ulcers with cross fissures. Between the ulcers are large knobs of hyperplastic swollen mucosa (pseudopolyps). (Courtesy of I. Laufer, Philadelphia, Pa.)

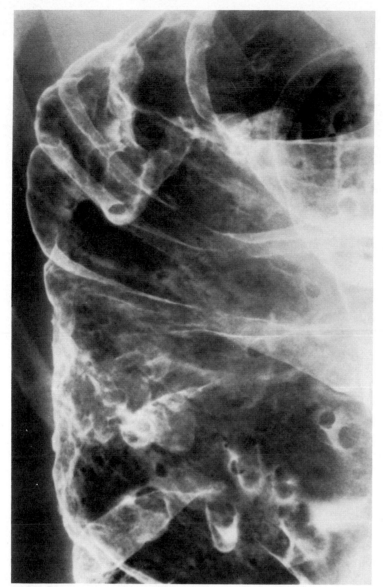

FIG. 10.25. PSEUDOPOLYPS IN CROHN'S COLITIS—PRIMARY AIR ENEMA
Detail film of the cecum demonstrating multiple tags of hyperplastic mucosa. (Reproduced by permission from Laufer, I.: *Double Contrast Gastrointestinal Radiology*. W. B. Saunders, Philadelphia, 1979.)

enteritis. In contrast to ulcerative colitis, it is a disease of the right colon; the entire colon is usually not involved, and the rectum is frequently spared. Segmental involvement and skip lesions are common. The ulceration is greatly varied, and coarse nodularity is frequently seen; the mucosa between the ulcers may be normal. Fistulas, sinuses, and strictures are not uncommon. The hallmarks of Crohn's disease of the colon are variability, discontinuity, and asymmetry.

DIFFERENTIAL DIAGNOSIS

The response of the colon to a given insult is limited. Initially, the bowel wall may respond by becoming inflamed and edematous. If the mucosa is injured sufficiently, it may undergo loss of integrity manifested by ulceration. The size, shape, degree, and extent of ulceration may vary from case to case, but there is a finite limit to the various possibilities. Finally, the wall may heal by fibrosis; the extent of healing will correspond to the site and degree of injury.

There are many possible sources of insult to the colon. Included are: various infectious agents, including amebic, salmonella, and shigella dysentery; tuberculosis; lymphogranuloma venereum, and schistosomiasis. Uremic colitis, allergic purpura, and antibiotic colitis are other potential exciting agents. It should be emphasized that the appearance of the "ulcerating colitis" that develops in any of these conditions may be very similar. Each of these entities has been discussed elsewhere in this text.

Another form of colitis has been termed "functional." For many years, a wide variety of diagnoses have been used to define what is basically a hyperactive large bowel disorder. Functional, spastic, and mucous colitis are best kept under the overall diagnostic label of irritable colon syndrome. That syndrome is discussed in the section on diverticular disease of the colon because the etiologic mechanism seems to be the same in both entities.

One entity that deserves special mention is a colitis that develops proximal to an obstructing lesion of the large bowel, either benign or malignant. Although resembling idiopathic ulcerative colitis, it more appropriately belongs under the category

TABLE 10.1

DIAGNOSTIC FEATURES TO AID IN DIFFERENTIATING ULCERATIVE FROM CROHN'S COLITIS

Features	Ulcerative Colitis	Crohn's Colitis
Age at onset	Childhood or, more often, early adult life	Early adult life
Distribution of disease in colon	Left side and rectum, or entire colon	Segmental involvement (usually right sided), or entire colon
Rectal involvement	Common—85%	Not common—25–40%
Rectal bleeding	Common	Infrequent
Type of ulcers	Early ulcers are tiny and spiculated; later ulcers are deeply undermined and "collar button"	Early ulcers are very small and rarely visible by x-ray but are associated with detectable nodularity and edema of bowel wall; later, ulcers tend to be deep and irregular in size, shape, and distribution
Small bowel involvement	May see "backwash ileitis" for a few centimeters but not true regional ileitis	Coexistence of small bowel involvement is a significant feature
Skip lesions	Not a feature	A diagnostic feature
Colon wall involvement	Circumferential and symmetrical	Asymmetrical
Fibrous thickening of colon wall	Not present	Classical transmural thickening
Stricture formation	Uncommon and late	Frequent and early
Intra-abdominal and pelvic sinus tracks and fistulas	Very rare	Common
Histologic changes	Mucosal and submucosal mainly	Begins in submucosa, but transmural inflammatory response and thickening classically develop
Noncaseating granulomas	Not a feature	May be found in about one-half of cases
Toxic megacolon	A definite complication	Rare, but does occur
Carcinoma	A definite complication	Rare, but does occur
Recurrence after surgery	Total colectomy is curative	Definite risk of recurrence after segmental resection, especially if there is coexisting small bowel disease

of ischemic colitis. This entity, as well as the vascular changes in ulcerative and Crohn's colitis, is discussed in Chapters 12, 13, and 17.

The commonest forms of colitis are "idiopathic" and "Crohn's"; accordingly, the radiologist is most frequently called upon to make the distinction between these two entities. In approximately three-fourths of the cases, a differential diagnosis can be made by utilizing all available information. A patient with colitis of the descending colon, sigmoid, and rectum who also has bloody diarrhea, typical sigmoidoscopic findings, and no radiographic sign of regional enteritis allows a straightforward diagnosis of ulcerative colitis. Similarly, a known case of regional enteritis with subsequent development of right-sided or segmental colitis can be diagnosed as Crohn's disease of the colon. However, in about one-quarter of the cases, there is a significant overlap of radiographic findings; this is not surprising for there may be a similar overlap in the clinical and pathologic findings as well. Table 10.1 lists various characteristics which may aid in a differential diagnosis.

BIBLIOGRAPHY

Ettinger, A.: Focal granulomatous colitis. Gastroenterology, *58*: 189, 1970.

Laufer, I.: *Double Contrast Gastrointestinal Radiology with Endoscopic Correlation.* W. B. Saunders, Philadelphia, 1979.

Laufer, I., and Hamilton, J.: The radiological differentiation between ulcerative and granulomatous colitis by double contrast radiology. Am. J. Gastroenterol., *66*: 259, 1976.

Lockhart-Mummery, H. E., and Morson, B. C.: Crohn's disease of the large intestine. Gut, *5*: 493, 1964.

Margulis, A. R., Goldberg, H. I., Lawson, T. L., *et al.*: The overlapping spectrum of ulcerative and granulomatous colitis: A roentgenographic pathologic study. Am. J. Roentgenol., *113*: 325, 1971.

Marshak, R. H.: Granulomatous disease of the intestinal tract (Crohn's disease). Radiology, *114*: 32, 1975.

Weedon, D. D., Shorter, R. G., and Ilstrup, D. M.: Crohn's disease and cancer. N. Engl. J. Med. *289*: 1099, 1973.

Wolf, B. S., and Marshak, R. H.: Granulomatous colitis (Crohn's disease of the colon). Am. J. Roentgenol., *88*: 662, 1962.

11

Unusual Inflammatory Lesions

JACK WITTENBERG, M.D.

PSEUDOMEMBRANOUS COLITIS (ANTIBIOTIC-INDUCED COLITIS)

Pseudomembranous colitis is an uncommon but potentially serious complication of antibiotic therapy. Its development has been observed in association with the well-established drugs such as tetracycline, penicillin, and ampicillin as well as with newer, wide spectrum agents such as lincomycin and clindamycin. While most commonly induced by the oral consumption of these antibiotics, the disease has also been induced by their intravenous administration. The interval between initiation of antibiotic therapy and clinical symptoms may vary from 1 day to 1 month; the average duration is approximately 2 weeks. The onset of symptoms may also occur following the cessation of antibiotic therapy.

Severe, often debilitating diarrhea with or without blood is the hallmark of pseudomembranous colitis. Abdominal cramps, tenderness, and occasionally signs of peritonitis are associated with the diarrhea. In unremitting cases, hypoprotein-emia, edema, ascites, and shock may follow.

The diagnosis must be considered in any patient receiving antibiotics who suddenly experiences copious diarrhea and any of the above signs. Proctosigmoidoscopy should be employed as the initial diagnostic procedure since a characteristic appearance of friable, edematous mucosa with yellowish-green exudate and/or white, patchy, raised 1–6 mm plaque-like lesions scattered over the mucosal surface provides confirmatory evidence (Fig. 11.1). In more severely affected patients, a confluent, purulent, pseudomembrane enveloping the entire mucosal surface may be observed. Histologically, this pseudomembrane is composed of mucus, fibrin, white blood cells, and bacteria. Shallow mucosal ulcerations may accompany any of these stages; they rarely are deep enough to affect the submucosa.

Plain films of the abdomen in severe cases frequently demonstrate moderate, but diffuse, gaseous distention of the colon. While the colonic alterations may be

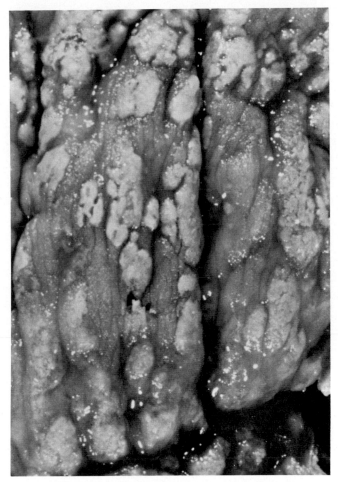

FIG. 11.1. PSEUDOMEMBRANOUS COLITIS

Mucosal view of resected sigmoid colon demonstrates the small, slightly raised plaques with intervening areas of edematous mucosa (Courtesy of Dr. Ervin Philipps, Boston, Mass.)

indistinguishable from toxic megacolon, the diffuseness of the haustral distortions and the extreme thickness of the bowel wall may provide a clue to the presence of pseudomembranous colitis. The latter finding is often best observed as either unusually wide, vertical interhaustral folds oriented perpendicular to and completely crossing the long axis of the bowel or deeply indented, rounded, soft tissue densities along the margin distorting the haustral contour (Fig. 11.2).

Since a barium enema is contraindicated in severe pseudomembranous colitis, careful clinical evaluation must be invoked before its performance. A wide spectrum of roentgenographic findings which overlap with those observed in other inflammatory diseases of the colon have been described; however, observation of alterations consistent with the plaque-like lesions previously described may allow a presumptive diagnosis in the proper clinical setting. When seen in profile, these tiny plaques produce an appearance of discrete 2–3 mm filling defects often distributed circumferentially about the margin of the colon (Fig. 11.3). While confusion may exist initially as to whether this serrated marginal pattern represents ulcers with

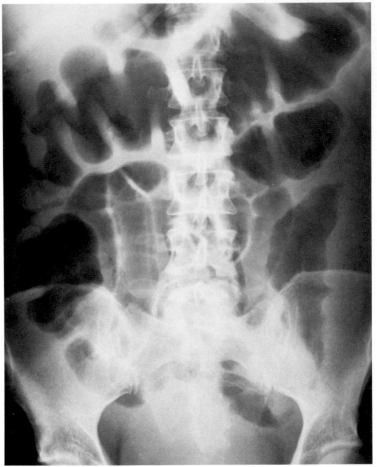

FIG. 11.2. PSEUDOMEMBRANOUS COLITIS

Moderately severe ileus affecting the entire intestine is present. The dilated transverse colon demonstrates very thick, interhaustral markings and mild irregularity of the haustral contours due to extensive edema.

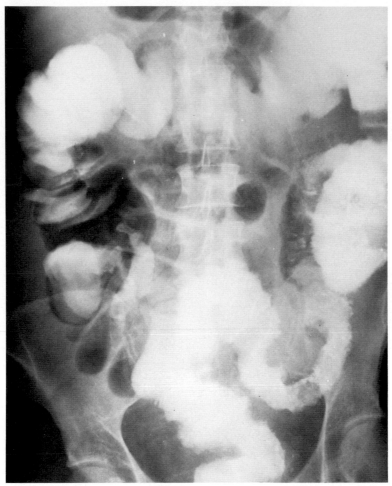

FIG. 11.3. PSEUDOMEMBRANOUS COLITIS
Distortion of the haustra is evident throughout the entire colon. The descending and sigmoid segments show marginal serrations simulating an ulcerative process but in this case are a result of barium interspersed between elevated pseudomembranous plaques.

surrounding edema or the consequence of barium interposed between small filling defects, an *en face* view of the lesions clearly demonstrates the existence of these small oval filling defects, often without coexistent ulceration (Fig. 11.4).

The differential diagnosis of these plaque-like lesions includes lymphosarcoma and familial polyposis; rarely are pseudopolyps as small and uniform in size. When these characteristic lesions are absent and mucosal and haustral distortions exist, the disease is often radiologically indistinguishable from the more common inflammatory diseases of the colon and a specific diagnosis must rest with clinical correlation.

NONGRANULOMATOUS BACTERIAL COLITIS (INFECTIOUS COLITIS)

Salmonellosis and Shigellosis

The most common etiology of the bacterial colitides can be attributed to organisms

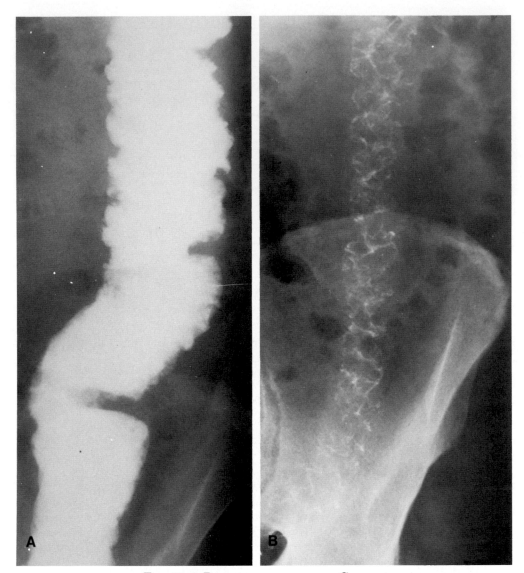

FIG. 11.4. PSEUDOMEMBRANOUS COLITIS
(A) The descending colon demonstrates slight marginal irregularity in the pre-evacuation film. (B) Following evacuation, the same segment shows distortion and prominence of folds but no definite ulcers. (Courtesy of Herbert Gramm, M.D., Boston, Mass.)

of either salmonella or shigella. Salmonellosis most frequently occurs in a self-limiting form, commonly known as "food-poisoning," and complete recovery is made within 4–5 days often without the necessity for any radiologic investigation. The more fulminant cases of salmonellosis and shigellosis have their greatest incidence in the previously debilitated individual. In such cases, salmonellosis usually involves the terminal ileum, but in approximately one-third of patients the colon may also be involved. Shigellosis (bacillary dysentery), on the other hand, preferentially affects the colon and usually spares the terminal ileum. While rarely observed in the northern hemisphere, it may be the cause of epidemics of severe, debilitating diarrhea in tropical and subtropical climates.

The ingestion of contaminated foods is the most frequent source of the infection with either organism. Acute, self-limited salmonellosis occurs following the ingestion of spoiled foods containing a thermostable endotoxin produced by the bacterium. The source of the more fulminant forms of either infection is usually the ingestion of eggs, meat, or milk of infected animal carriers or food contaminated by human carriers. Fecal contamination of water supplies or transmission by flies, cockroaches, or other insects provides the source of epidemics in less advanced societies.

The incubation period varies from several hours to several weeks. Diarrhea is the most characteristic sign and in severe infections the volume of fluid losses may become life-threatening. Pathologically the mucosa and submucosa demonstrate edema, hyperemia, hemorrhage, and leukocytic infiltration. Both mucosal ulceration and bowel wall thickening are observed. Shigellosis may progress to a subacute or chronic stage with periods of exacerbation and remission and in such form may be indistinguishable both clinically and roentgenographically from ulcerative or Crohn's colitis.

A paralytic ileus pattern is the most common plain film manifestation. Small bowel distention predominates in salmonellosis while shigellosis shows large amounts of colonic gas as well as fluid levels. Free intraperitoneal gas is more commonly described in salmonellosis because of its tendency for deep ulcerations and perforation.

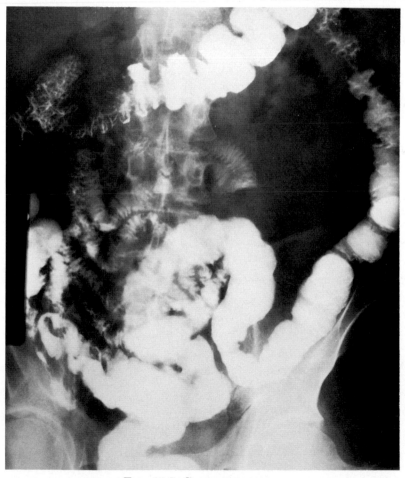

FIG. 11.5. SALMONELLOSIS
Spasm and haustral distortion are evident segmentally in the colon. Spot-films of the rectosigmoid showed incomplete distensibility with tiny ulcers.

The radiographic abnormalities observed by barium examination are related to the severity and stage of the colonic involvement. In the acute, severe form, a pancolitis is present and deep, collar button ulcers may predominate. In less severe infestations, total or segmental involvement is seen with the rectum variably involved clinically (Fig. 11.5). While segmental disease affects any part of the colon, the descending colon is the most frequently involved. Superficial ulcerations may be present but more commonly coarse, nodular, edematous folds are observed (Fig. 11.6). Invariably nonspecific findings such as spasm, haustral distortion, and excess fluid accompany either of these mucosal changes.

The differentiation between salmonella and shigella colitis based on roentgenographic changes in the colon is impossible. However, involvement of the terminal ileum strongly favors the former. Similarly, the differentiation between idiopathic ulcerative colitis, Crohn's disease, or other granulomatous colitides such as tuberculosis or amebiasis is rarely possible and bacteriologic investigation in unclear cases remains the source of a specific diagnosis. These causative agents must be assiduously and meticulously sought since steroid therapy appropriate to the noninfectious colitides is obviously contraindicated in the infectious type.

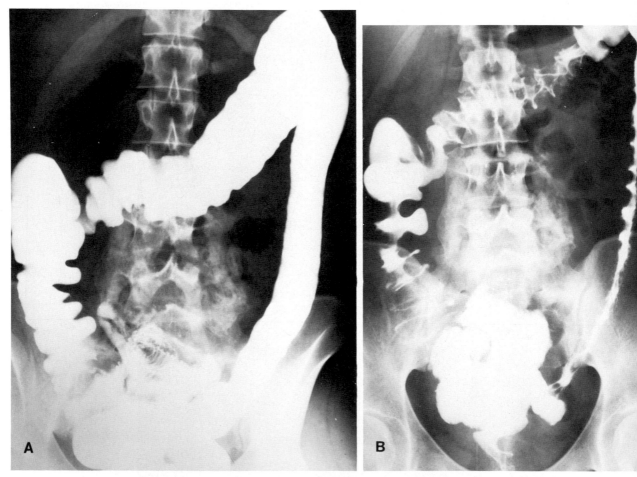

FIG. 11.6. SALMONELLOSIS

(A) Before evacuation the colon presents both right-sided haustral distortion and left-sided tubulation. (B) Following evacuation the contour distortion persists with evidence of nodular, edematous mucosal folds in the transverse and descending colon.

AMEBIASIS

Natural History and Clinical Features

Amebiasis is a disease caused by infestation with the protozoan, *Entamoeba histolytica.* Man is infected when he ingests a viable cyst in food or drink contaminated by fecal material, frequently from the fingers of food handlers. The cyst then dissolves in the alkaline small intestine and the released trophozoites pass into the cecum where they may invade the mucosa. The trophozoites rapidly multiply and can invade the remainder of the colon, can be excreted in the feces, or can seed the bloodstream to lodge in other organs. The most common extracolonic sites of involvement are the liver and the lung.

It is estimated that 20% of the world's population carry the parasite, the largest incidence being in less well developed, tropical climates. Only a small number of the carriers, however, develop the invasive form of amebiasis. Transformation of the organism from the cyst to the invasive trophozoite form is related to the virulence of the strain and alterations in the host defensive mechanisms. Invasive amebiasis usually manifests itself as a segmental or diffuse colitis; far less common forms include typhloappendicitis, an ameboma, or fulminating colitis. The clinical symptoms depend on the severity of the infestation and vary from mild abdominal pain and diarrhea to severe, colicky, debilitating pain with bloody, copious diarrhea; this latter form may be fatal.

When the trophozoites invade mucosa, they produce tiny areas of inflammation which rapidly undergo necrosis. The intervening normal mucosa becomes involved as the areas of necrosis coalesce, and the ulcers may penetrate into the submucosa. Part of the host response includes the formation of granulation tissue in an attempt to wall off the infection. The overall picture is therefore one of mucosal ulceration with bowel wall thickening by granulation tissue. As the disease progresses into its chronic form, fibrosis causes shortening of the colon.

The diagnosis is suspected by endoscopic visualization of edematous mucosa which contains whitish ulcerations. Positive identification is made by recognition of the trophozoite in the mucus covering the ulcers. The organism may also be demonstrated in the stool, but handling and incubation of the stool must be carefully done. For reasons that are not clear, it is claimed that the organism will be absent from the stool for up to 1 month following the performance of a barium enema examination.

Several amebecides are available for treatment of the disease, and complications are rare. Perforation, fistula formation, or sinus tracks almost never occur and large bowel obstruction or severe hemorrhage is also quite unusual.

Roentgen Findings

Plain films of the abdomen are usually unrevealing except in the fulminant form of the disease when an appearance of toxic megacolon, indistinguishable from that caused by other etiologies, may be observed. The dilatation on a supine film invariably involves the transverse colon where haustral distortion and pseudopolyps may be detected (Fig. 11.7).

The barium enema reveals a variety of changes including mucosal edema or nodularity (Fig. 11.8), haustral thickening and spasm (Fig. 11.9). Ulcerations are frequently superficial but in severe cases may develop into deeply penetrating, collar button forms. Either a diffuse pancolitis or a segmental involvement may be observed. When segmental, the involvement is usually in order of frequency: the rectosigmoid, cecum (Fig. 11.10) and the ascending colon (Fig. 11.11). Typhloappendicitis occurs when segmental involvement of the cecum secondarily leads to

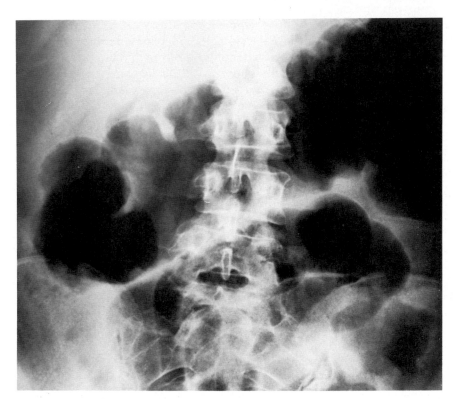

FIG. 11.7. AMEBIASIS
Toxic dilatation of transverse colon in amebiasis.

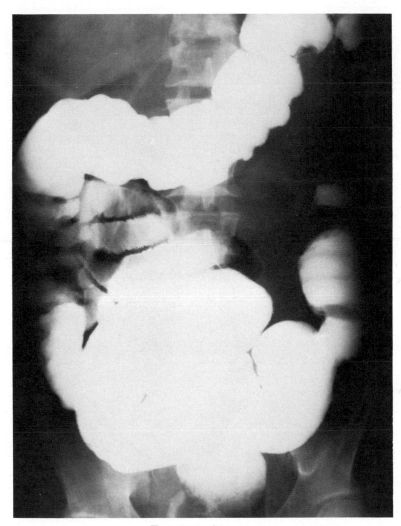

FIG. 11.8. AMEBIASIS
The haustral distortion is evident in the transverse colon and particularly marked
on the inferior surface where large nodular indentations are present.

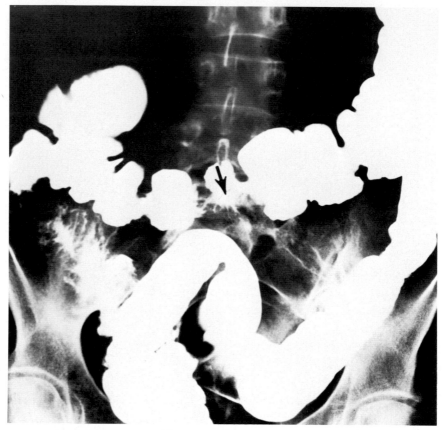

FIG. 11.9. AMEBIASIS
The ascending colon is contracted and was hyperactive at fluoroscopy. An area of
irregular narrowing with ulceration is present in the transverse colon (arrow).

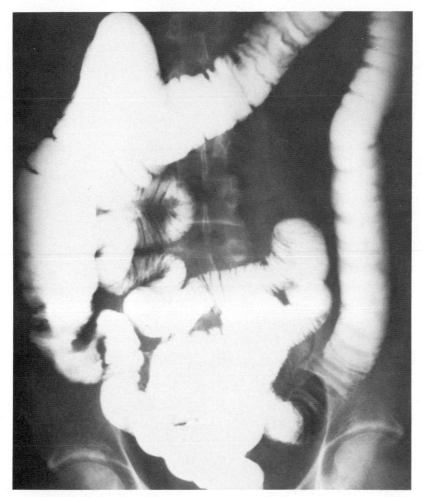

Fig. 11.10. Amebiasis
Segmental cecal involvement demonstrating limited distensibility with thickening
of the ileo-cecal valve. The remainder of the colon and ileum is normal.

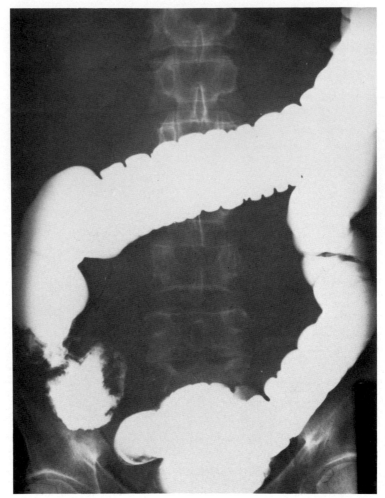

FIG. 11.11. AMEBIASIS
The ascending colon and cecum are narrowed and mildly shortened.

appendicitis. However, primary involvement of the appendix may be also observed. An ameboma is a focal lesion of the colon which results from marked thickening of the entire circumference of the bowel wall. Radiographically, this results in a luminal mass or an annular lesion which lacks distensibility and may have angular margins, resembling an apple core form of carcinoma. The presence of an ameboma can be suspected when accompanying inflammatory abnormalities are seen elsewhere in the colon or by observation of the lack of consistency of the shelf-like angular margins. If suspected, antiamebic therapy can induce a rapid reversal of an ameboma to a normal configuration.

Differential Diagnosis

Since the ileum is uncommonly affected by amebiasis, ileal disease, especially if extensive, favors Crohn's disease. In those patients in whom the disease is limited to the colon, transverse and longitudinal ulcerations, eccentric involvement of the colonic wall or fistula formation strongly favor Crohn's disease. Ulcerative colitis and amebiasis may also be indistinguishable; however, skip areas commonly seen in amebiasis are uncommon in ulcerative colitis.

Primary and metastatic carcinomas are also sometimes considered in the differential diagnosis particularly in the cecal area. A carcinoma is usually more eccentric, rigid, and irregular with gross mucosal destruction. In amebiasis, the lesion is longer and more symmetrical; there is evidence of irritability and spasm and the mucosa is altered but not destroyed.

TUBERCULOSIS

While bovine mycobacterium tuberculosis is a vanishing disease in the United States, this is not true in the remainder of the world where less attention is paid to the pasteurization of milk. When encountered in the United States, the disease invariably occurs in a patient with pulmonary tuberculosis although the manifestation of the intestinal disease may not coincide with that of the pulmonary disease. Gastrointestinal tuberculosis has its greatest incidence in those patients with cavitating pulmonary lesions and positive sputum; the ingestion of the latter leads to seeding of the gastrointestinal tract.

Clinical Features

Tuberculous involvement of the gastrointestinal tract may be asymptomatic even when changes can be demonstrated by barium examination. When symptomatic, a wide variety of nonspecific complaints such as weight loss, fever, anorexia, right lower quadrant pain, and diarrhea are encountered.

The diagnosis may be suggested from the x-ray appearance of the colon, but is definitively established through the culture of excreta or the demonstration of caseating tubercles or organisms from surgically resected tissues. Complications such as obstruction or perforation may be the initial presenting gastrointestinal symptoms in this low-grade infection.

Pathology

The organism lodges in the depths of the mucosal glands and in the submucosa; from here, it passes to the mesenteric lymph nodes. The ensuing inflammatory response and endarteritis leads to mucosal ischemia and ulceration that may extend to the serosa. A combination of the inflammatory changes, fibrosis, and lymphatic obstruction leads to the formation of a thick, fixed, colonic wall. Occasionally, a localized mass, the tuberculoma, results.

Roentgen Findings

Calcification of mesenteric nodes is rarely observed. The insidious nature of the disease may result in the presentation of the patient with perforation (Fig. 11.12) or small bowel obstruction (Fig. 11.13). The most frequent segment of the colon to be involved is the cecum (Fig. 11.14). The next most frequent colonic segments affected are the ascending and transverse colon, invariably in continuity with the cecum (Fig. 11.15, A and B). In acute stages it may be difficult to fill the cecum adequately because of sustained spasm. The ileum also will show a hyperirritable state with narrowing and possibly ulcers.

In the more chronic form of the disease, the cecal changes reflect the pathologic state. As healing and fibrosis occur, the cecum becomes distorted, rigid, and shortened. The ileocecal valve is well seen secondary to its thickened, stiff lips, and the terminal ileum frequently appears narrowed, not unlike its appearance in regional ileitis. Occasionally, both the acute and chronic stages of the disease are best appreciated on a small bowel follow-through study.

In those cases where areas of the colon other than the cecum are involved, the

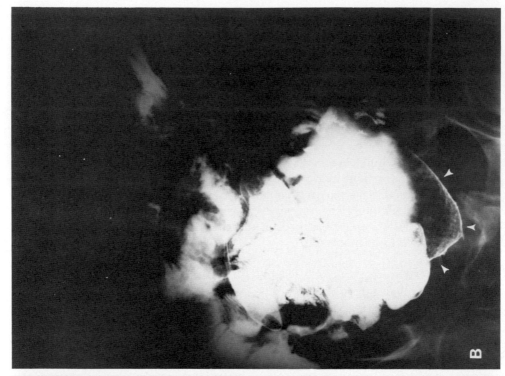

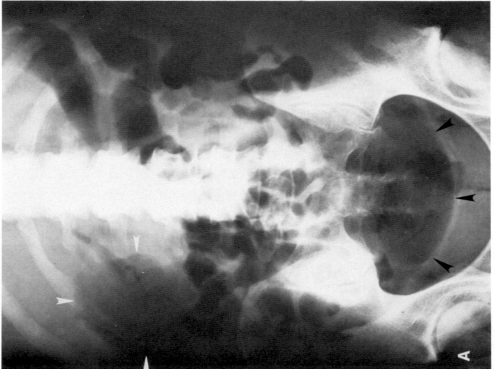

(A) Patient with pulmonary tuberculosis undergoing treatment who entered the hospital because of diarrhea. Collections of free abdominal gas are shown on the supine film in both the right subhepatic area (white arrows) and pelvis (black arrows). (B) Barium enema demonstrates shrunken cecum, narrowed distal ileum and barium outlining the peritoneal cavity (arrows). The perforation was thought to originate from the distal ileum.

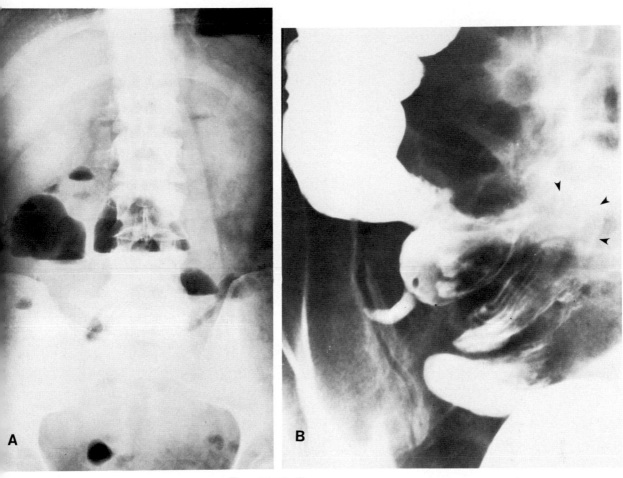

FIG. 11.13. TUBERCULOSIS

(A) Patient with previously treated cecal tuberculosis with a pattern of small bowel obstruction. (B) Emergency barium enema shows marked narrowing of the cecum and ascending colon with an angulated terminal ileum (arrows) which, at operation, was responsible for the small bowel obstruction.

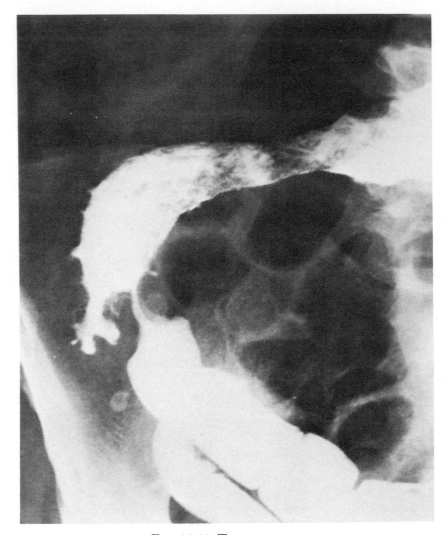

FIG. 11.14. TUBERCULOSIS

A detail film demonstrates extensive contraction of the cecum and right colon. The last few centimeters of ileum are narrowed.

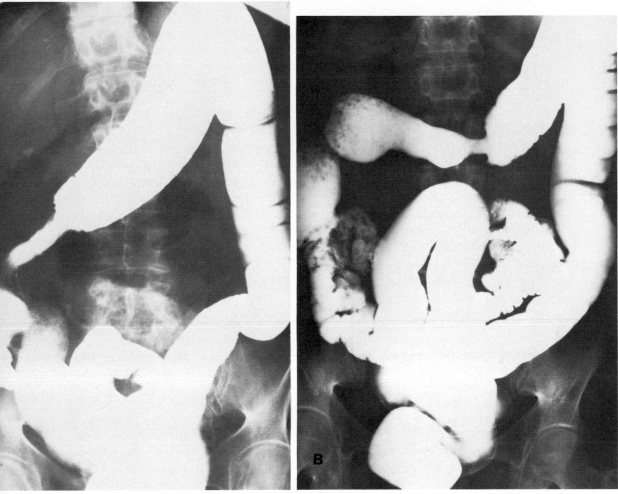

FIG. 11.15. TUBERCULOSIS
(A) Narrowing of ascending and proximal transverse colon. (B) Extensive involvement of the colon from the cecum to the distal transverse colon.

appearance is not unlike that of a benign stricture. Finally, in those very rare cases of total colon involvement, the appearance is identical to ulcerative colitis. The differential diagnosis has been considered under amebiasis.

SCHISTOSOMIASIS

Natural History

The schistosomes, or blood flukes, consist of *Schistosoma mansoni*, *S. japonicum*, and *S. haematobium*. It has been estimated that at least 10% of Puerto Rican school children in New York City are infected with this parasite, mainly *S. mansoni*.

The organism, after partial maturation in the snail, enters the body by penetrating the intact skin and is carried by the venous blood to the right heart, through the lungs, to the left heart, and into the systemic circulation. Only the larvae which reach the portal venous bed develop into mature worms. The adult worms may reside within the portal venous bed for 20–30 years. The mature worms migrate against the portal venous blood flow into the smaller venules of the inferior mesenteric vein where the female deposits her ova. Those ova that penetrate into the lumen of the bowel are passed from the body and continue the life cycle. Some of the ova may be washed back into the venous stream, and return to the liver where they can cause cirrhosis and portal hypertension. Some ova may also re-enter the systemic circulation, and reach the lungs where they can incite vasculitis and fibrosis.

Pathology Related to Roentgen Findings

Ova which lodge in the bowel wall stimulate an inflammatory response, the severity of which determines the roentgen pattern. The descending and sigmoid colons are the most frequent sites of disease, but any portion of the colon may be involved. The earliest changes are spasm, disturbed motility, and a loss of haustral pattern. The mucosa is edematous and may show tiny ulcerations. The appearance of this stage of the disease may simulate ulcerative colitis. The lesion progresses to either stricture formation or the formation of a localized intramural mass which projects into the lumen. The differentiation from a nonspecific benign stricture or from a carcinoma of the colon may be impossible.

FUNGUS DISEASE

Histoplasmosis, mucormycosis, actinomycosis, and monilia are among the fungi that may cause pathologic lesions in the colon. They may arise primarily in the bowel, or they may invade the colon from another site in the body. For example, histoplasmosis usually starts in the lungs. Fungus infection most frequently occurs in chronically ill, debilitated patients, and is a poor prognostic omen.

The fungi are capable of invading the bowel wall and vessels, producing an intense, localized inflammatory reaction. The bowel wall may be irritable and spastic. Mucosal ulcers are usually not seen unless they are large; the mucosal folds may appear thickened and irregular. The late stage is one of narrowing of the bowel lumen by an irregular masslike lesion of inflammatory tissue with an x-ray appearance suggesting carcinoma. The correct diagnosis is rarely made in the preoperative or premortem period.

LYMPHOGRANULOMA VENEREUM

Lymphogranuloma venereum is caused by a large virus belonging to the psitticosis group and is spread by venereal contact. In the male, the disease is manifested by a primary genital sore followed by inguinal adenitis, the so-called bubo. In the female, the primary lesion occurs in the vagina or on the cervix, and rectal strictures are much more common.

The virus may reach the perirectal lymphatics by way of the prostatic gland drainage in the male, or by way of the rectovaginal septum in the female and establish a lymphangitis; the resulting fibrosis leads to a rectal stricture. The disease occurs with almost equal frequency in males and females in the sexually active age group. Symptoms include rectal bleeding, tenesmus, and a change in bowel habits including diarrhea and constipation. Diagnosis may be established by the Frei intradermal skin test or by a complement fixation test.

Although the rectum is the first and usually the only portion of the colon affected, other segments or even the entire colon may be involved. The bowel is spastic and irritable, as in any colitis, and shows a loss of haustral pattern. The mucosa is boggy and edematous and ulcerations may be present. The colon quickly returns to a normal appearance if therapy is instituted at this time.

The disease usually presents as a rectal stricture beginning just above the anus and varying in length from 2–25 cm. The diseased segment is narrowed, fixed, and irregular. The lumen may become so narrowed that it resembles a string. The proximal margin of the adjacent normal colon, which is dilated, frequently narrows in a smooth conical fashion. The mucosa is irregular with multiple shaggy ulcers (Fig. 11.16). Fistulas and sinus tracks of varying lengths, shape, and configuration are frequently present. Communication with perirectal abscess cavities or with the lower vagina or perianal skin is not uncommon. Other causes of colonic strictures such as radiation injury, ulcerative colitis, amebiasis, tuberculosis, or carcinoma must be considered in the differential diagnosis.

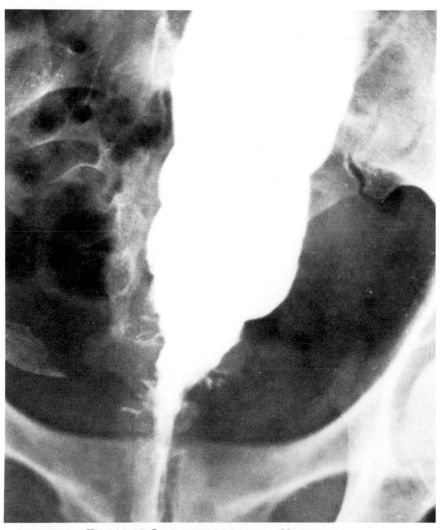

FIG. 11.16. LYMPHOGRANULOMA VENEREUM
There is a long rectal stricture with multiple deep ulcers.

BIBLIOGRAPHY

Annamunthodo, H., and Marryatt, J.: Barium studies in intestinal lymphogranuloma venereum. Br. J. Radiol., *34*: 53, 1961.

Cardoso, J. M., Kimura, K., Stoopen, M., Cervantes, L. F., Elizondo, L., Churchill, R., and Moncada, R.: Radiology of invasive amebiasis of the colon. Am. J. Roentgenol., *128*: 935, 1977.

Chait, A.: Schistosomiasis mansoni: Roentgenologic observations in a nonendemic area. Am. J. Roentgenol., *90*: 688, 1963.

De Feo, E.: Mucormycosis of the colon. Am. J. Roentgenol., *86*: 86, 1961.

Farman, J., Rabinowitz, J. G., and Meyers, M. A.: Roentgenology of infectious colitis. Am. J. Roentgenol., *119*: 375, 1973.

Goldberg, H. I., and Reeder, M. M.: Infections and infestations of the gastrointestinal tract. In *Alimentary Tract Roentgenology*, 2nd ed., Vol. 3, edited by A. R. Margulis and H. J. Burhenne. C. V. Mosby Co., St. Louis, 1973.

Perez, C. A., Sturim, H. S., Kouchoukos, N. T., and Kamberg, S.: Some clinical and radiographic features of gastrointestinal histoplasmosis. Radiology, *86*: 482, 1966.

Stanley, R. J., Melson, G. L., and Tedesco, F. J.: The spectrum of radiographic findings in antibiotic-related pseudomembranous colitis. Radiology, *111*: 519, 1974.

Weinfeld, A.: The roentgen appearance of intestinal amebiasis. Am. J. Roentgenol., *96*: 311, 1966.

12

Ischemic Colitis

JACK WITTENBERG, M.D.

INTRODUCTION

Segmental vascular disease of the colon is a relatively new pathologic entity, having been first elaborated in the early 1960's. Despite this rather recent description, a great deal of etiologic and pathologic information has been accumulated which provides justification for singling out this disease as an entity distinct from the more common inflammatory diseases of the colon. While originally ascribed to arteriosclerotic occlusive disease concomitantly affecting the inferior mesenteric artery and the superior mesenteric artery resulting in a perfusion deficit at their junction at or near the splenic flexure (watershed area), recently available angiographic evidence has made this theory untenable. It has become clear that the ischemic process most commonly affects the colon in the distribution of either the superior mesenteric artery or the inferior mesenteric artery circulation, with involvement of the latter vascular network approximately 5 times more common than the former. In the majority of patients, the major mesenteric arterial and venous branches have been shown to be patent and the pathophysiologic event is presumed to be regional alterations in the vasa recta of the colonic wall. Certainly, a prototype for intestinal ischemia resulting from small vessel perfusion abnormalities exists in the separate entity of extensive nonocclusive ischemia of the intestine in which these pathophysiologic events have been more clearly elucidated.

The recent observations of the absence of major vascular occlusion in ischemic colitis has raised the question of whether this disease may just be a variant of ulcerative colitis or Crohn's colitis occurring in an elderly population. However, accumulated clinical and pathologic observations argue strongly against this explanation. Unlike ulcerative colitis and Crohn's colitis, spontaneous ischemic colitis invariably affects the older aged population, does so in an acute fashion and then follows a short, generally mild clinical course. The lesion can be observed by barium enema to reverse rapidly and rarely recurs. When the rare stricture follows an acute episode, it does so within 2–4 weeks. Ischemic colitis largely affects the colon at or beyond the splenic flexure, but unlike ulcerative colitis is segmental in nature sparing the rectum in the majority of patients. Unlike Crohn's colitis which is a transmural disease, ischemic colitis predominantly involves the mucosal and submucosal layers of the bowel wall. The rapidity with which ischemic colitis reverses itself, leaving no evidence of colonic deformity, is also uncharacteristic of Crohn's colitis. However, it should be emphasized that when judged by clinical, roentgenographic *or* pathologic criteria, ischemic colitis may be indistinguishable from these other more common entities. Therefore, the diagnosis of this entity can only be reliably made after integration of historical, roentgenographic, and histologic data.

Somewhat more clear-cut in its definition of a vascular etiology is iatrogenically induced ischemia which occurs following abdominal aortic aneurysmectomy or abdominoperineal resection for distal colonic carcinoma. In either of these operations, the inferior mesenteric artery or its branches may be transected and collateral circulation may not be sufficient to maintain adequate vascular perfusion. The roentgenographic and pathologic features of these ischemic processes are indistinguishable from those of spontaneous ischemic colitis. As well, the clinical evolution of the ischemic disease is very similar in that a benign clinical course often ensues with complete reversal of the colonic lesion.

CLINICAL FEATURES

Ischemic colitis shows no sex predilection; it appears to affect caucasians much more commonly than Negroes for reasons that are unclear. The major symptom is left lower quadrant pain, mild in intensity but abrupt in onset. Two-thirds of patients will have diarrhea. Approximately one-half of all patients report bright red blood accompanying the diarrhea and in about 40% of the remainder the stool will be guaiac-positive. These composite findings may be accompanied by mild rebound tenderness and clinically simulate diverticulitis, which is the commonest admitting diagnosis. Since the rectum may be involved with the ischemic process, sigmoidoscopy can be of value in the differential diagnosis. In the small group of patients who have severe pain, unremitting diarrhea and/or unremitting rebound tenderness, the threat of transmural colonic infarction requires emergency operative intervention. However, in most instances, the pain and diarrhea will quickly abate and no more than supportive medical therapy will be required.

ROENTGEN FINDINGS

Plain Film of the Abdomen

The plain film of the abdomen often shows a mild or moderate increase in the volume of gas in the large and small bowel but rarely suggests mechanical obstruction (Fig. 12.1). The rare fulminant case may show a roentgenographic appearance of toxic megacolon indistinguishable from that caused by other etiologies (Fig. 12.2). The colonic gas provides an excellent contrast medium for carefully inspecting the margins of the bowel when ischemic colitis is clinically suspected. In the exudative phase of the disease, multiple, smooth, soft tissue densities protruding into the lumen of the bowel may be detected and allow a presumptive diagnosis in the appropriate clinical setting (Figs. 12.1 and 12.2). These "thumbprints" will be present on the plain film in approximately one-fifth of patients with ischemic colitis. The intramural process frequently narrows the lumen and causes the colonic outline to appear ahaustral and rigid (Figs. 12.3 and 12.4). Intramural gas rarely accompanies colonic ischemia; when present the gas occurs in linear collections (Fig. 12.5) unlike the cystic accumulations seen in pneumatosis coli (Fig. 12.6).

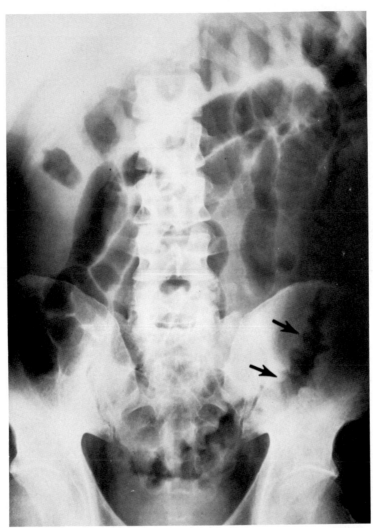

FIG. 12.1. PARALYTIC ILEUS ACCOMPANYING ISCHEMIC COLITIS
There is a mild increase in the volume of gas in both the small and large intestines. Despite the extensive exudative disease (arrows) evident in the narrowed descending and sigmoid colon, there is no proximal colonic dilatation.

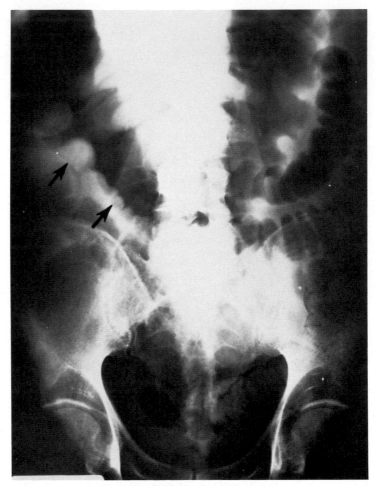

FIG. 12.2. TOXIC MEGACOLON

The dilatation of the transverse colon with soft tissue densities protruding into its lumen (arrows) create a pattern of toxic megacolon. In this 60-year-old man, the soft tissue masses represented submucosal hemorrhage of ischemic colitis rather than pseudopolyps.

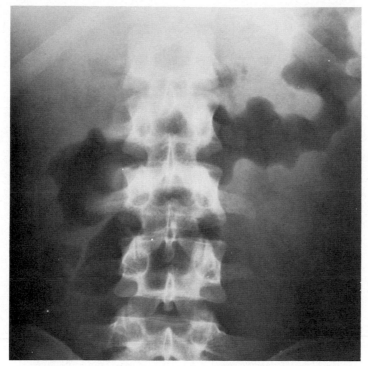

FIG. 12.3. ISCHEMIC COLITIS OF TRANSVERSE COLON

The transverse colon shows a distorted haustral pattern and rigidity of the bowel wall.

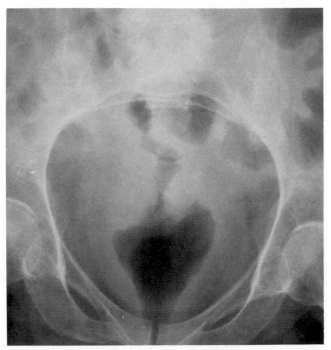

FIG. 12.4. ISCHEMIC COLITIS OF RECTOSIGMOID COLON

A short segment of the proximal rectum and distal sigmoid colon demonstrate the marked narrowing and haustral distortion. The narrowing is a consequence of both spasm and the intramural process.

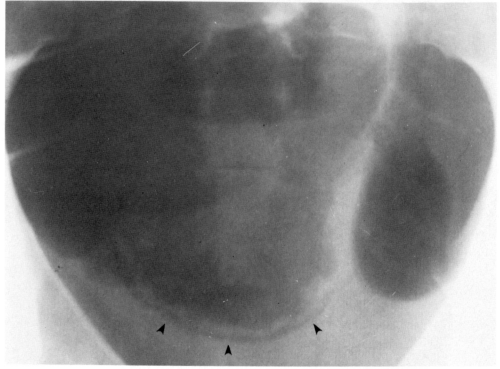

FIG. 12.5. PNEUMATOSIS IN ISCHEMIC CECUM

A linear collection of gas is apparent in the tip of the cecum (arrows). While the disease extended to the mid-ascending colon, this was the only segment to contain intramural gas.

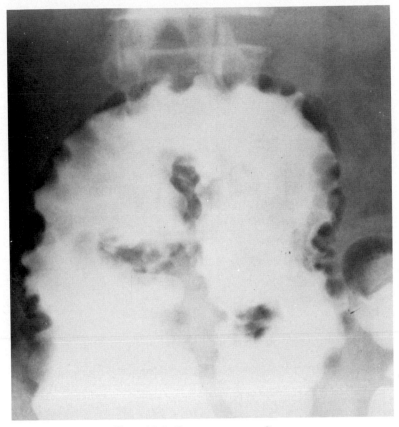

FIG. 12.6. PNEUMATOSIS COLI

The gas collections of pneumatosis coli are typically smooth and rounded and project beyond the bowel wall. Note how they also produce impressions on the barium column which could be confused with "thumbprinting."

Barium Enema

A barium enema, which is the radiographic procedure of choice in any patient with suspected ischemic colitis, will show evidence of an inflammatory process in over three-fourths of the patients. Occasionally, the plain film will demonstrate evidence of localized perforation and the enema should be performed with a water-soluble contrast agent. In addition to providing evidence of the underlying pathologic lesion, an immediate barium enema provides information as to the extent and distribution of the lesion if surgery is contemplated or it may detect coexistent colonic obstruction as the precipitant of the ischemic episode (Fig. 12.7).

The primary radiographic features of ischemic colitis have been shown to be the result of bleeding and edema in the bowel wall or sloughing of mucosa. The radiographic counterparts are, in the former, multiple, smooth, rounded, filling defects indenting the barium column, "thumbprinting" (Fig. 12.8); and in the latter, diffuse, tiny ulcerations (Fig. 12.9). The exudative process may take two additional forms: (1) multiple, parallel, thin transverse filling defects (transverse ridging) probably the result of blood dissecting in the colon wall (Fig. 12.10) or (2) thickening and blunting of mucosal folds (Fig. 12.11). The ulcerative phase infrequently demonstrates a cobblestone appearance on postevacuation films (Fig. 12.12). Nonspecific but common coincidental findings in all phases of ischemia include luminal narrowing, bowel wall rigidity, and loss of haustration (Fig. 12.13).

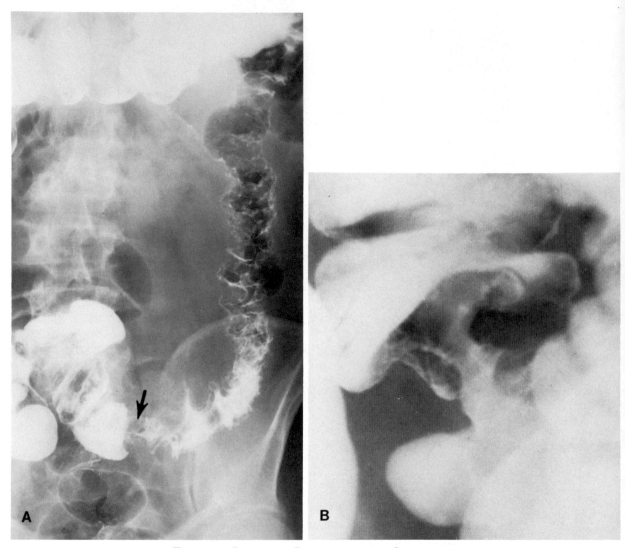

FIG. 12.7. ISCHEMIA PROXIMAL TO A CARCINOMA

The ischemic process involves the descending and proximal sigmoid colon. The
arrow (**A**) designates the position of the annular constricting carcinoma which is
shown in (**B**).

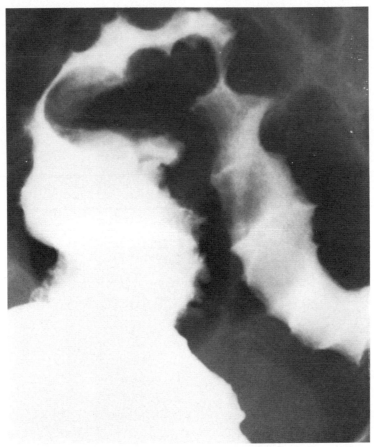

FIG. 12.8. ISCHEMIC COLITIS WITH HEMORRHAGE

Spot-film taken during the filling phase of a barium enema. The smooth indentations ("thumbprints") are the result of hemorrhage and/or edema in the submucosa.

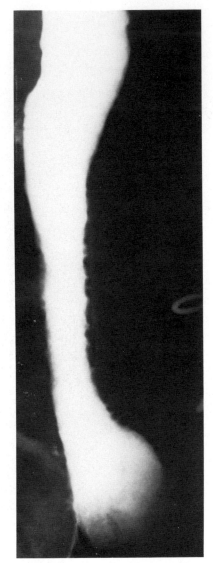

FIG. 12.9. ISCHEMIC COLITIS WITH ULCERATION
Shallow, thin mucosal ulcers are present in the descending colon, largely on the
lateral side. Deeper or collar button ulcers are not frequently seen in ischemic colitis.

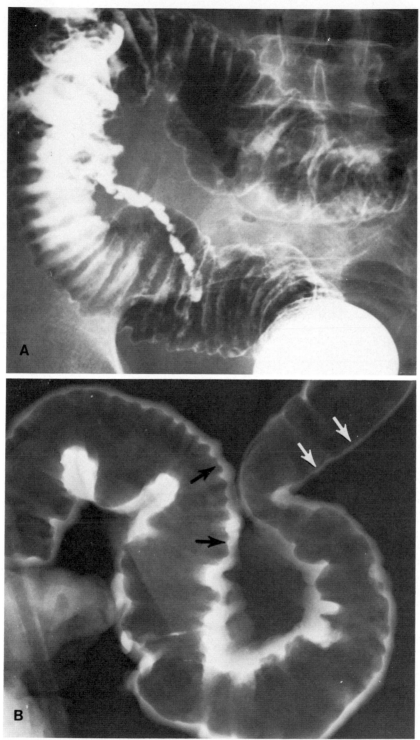

FIG. 12.10. ISCHEMIC COLITIS WITH TRANSVERSE RIDGING
(**A**) Multiple, transverse filling defects with slightly undulating margins affect most of the sigmoid colon. (**B**) The resected specimen from (**A**) filled with air demonstrates the same transverse markings along with the thickening of the bowel wall itself (black arrows) contrasting with the normal wall thickness (white arrows).

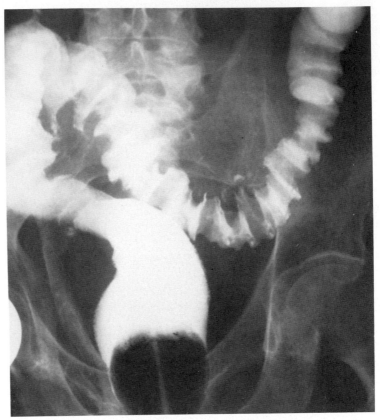

FIG. 12.11. ISCHEMIC COLITIS WITH MUCOSAL DISTORTION

An ischemic segment of sigmoid colon shows thickened, blunted mucosal folds.
The appearance simulates the muscle hypertrophy of diverticular disease.

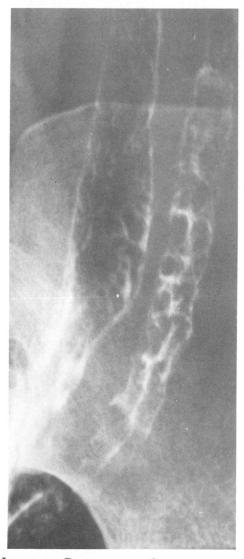

FIG. 12.12. ISCHEMIC COLITIS WITH COBBLESTONE APPEARANCE
Occasionally ischemic colitis creates a criss-crossing pattern of ulcerations which
is indistinguishable from the cobblestone appearance of Crohn's colitis.

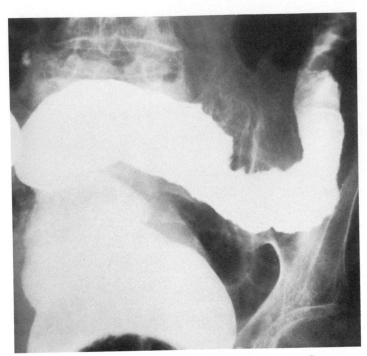

FIG. 12.13. NONSPECIFIC CHANGES IN ISCHEMIC COLITIS

The narrowing, rigidity, and irregularity of the sigmoid colon are nonspecific signs the interpretation of which would require historical and histologic correlation. In those patients in whom a diagnosis remains in doubt, a follow-up examination which demonstrates a rapid reversal to normal suggests an ischemic process.

The distribution of lesions observed in a group of 52 patients is shown in Fig. 12.14. It is noteworthy that the ischemic process involved the rectum (Fig. 12.15) in 19% of this group. The average length of involved colon by radiographic evaluation was approximately 42 cm. Patients with diseased segments greater than 50 cm had the poorest prognosis.

Occasionally, the luminal narrowing appears as an annular, constricting lesion on the initial examination and raises the suspicion of a carcinoma. In these patients, a repeat examination within 1 week will allow differentiation between a malignant and ischemic process since the latter process will invariably be altered from its original appearance (Fig. 12.16). In the patient with an unequivocal diagnosis who follows a benign clinical course, early hospital discharge is suitable as long as subsequent barium enema is performed in 2–3 weeks (Fig. 12.17). This will substantiate radiographically the benign evolution of the lesion and/or uncover the less than 5% of patients with stricture as a complication (Fig. 12.18).

PATHOLOGY

Acute ischemic colitis is characterized by mucosal necrosis with submucosal edema and hemorrhage, producing a variegated, cobblestone appearance to the luminal surface (Fig. 12.19). If transmural infarction occurs, greenish patches of gangrene will be apparent on the serosal surface. Microscopically, as might be expected in the older age group, a spectrum of arteriosclerotic changes can be observed in the vasa recta. The severity of such changes, however, is not clearly different from those which are present in a similar aged population without ischemic colitis and these observations support the thesis that a functional component may

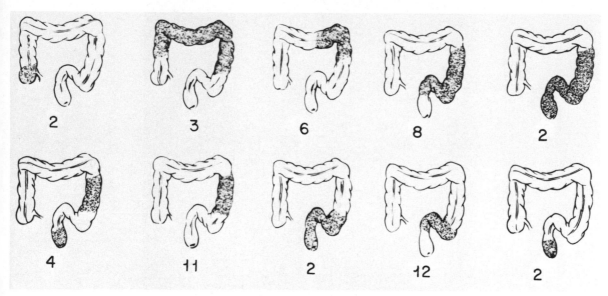

FIG. 12.14. DISTRIBUTION OF ISCHEMIC COLITIS IN 52 PATIENTS
The segmental involvement and approximate length of colonic ischemia is shown
in 52 patients. Rectal involvement is present in 19% of patients.

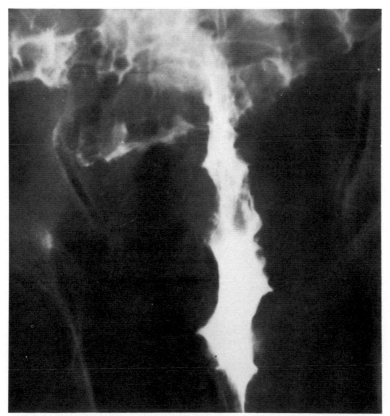

FIG. 12.15. ISCHEMIC COLITIS OF RECTUM
Marked narrowing and "thumbprinting" of the rectum in a patient with extensive
disease extending to the sigmoid colon. Frequently the rectal disease is not evident
by barium enema and is only detected by proctoscopy.

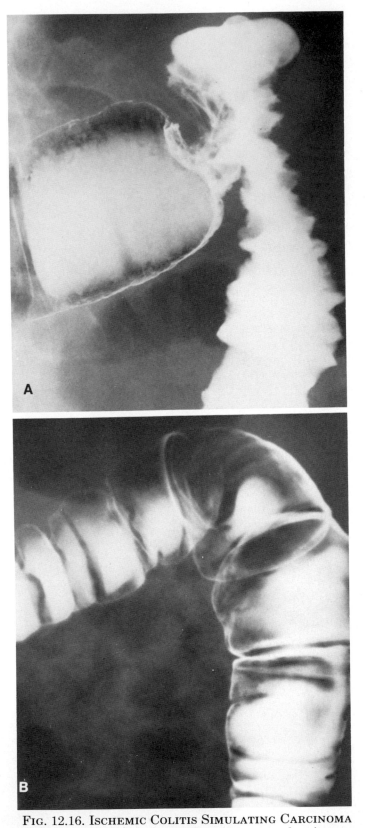

FIG. 12.16. ISCHEMIC COLITIS SIMULATING CARCINOMA

(A) The annular narrowing of the distal transverse colon just proximal to the ischemic segment of splenic flexure raised the question of a coexistent carcinoma. (B) An examination performed 8 days later demonstrates complete reversal to normal. The narrowing was most likely due to sustained spasm.

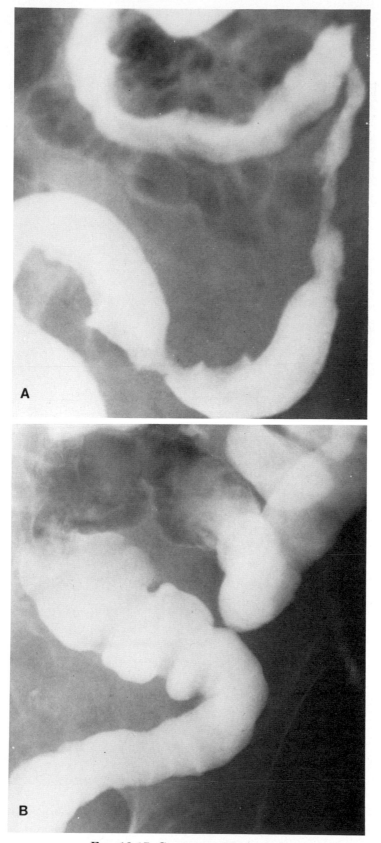

FIG. 12.17. COMPLETE HEALING

The ischemic segment in (**A**) was re-examined in 18 days (**B**) and demonstrated no residual disease.

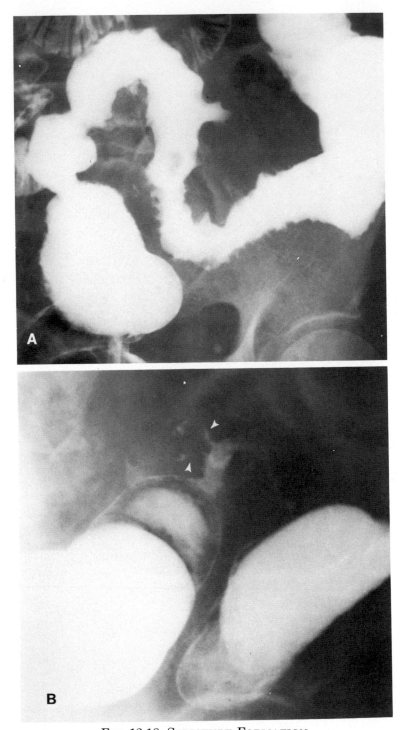

FIG. 12.18. STRICTURE FORMATION

After 19 days the ischemic segment in (**A**) healed but with a short, narrow stricture in the mid-sigmoid colon (**B**). Two sinus tracks (arrows) are also evident.

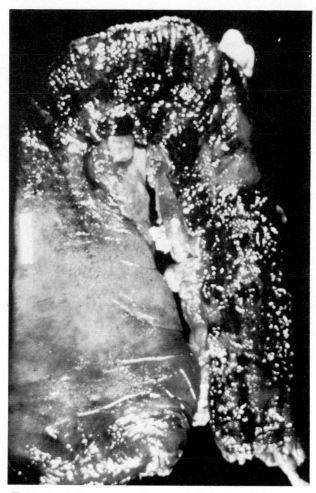

FIG. 12.19. ISCHEMIC COLITIS OF SIGMOID COLON
The characteristic multiple, raised, smooth, hemorrhagic areas of an ischemic
segment of sigmoid colon are illustrated.

be an important contributing factor. The increased frequency with which capillary
and venous thrombi have been noted within the ischemic segments has given rise to
an alternative explanation that an intravascular coagulation syndrome, occurring
principally in the gut, is the basis of the ischemia. However such observations have
also been made in other acute inflammatory colonic processes, and it is not clear
whether this is the cause or the result of the disease process itself.

DIFFERENTIAL DIAGNOSIS

Iatrogenically induced disease must be considered in any patient with previous
colonic or abdominal vascular surgery (Figs. 12.20 and 12.21). A variety of diseases
may be accompanied by hemorrhage or other exudative processes within the bowel
wall and their differentiation by radiographic criteria is impossible. Historical or
laboratory information may be available in excluding bleeding diathesis such as may
occur with hemophilia, Henoch-Schoenlein purpura, idiopathic thrombocytopenic
purpura, anticoagulation overdose, or hemolytic-uremic syndrome. Infrequently, the
colon is the first site of an ischemic episode occurring in primary arteritides so that
invariably a previous history will allow this consideration to be excluded. Intravas-

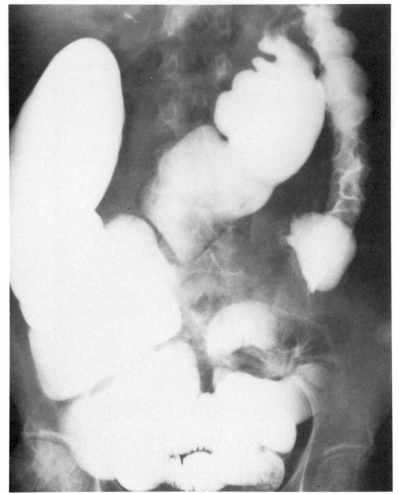

FIG. 12.20. ISCHEMIC COLITIS FOLLOWING ABDOMINOPERINEAL RESECTION
This patient underwent an abdominoperineal resection of an adenocarcinoma of the distal colon 3 months previously. Characteristic signs of ischemia are present distal to the splenic flexure. Note sparing of the very distal segment which may be explained by collateral vessels available from the abdominal wall about the colostomy site.

cular occlusion occurring in patients with sickle-cell disease will produce an ischemic process radiographically indistinguishable from the spontaneous form (Fig. 12.22). Finally, drugs used for oral contraception may cause a segmental colitis consistent with an ischemic process and differ clinically only in the younger group of patients that are affected.

Mechanical factors precipitating an ischemic episode must always be considered particularly in the age group under consideration which also suffers from the highest incidence of volvulus and carcinoma. Frequently, the episode of volvulus will be sustained so that its contribution will be clear-cut (Fig. 12.23). It is important that

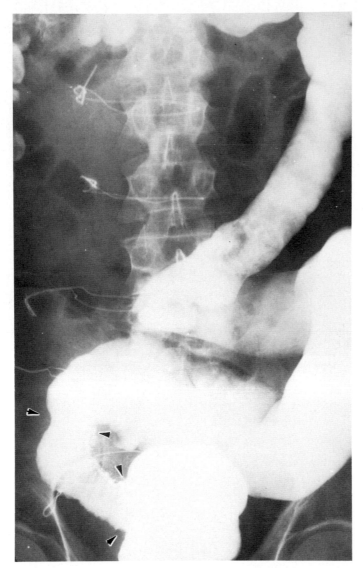

FIG. 12.21. ISCHEMIC COLITIS FOLLOWING ABDOMINAL ANEURYSMECTOMY

Seven days following repair of an abdominal aortic aneurysm, this emergency examination was performed because of bright red, rectal bleeding. A short segment of distal sigmoid colon (arrows) demonstrates signs of ischemia which were confirmed by sigmoidoscopy. A repeat barium enema after seven days of conservative therapy demonstrated reversal to normal.

an obstructing carcinoma be carefully sought since the presence of the more extensive ischemic lesion may distract an observer from detecting a coexistent cancer.

While direct colonoscopic observation and biopsy may allow a differentiation of ischemic colitis from ulcerative colitis and Crohn's colitis, it is to be emphasized that there is a considerable overlap in both the gross and histologic appearance. In such situations, the acute, self-limiting, nonrecurring characteristics of ischemic colitis should differentiate it from the more indolent, recurring features of these two more common inflammatory diseases.

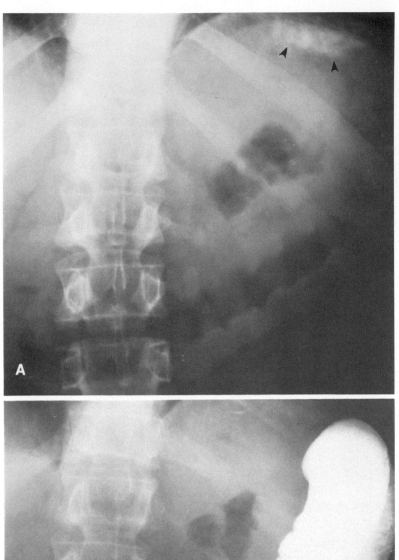

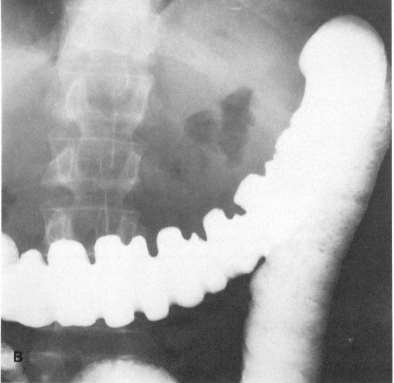

FIG. 12.22. ISCHEMIC COLITIS IN SICKLE-CELL DISEASE
(A) Soft tissue densities protruding into the lumen of the distal transverse colon
are evident in this patient with homozygous sickle-cell disease. Calcification beneath
the diaphragm (arrows) is consistent with an infarcted spleen. (B) The barium
enema demonstrates the disease to be limited to the distal transverse colon and the
abnormality resolved spontaneously on conservative therapy.

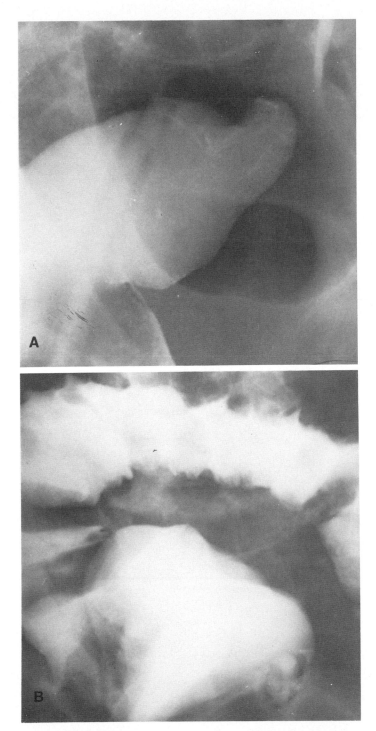

FIG. 12.23. ISCHEMIC COLITIS FOLLOWING VOLVULUS
(A) Complete obstruction due to a volvulus of the distal sigmoid colon. (B) Examination performed 3 days later demonstrates ischemic changes of the sigmoid colon.

BIBLIOGRAPHY

Morson, B. C.: Pathology of ischemic colitis. Clin. Gastroenterol., *1:* 765, 1972.

Ochsner, J. L., Cooley, D. A., and DeBakey, M. E.: Associated intraabdominal lesions encountered during resection of aortic aneurysms: Surgical considerations. Dis. Colon Rectum, *3:* 485, 1960.

Schwartz, S. S., and Boley, S. J.: Ischemic origin of ulcerative colitis associated with potentially obstructing lesions of colon. Radiology, *102:* 249, 1972.

Schwartz, S. S., Boley, S. J., Robinson, K., Krieger, H., Schultz, L., and Allen, A. C.: Roentgeno-logic features of vascular disorders of the intestines. Radiol. Clin. North Am., *2:* 71, 1964.

Wittenberg, J., Athanasoulis, C. A., Shapiro, J. H., and Williams, L. F., Jr.: A radiological approach to the patient with acute, extensive bowel ischemia. Radiology, *106:* 13, 1973.

Wittenberg, J., Athanasoulis, C. A., Williams, L. F., Jr., Paredes, S., O'Sullivan, P., and Brown, B.: Ischemic colitis. Radiology and pathophysiology. Am. J. Roentgenol., *123:* 287, 1975.

Wittenberg, J., O'Sullivan, P., and Williams, L. F., Jr.: Ischemic colitis after abdominoperineal resection. Gastroenterology, *69:* 1321, 1975.

13

Angiography of the Colon

CHRISTOS A. ATHANASOULIS, M.D.

INTRODUCTION

The main applications of angiography in patients with colonic disorders are three: (1) Diagnosis of primary vascular disease which may affect anatomic integrity and/ or function of the colon. (2) Diagnosis of colonic disorders which may secondarily involve blood vessels. (3) Management of some of the above conditions with angiographic methods. The arteriographic demonstration of an embolic occlusion of the mesenteric artery or its branches is an example of the first application. The diagnosis of tumors or inflammation based on angiographic patterns of the vessels secondarily affected by these conditions constitutes an example of the second application. The third and newest application is therapeutic. It is exemplified by the intra-arterial infusion of vasodilatory drugs for the management of bowel ischemia and the infusion of vasopressin or the use of transcatheter embolization for the control of colonic bleeding.

The distinction between primary vascular disorders and those indirectly involving blood vessels is not always possible. The cause and effect relationship between ischemia and inflammation can not be sharply defined. These problems, already discussed in Chapters 9, 10, 11, and 12, have resulted in a nonuniform and rather confusing terminology of colonic vascular disorders. The reasons are multiple but the following three factors are the most pertinent: (1) Morphologically, the splanchnic vasculature can respond to various pathologic conditions in a limited number of ways. Overlap of angiographic changes should therefore be expected among various disorders. (2) Physiologically, the splanchnic vascular bed is complex and influenced by numerous extrinsic, intrinsic, local and/or systemic factors. Our knowledge lacks a unifying concept of this complex circulation. (3) Angiographically the degree of resolution is too limited to allow a comprehensive study of the small colonic vessels. It is therefore with these limitations in mind that angiography of colonic disorders will be approached in this chapter.

METHOD

Abdominal aortography and selective mesenteric arteriography are performed percutaneously according to the Seldinger and Ödman techniques.

The superior mesenteric, inferior mesenteric, and celiac arteries should be studied for complete angiographic evaluation of the colon. The sequence of selective injections will be dictated by the clinical problem. For instance, in a patient with rectal bleeding of unknown origin, the superior mesenteric arteriogram is performed first, because in 75% of such patients the bleeding site is angiographically found in the right colon. If, on the other hand, bleeding is the result of resection via the colonoscope of a polyp in the descending colon, an inferior mesenteric arteriogram may be all that is necessary for demonstration of the bleeding site and treatment with intra-arterial vasopressin.

It has been suggested that the inferior mesenteric artery should be the first vessel to be studied before the urinary bladder fills with contrast medium thus obscuring the rectosigmoid vessels. This may have merit in patients who have no indwelling catheter in the bladder or those who are unable to void during the examination.

Serial filming should be extended for 25–30 sec so that all three phases, arterial, capillary, and venous, are depicted. Direct serial magnification arteriography is a prerequisite for the evaluation of small vascular malformations. Pharmacoangiography using 25–50 mg of intra-arterial tolazoline hydrochloride enhances the venous phase. This, however, should be avoided in the patient evaluated for bleeding as some of the diagnostic features of angiodysplasia, for example, are based on the time sequence of vein opacification. This sequence can be altered with the use of a vasodilator.

The veins draining the colon may also be studied with direct catheterization of the portal vein and its tributaries using the percutaneous transhepatic route. The potential of this method in the evaluation of colonic disorders has not been explored yet.

Complications of percutaneous arteriography of colonic disorders are the same as those with percutaneous transfemoral artery catheterization of any visceral vessel, namely 0.03% death, 0.1% serious, and 1% minor.

ANATOMY

Large Arteries

The normal anatomy of large vessels of the colon must be known before abnormalities can be appreciated. The reader is referred to Chapter 2 for a description of the pertinent anatomy of these vessels.

Variations from the normal are also worth considering not only for theoretical but for practical reasons as well. Fig. 13.1 serves to illustrate this point. The middle colic artery originates not from the superior mesenteric but rather from the celiac artery. Thus, in this patient the angiographic study of the colon would have been incomplete without a celiac axis arteriogram. Other relevant variations of the colonic arteries

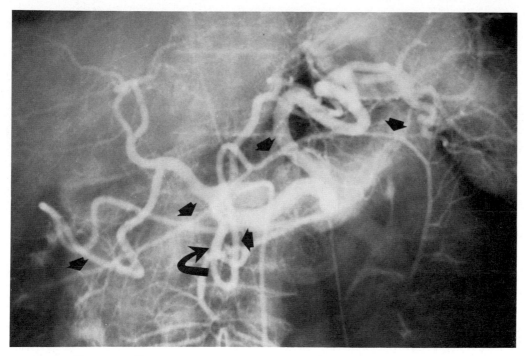

FIG. 13.1. VARIATION OF THE MIDDLE COLIC ARTERY ORIGIN
Celiac axis arteriogram. The dorsal pancreatic artery (curved arrow) gives origin to the middle colic artery (arrowheads).

include: (1) origin of the middle colic from a replaced right hepatic artery stemming from the superior mesenteric artery; (2) accessory middle colic arising either from the superior mesenteric or the dorsal pancreatic, a branch of the splenic artery (Fig. 13.2); and (3) right colic origin from the middle colic (30%), the ileocolic (12%), and not present (18%).

Small Vessels

From secondary or tertiary arterial arcades arise the vasa recta which reach the bowel wall at the tenia mesocolica and then divide into short and long branches continuing subserosally. These branches pierce through the muscularis and form a rich vascular plexus in the submucosa which ramifies on the inner surface of the muscularis mucosa. Arterial branches arise from the submucosal plexus and extend to the base of the mucosa where they branch extensively and lead directly into channels that pass to the surface capillary plexus. Seen from the mucosal surface this capillary plexus assumes a honeycomb appearance due to the vascular channels that surround the luminal openings of the vertically arranged crypts of Lieberkühn (Plate 13.1, A, p. 346).

This extensive arteriolar and precapillary network together with the precapillary sphincters constitute the resistance vessels largely responsible for the autoregulatory control of intestinal blood flow. Blood flow changes at this microcirculatory level are probably responsible for the low flow states which will be discussed later in this chapter.

ISCHEMIA

Ischemia of the colon is presently the most common vascular disorder of the

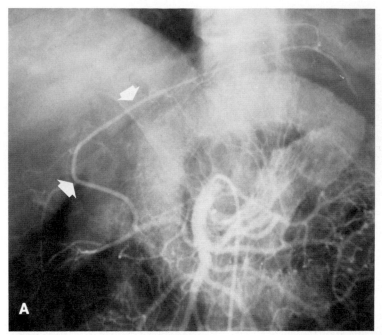

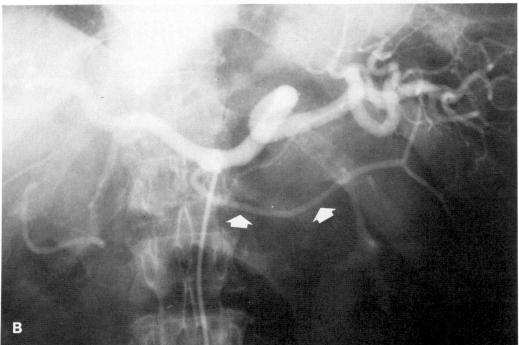

FIG. 13.2. ACCESSORY MIDDLE COLIC ARTERY

(A) Superior mesenteric arteriogram. The arrowheads point to the middle colic artery supplying the transverse colon. (B) Celiac axis arteriogram in the same patient as in (A). An accessory left branch of the middle colic artery takes origin from the dorsal pancreatic artery (arrowheads).

intestines. Possible factors predisposing to colon ischemia are: (1) inherently lower blood flow to the colon as compared to the small bowel; (2) reduced blood flow to the colon during functional motor activity—this is contrary to increased blood flow to the small bowel during digestion and peristalsis; (3) blood flow changes in response to changes in environment, eating a meal or emotionally stressful situations; and (4) colon blood flow mostly affected by autonomic stimulation.

Reduction of blood flow may be due to morphologic changes in the mesenteric vasculature—atheroma, emboli, vasculitis, or to generalized poor perfusion—shock, cardiac decompensation, etc. However, whatever the cause or predisposing factor may be, the end result of ischemia is the same, namely a spectrum ranging from reversible morphologic and functional changes to transmural necrosis of the bowel wall.

Ischemic lesions of the colon may be classified into two general categories: (1) occlusive vascular disease; and (2) nonocclusive ischemia or low flow states.

Occlusive Vascular Disease

Superior Mesenteric Vessels

The cecum, ascending and right transverse colon along with a portion of the distal small bowel may become ischemic as a result of blood flow obstruction by an embolus or thrombus. Venous thrombosis accounts for less than 10% of instances of acute occlusive ischemia. In addition to the idiopathic form, occlusion of the mesenteric vein or its tributaries may be secondary to obstruction of venous outflow by abdominal tumors or stagnation of blood in patients with portal hypertension.

The clinical symptoms vary depending on the extent and severity of ischemia. They include any or all of the following: vomiting, diarrhea, abdominal pain, and blood in the stool. Leukocytosis is common but not specific.

A plain film of the abdomen at this stage may suggest the diagnosis of extensive infarction by revealing the absence of gas, submucosal edema, or hemorrhage in the bowel wall or gas in the portal vein. More important is that other conditions such as a perforated viscus can be excluded.

The definitive diagnosis is established with angiography which should be performed as soon as the disease is clinically suspected. Midstream abdominal aortography in both the anteroposterior and lateral planes should be performed followed by superior mesenteric arteriography. The former will provide information about the origin of the mesenteric vessels; the latter about the presence of multiple occlusions, the extent of collateral vessel development, and the patency of mesenteric veins.

Obstruction of the superior mesenteric artery resulting in bowel ischemia is equally divided between acute thrombosis on the basis of an atheroma and embolism. Thrombosis involves the origin or proximal segment of the superior mesenteric artery whereas emboli lodge more distally at bifurcations (Figs. 13.3 and 13.4).

Collateral Flow to an Occluded Superior Mesenteric Artery

Occlusion or a hemodynamically significant stenosis at the origin of the superior mesenteric artery results in collateral flow developing through the pancreaticoduodenal arcades and the marginal anastomotic artery of the colon (marginal artery of Drummond). The dorsal pancreatic-superior mesenteric artery anastomosis may also become functional. The marginal or meandering branch of the inferior mesenteric artery is the most common collateral pathway terminating in the middle colic artery (Figs. 13.3 and 13.5).

Neither of the above mentioned collateral pathways can effectively reconstitute

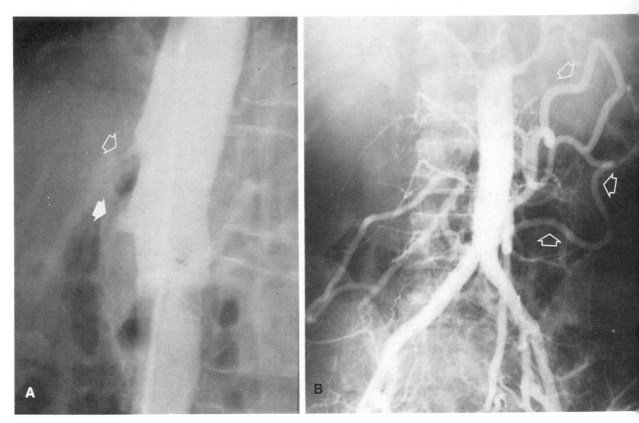

FIG. 13.3. THROMBOTIC OCCLUSION OF THE CELIAC AXIS AND THE SUPERIOR
MESENTERIC ARTERY

(A) Midstream abdominal aortogram, lateral projection. The open arrowhead
points to the origin of the occluded celiac axis. The arrowhead points to the occluded
origin of the superior mesenteric artery. (B) Midstream abdominal aortogram,
anteroposterior projection. Same patient as in (A). The arrowheads point to an
enlarged meandering vessel which serves as a collateral pathway between the
inferior mesenteric and the superior mesenteric artery, distal to the point of
occlusion.

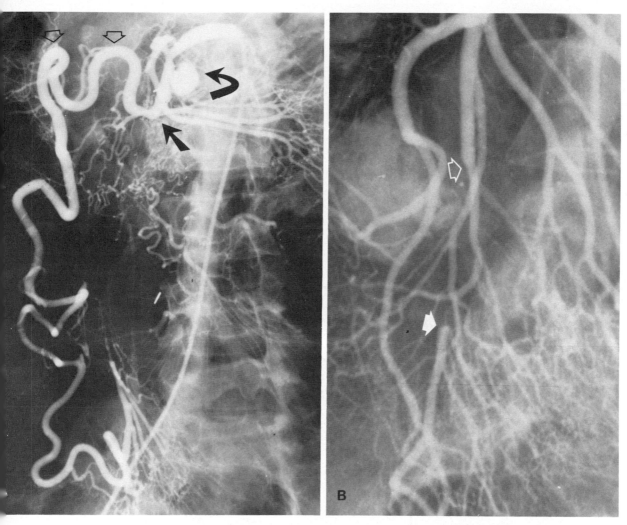

FIG. 13.4. EMBOLIC OCCLUSIONS OF SUPERIOR MESENTERIC ARTERIAL BRANCHES
(**A**) Superior mesenteric arteriogram in a patient with abdominal pain and diarrhea. The straight arrow points to the occluded superior mesenteric artery. Collateral flow to the distal branches of the superior mesenteric artery has developed via the enlarged middle colic artery (open arrowheads). The curved arrow points to a false aneurysm of the proximal superior mesenteric artery, the result of previous operative embolectomy. (**B**) Embolic occlusion of a small branch of the superior mesenteric artery. This is on a different patient than the one shown in (**A**). Superior mesenteric arteriogram was performed because of diarrhea and abdominal pain 2 weeks following coronary angiography. The open arrowhead shows the point of occlusion and the arrowhead a reconstituted branch distally. Symptoms subsided with no operation.

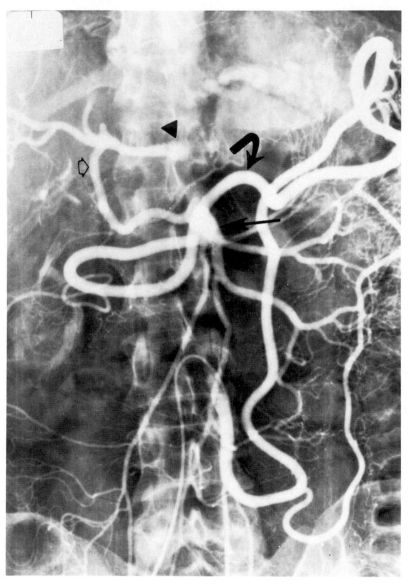

Fɪɢ. 13.5. Cᴏʟʟᴀᴛᴇʀᴀʟ Fʟᴏᴡ ᴛᴏ ᴀɴ Oᴄᴄʟᴜᴅᴇᴅ Sᴜᴘᴇʀɪᴏʀ Mᴇsᴇɴᴛᴇʀɪᴄ Aʀᴛᴇʀʏ
    Inferior mesenteric arteriogram on a patient with occluded superior mesenteric
and celiac arteries. Blood flow to the superior mesenteric artery (straight arrow) is
reconstituted via the left colic-middle colic arterial pathways (curved arrow). The
arrowhead points to the celiac axis which is reconstituted via the pancreaticoduo-
denal-gastroduodenal pathway (open arrowhead). (Reproduced with permission
from Marshak, R. H., and Lindner, A. E.: *Radiology of the Small Intestine*, 2nd Ed.
W. B. Saunders, Philadelphia, 1976.)

blood flow, if the point of obstruction is distal to the origin of the middle colic artery. In this instance, small collateral vessels form from adjacent jejunal branches in an attempt to breach the occlusion.

Inferior Mesenteric Vessels

The inferior mesenteric artery is frequently occluded at its origin from atheromatous deposits. However, infarction of the left colon from thrombosis or embolization is rare due to the abundant collateral supply from the middle colic or the hemorrhoidal arteries.

Infarction of the left colon occurs in 2–5% of patients undergoing aortoiliac reconstruction. In addition to the interruption of the inferior mesenteric artery other factors which may contribute to this complication include: (1) compromise of collateral blood flow; (2) direct trauma to the left colon; (3) thrombosis of the inferior mesenteric vein; and (4) intraoperative hypotension in combination with any of the above.

The reported incidence of this complication is 2.5%. However, the mortality among patients who develop this problem may be as high as 6.5%. Therefore, we consider aortography an essential study in the pre- and postoperative evaluation of patients with abdominal aortic aneurysms or aortoiliac occlusive disease (Fig. 13.6).

Collateral Flow to an Occluded Inferior Mesenteric Artery

In the presence of a hemodynamically significant stenosis or obstruction at the origin of the inferior mesenteric artery collateral flow is supplied from the marginal anastomotic artery, middle colic-left colic arcade, the arc of Riolan and from anastomoses between the superior hemorrhoidal—a branch of the inferior mesenteric—and the middle and inferior hemorroidal arteries—branches of the internal iliac vessels (Fig. 13.7).

"Aortoiliac Steal"

This term has been applied to describe large or small bowel infarction following aortoiliac grafting with interruption of the inferior mesenteric artery. It has been postulated that because of the reconstruction, blood flow to the extremities improves at the expense of the mesenteric circulation, therefore the term "steal." I propose that both the term and the explanation are incorrect. Preoperative or postoperative aortography in such patients has shown that both the celiac and superior mesenteric arteries are occluded or their lumens considerably compromised. Blood supply to the entire bowel is therefore from the marginal branch of the inferior mesenteric artery. Interruption of this vessel would result in ischemia and gangrene (Fig. 13.6).

Ischemic Proctitis

There have been patients with isolated ischemic changes of the rectum seen on sigmoidoscopy. Pain is the typical presenting symptom. Aortography has demonstrated an occluded or markedly stenotic origin of the inferior mesenteric artery. Relief from pain following bypass of the occluded inferior mesenteric artery segment has been reported. This entity is to be distinguished from "ischemic colitis" which is not associated with vascular occlusion and which is discussed in Chapter 12.

Miscellaneous Conditions, Potential Causes of Occlusive Ischemia

There are a variety of conditions which may primarily or secondarily involve the mesenteric blood vessels thus reducing blood flow and causing ischemia. These include the following.

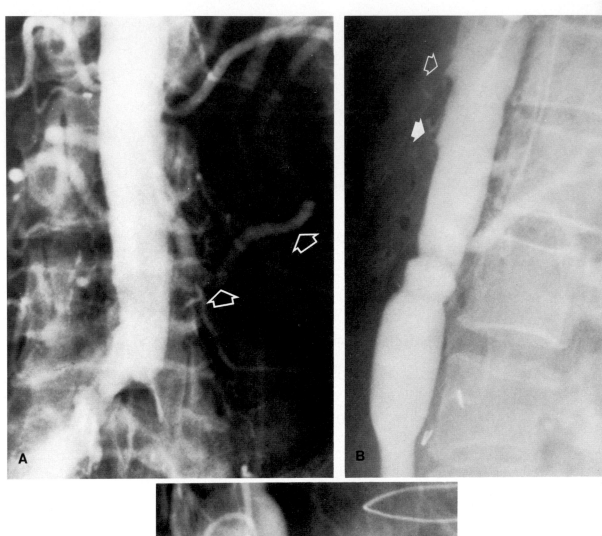

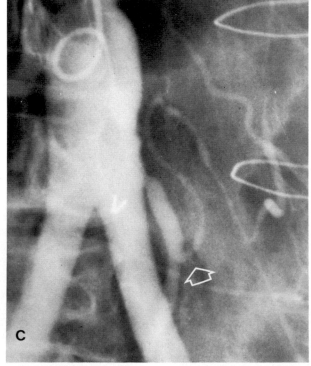

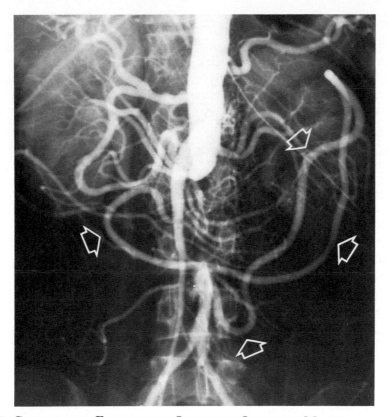

FIG. 13.7. COLLATERAL FLOW TO AN OCCLUDED INFERIOR MESENTERIC ARTERY
Translumbar aortogram. The aorta is occluded. The middle-left colic arterial pathway (arrowheads) reconstitutes blood flow to the inferior mesenteric artery and the distal aorta.

FIG. 13.6. COLON INFARCTION FOLLOWING AORTOFEMORAL RECONSTRUCTION
(A) Preoperative aortogram. Study performed elsewhere shows an enlarged left colic artery (arrowheads). Despite the fact that no lateral view was obtained, the enlarged colic artery should have signaled the possibility of superior mesenteric artery occlusion. The patient underwent aortofemoral bypass graft procedure with reimplantation of the inferior mesenteric artery. Twenty-four hours later he developed abdominal pain, fever, and leukocytosis. (B) Postoperative aortogram lateral projection. The open arrowhead points to the occluded celiac axis. The arrowhead points to the occluded superior mesenteric artery. (C) Postoperative aortogram anteroposterior view. The re-implanted inferior mesenteric artery is opacified. However, the large left colic artery is no longer visualized (arrowhead). Occlusion of this blood vessel at surgery in the presence of compromised superior mesenteric arterial blood flow resulted in bowel infarction.

Aortic dissection

Aortic dissection may involve the origins of the mesenteric vessels and lead to bowel infarction. The mechanism is either due to narrowing of the lumen of the mesenteric branches by the dissection or to the formation of a false channel for aortic flow which does not open into the mesenteric vessels. Aortography is the only method available to establish the diagnosis and delineate the extent of the dissection.

Volvulus or hernia incarceration

Intestinal blood flow can be compromised because of strangulation following volvulus or hernia incarceration. In most instances the diagnosis will be suspected on the basis of clinical and plain film findings. However, at times the volvulus is not recognized and angiography may be performed to diagnose occlusive or nonocclusive intestinal ischemia. In these instances, familiarity with the spiral arrangement that mesenteric vessels assume in the presence of a volvulus or hernia will lead to the correct diagnosis and appropriate management (Fig. 13.8).

Vasculitis

Polyarteritis nodosa, lupus, scleroderma, rheumatoid arthritis, and dermatomyositis have all been known to produce a necrotizing arteritis which may involve mesenteric vessels. Typically, there is segmental involvement of small and medium sized branches with perivascular inflammation and fibrinoid necrosis. This may lead to rupture, aneurysm formation and/or thrombosis, all detectable with magnification selective arteriography.

A very characteristic nodularity and beaded appearance has been angiographically observed with involvement of the colic arteries by periarteritis nodosa. The angiographic findings are the result of aneurysmal dilatations associated with areas of intramural dissections. These changes can lead to intra-abdominal or retroperitoneal hemorrhage and intestinal infarction (Fig. 13.9).

Infarction without Major Vessel Occlusion (nonocclusive ischemia—low flow states)

In about 50% of the patients with intestinal infarction, no major mesenteric vessel occlusion is found at surgical exploration or post mortem. Thus, the term nonocclusive bowel ischemia. Within this group it is important to distinguish between two completely different entities. First, is acute extensive nonocclusive mesenteric ischemia which involves the superior mesenteric vascular bed, therefore small bowel and the right half of the colon. Second, is so-called "ischemic colitis." Distinction between these two entities is fundamental because the radiologic approach to the diagnosis, the treatment, the natural history, and the outcome is completely different.

Acute Extensive Nonocclusive Mesenteric Ischemia

As the term indicates angiographically and at surgery or autopsy the intestinal arteries and veins are patent in the presence of infarction. However, experimental and clinical studies have shown that in these patients there is profound constriction of the mesenteric arteries which may lead to bowel ischemia.

Acute mesenteric ischemia is likely to develop in patients over the age of 50 with any of the following predisposing conditions: (1) arteriosclerotic or valvular heart disease; (2) congestive heart failure with digitalis therapy and use of diuretics; (3) cardiac arrhythmias; (4) recent myocardial infarction; or (5) hypovolemia or hypotension of any etiology.

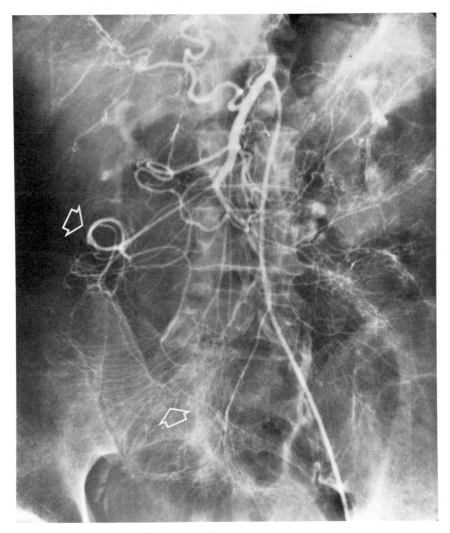

FIG. 13.8. CECAL VOLVULUS

Superior mesenteric arteriogram in a patient with abdominal pain and bloody
diarrhea. The branches of the ileocolic artery have assumed a whirl configuration
(arrowheads) the result of cecal volvulus.

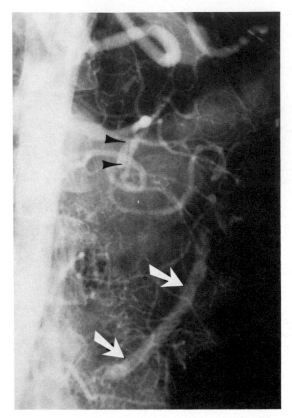

FIG. 13.9. PERIARTERITIS OF THE COLIC ARTERY

Midstream abdominal aortogram in a patient with intra-abdominal hemorrhage.
The white arrows point to a sausage-like structure representing dissection of the left
colic artery. The black arrowheads point to dissection of the left renal artery. At
exploration the left colic artery had ruptured with bleeding into the sigmoid
mesocolon. (Reproduced with permission from Bockus, H. L.: *Gastroenterology,* 3rd
Ed., Vol. 4. W. B. Saunders, Philadelphia, 1976.)

Abdominal pain is present in 75–98% of these patients. Unexplained abdominal
distention, nausea, vomiting, diarrhea, or rectal bleeding may be present. Signs of
peritoneal irritation or leukocytosis out of proportion to the physical findings are
signs of advancing intestinal necrosis.

Once the disease is clinically suspected, radiographs of the chest and the abdomen
should be obtained followed by emergency angiography, which is performed in place
of a "first-look" exploratory laporotomy. The angiographic features of low flow
states are mainly those of intense mesenteric constriction (Fig. 13.10). If at angiography occlusive disease is excluded and vasoconstriction is found, the catheter is left
in the superior mesenteric artery and papaverine hydrochloride is infused in an
attempt to reverse vasoconstriction and re-establish blood flow to the bowel. General
supportive measures especially volume replacement are established as early as
possible. Papaverine infusion is continued for approximately 24 hr when a repeat
arteriogram is performed. If there is no vasoconstriction and the clinical condition
has improved, the infusion is discontinued, otherwise a "second-look" abdominal
exploration is performed.

Because of the above described aggressive approach to the diagnosis and therapy
of low flow states, some improvement has been realized in the mortality rate which
had been approaching 90–100%.

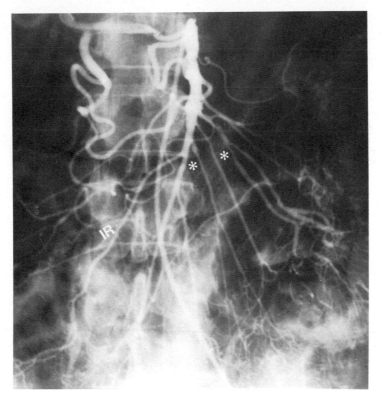

FIG. 13.10. NONOCCLUSIVE MESENTERIC ISCHEMIA—LOW FLOW STATE

Superior mesenteric arteriogram on a patient who following a myocardial infarct presented with abdominal pain and bloody diarrhea. The branches of the superior mesenteric artery are constricted. The sausage-like configuration of several jejunal arteries is typical of the angiographic appearance of mesenteric vascular constriction in low flow states.

Ischemic Colitis

The reader is referred to Chapter 12 for a detailed discussion of the etiology, pathophysiology, and radiologic manifestations of "ischemic colitis."

The term is not correct because "colitis" denotes inflammation and the milder of these reversible ischemic episodes are not inflammatory but hemorrhagic. However, in absence of a better term, "ischemic colitis" describes the condition classically shown by air or barium enema to produce smooth round indentations of the barium column, the so-called thumbprints, the result of submucosal edema and hemorrhage.

Angiography has little to offer in this group of patients. When performed, inferior mesenteric arteriography shows no arterial or venous occlusions but rather hypervascularity of the bowel wall with intense opacification of the draining veins (Fig. 13.11). These findings are not specific, simply indicating hyperemia at the site of the initial insult.

The initial problem in the management of patients with suspected "ischemic colitis" is therefore to distinguish them from patients with acute mesenteric ischemia. In general patients with the former have mild pain and minimal physical findings, while patients with the latter appear more sick, have more severe pain and often present a history of a pre-existing cardiac disorder. If acute mesenteric ischemia is suspected, angiography is performed first. If it is not believed to be present, a barium enema should be performed within 48 hr of the acute episode in

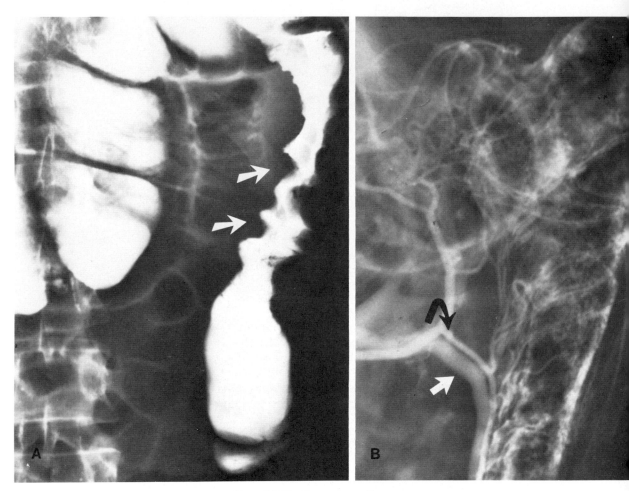

FIG. 13.11. ISCHEMIC COLITIS

(A) Barium examination of the colon in a patient with diarrhea and crampy abdominal pain. Spot-film of the splenic flexure. The arrows point to smooth indentations on the barium column the so-called thumbprints, the result of submucosal edema and/or hemorrhage. (B) Inferior mesenteric arteriogram, in the same patient, shows patent arteries (curved arrow), veins (straight arrow), and hypervascularity of the bowel wall. (Reproduced with permission from Bockus, H. L.: *Gastroenterology*, 3rd Ed., Vol. 4. W. B. Saunders, Philadelphia, 1976.)

order to establish the diagnosis of "ischemic colitis." If differentiation is not possible, an enema, performed with air alone, may be considered. If this study does not show changes indicative of ischemic colitis, then angiography should be carried out.

INFLAMMATORY BOWEL DISEASE

Increased vascularity, intense opacification of the bowel wall, and arteriovenous shunting or intense opacification of the draining veins are the typical angiographic findings of inflammation (Figs. 13.12 and 13.13). The increased vascularity in response to or in conjunction with inflammation can be best appreciated in injected specimens viewed under the dissecting microscope (Plate 13.1, B, p. 346). However, with today's degree of resolution angiography can not differentiate among various inflammatory conditions of the bowel especially in the early stages.

In later stages of progressive or recurrent inflammatory bowel disease there is one angiographic feature that has been observed more frequently with regional colitis (Crohn's disease) than with ulcerative colitis. This feature is tortuosity of the vasa recta as they pierce through the thickened muscularis and a reduction in the number of vasa recta in severely diseased and fibrosed bowel segments (Fig. 13.13).

Although nonspecific, the angiographic features of colonic inflammation should be known. There have been instances when rectal bleeding was the first manifestation of colitis. Angiography performed to localize the bleeding site revealed the features of the underlying inflammation.

One additional application of angiographic methods is the intra-arterial infusion of vasopressin for the control of bleeding complicating ulcerative or Crohn's colitis. Naturally this is a temporizing maneuver, but it is helpful in that it may change an emergency colectomy to a more elective operative intervention (Fig. 13.14).

COLITIS PROXIMAL TO COLONIC NEOPLASMS

Colitis has been noted to develop proximal to obstructing and nonobstructing carcinomas of the colon. It is now believed that this "colitis" is of ischemic origin. As a matter of fact it has been reported that 10% of patients with ischemic colitis have an associated carcinoma and that another 10% have some other condition interfering with normal colonic motility. This association must be kept in mind during radiologic examination of the colon (see Chapters 12 and 17).

VASCULAR PATHOGENESIS OF ENTERITIS AND COLITIS

It was mentioned earlier that the lines between bowel ischemia and inflammation are ill-defined. It has been suggested that secondary vascular occlusions may contribute to the pathology of regional enteritis and Crohn's colitis. Further, the colitis developing proximal to colonic carcinomas is now considered to be of ischemic origin. These observations have led to the proposal of a common vascular pathogenesis of the various forms of enteritis and colitis, the common pathogenetic feature being a disturbance of the arterial-venous-lymphatic complex and its controlling neural and metabolic factors.

TUMORS

Tumors of the colon are detected with barium studies and colonoscopy. Angiography is rarely indicated. The angiographic features of certain tumors are mentioned, because they may be encountered during angiographic examination of the colon for other reasons.

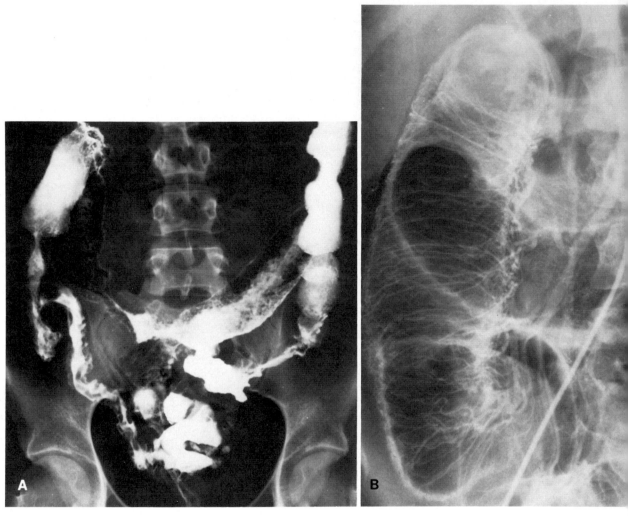

FIG. 13.12. ULCERATIVE COLITIS

A 31-year-old woman with diarrhea and occult rectal bleeding. (**A**) Barium examination of the colon shows changes of ulcerative colitis. (**B**) Superior mesenteric arteriogram. Detailed view of the right colon shows characteristic nontapered step ladder appearance of the vasa recta.

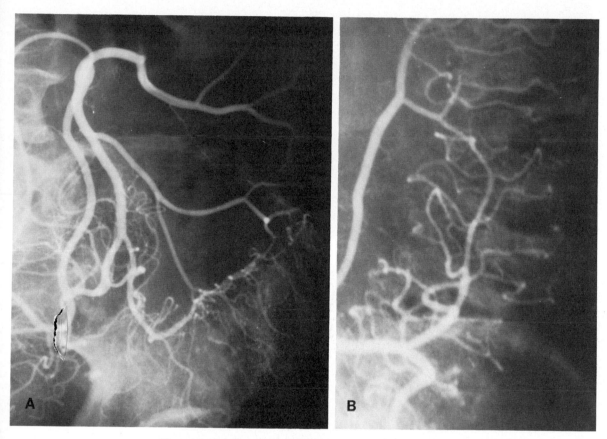

FIG. 13.13. CROHN'S DISEASE OF THE COLON

Inferior mesenteric arteriogram. The sigmoid colon is depicted in (**A**) and a detailed view of the descending colon in (**B**). In contrast with the appearance of ulcerative colitis (see Fig. 13.12) there is marked tortuosity of the vasa recta as they penetrate the bowel wall.

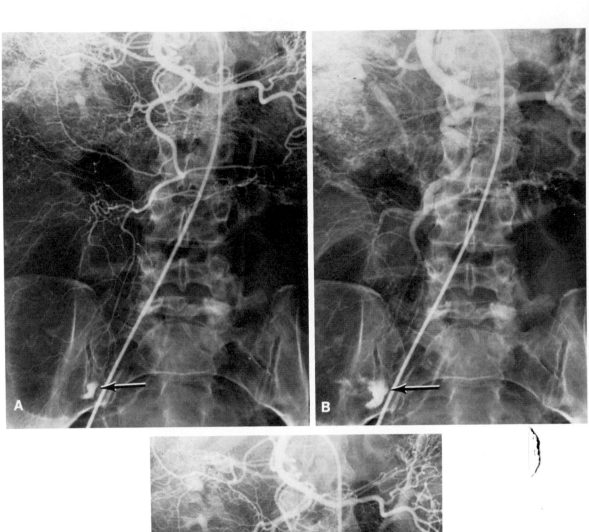

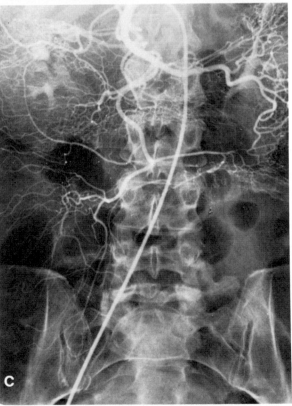

Benign tumors such as angiomas may vary in appearance from a small telangiectasia to large cavernous hemangiomas or arteriovenous malformations (Fig. 13.15). Villous adenomas are moderately vascular, exhibiting tumor vessels and stain, as are adenocarcinomas but to a lesser degree (Fig. 13.16). Carcinoid tumors exhibit as a characteristic finding—foreshortening of the mesentery with arterial and venous occlusions, the result of extensive desmoplastic reaction (Fig. 13.17).

Liver metastases from colonic carcinoma may be vascular or avascular. Tumors of the kidney and the pancreas may at times derive blood supply from the mesenteric vasculature, but this "parasitic" supply does not necessarily imply tumor invasion into the colon.

BLEEDING

The application of angiography in the evaluation of patients with rectal bleeding has considerably contributed to our understanding of colonic disorders which may cause massive hemorrhage.

New knowledge based on angiographic observations may be summarized as follows: (1) Angiodysplasia of the right colon has been established as a source of bleeding in elderly patients. (2) In elderly patients rectal bleeding is more frequently due to angiodysplasia than to diverticular disease. (3) Bleeding from a diverticulum is more likely to originate from the right colon, despite the preponderance of diverticula on the left. (4) Blind subtotal colectomy for rectal bleeding can hardly be justified in view of the radiologist's potential to localize the source and acutely control the bleeding with intra-arterial vasopressin.

Angiography may be performed (1) on an emergency basis for massive bleeding of sufficient magnitude to produce hypovolemia and require transfusions; or (2) electively for low grade recurrent blood loss. In the first instance barium studies can not and should not be performed before angiography. Rectosigmoidoscopy and colonoscopy should both be carried out, although colonoscopy is more difficult and may not be possible in an emergency situation. In the second instance angiography is performed only after meticulous barium studies of the upper and lower gastrointestinal tract and endoscopy have failed to reveal the source of bleeding or any other pathology.

Diverticular Bleeding

Mesenteric arteriography during the time of acute rectal bleeding may localize the bleeding diverticulum with the demonstration of contrast medium extravasation. The extravascular contrast pools within the confines of the diverticulum and forms a density persisting late into the venous phase of the arteriogram (Fig. 13.18).

FIG. 13.14. ULCERATIVE COLITIS; BLEEDING CONTROLLED WITH INTRA-ARTERIAL VASOPRESSIN

(A) Superior mesenteric arteriogram shows extravasation of contrast medium in the cecum (arrow). (B) During the late phase contrast extravasation persists (arrow). (C) Superior mesenteric arteriogram, during infusion of vasopressin, 0.2 U/min, shows constriction of mesenteric arterial branches and no extravasation. The bleeding was clinically controlled and the patient underwent elective colectomy. (Reproduced with permission from Baum, S., Athanasoulis, C. A., Waltman, A. C., and Ring, E. J.: Gastrointestinal hemorrhage, Part II: Angiographic diagnosis and control. In *Advances in Surgery*, Vol. 7, edited by J. D. Hardy, R. M. Zollinger, *et al.* © 1973, Year Book Medical Publishers, Inc., Chicago.)

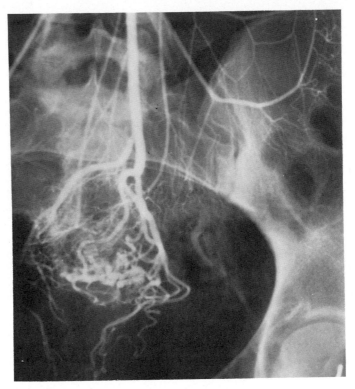

FIG. 13.15. ARTERIOVENOUS MALFORMATION OF THE RECTOSIGMOID
Inferior mesenteric arteriogram, in a young female with rectal bleeding, shows
arteriovenous malformation in the rectosigmoid region.

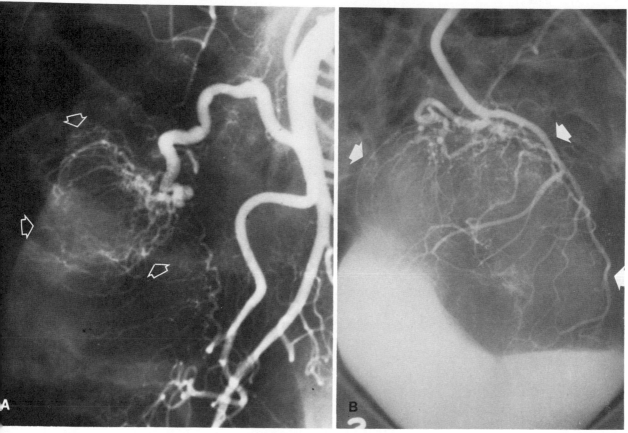

FIG. 13.16. ADENOCARCINOMA OF THE COLON

(A) Superior mesenteric arteriogram on a patient with carcinoma of the ascending colon. The arrowheads point to tumor vascularity. (B) Inferior mesenteric arteriogram on a different patient than the one shown in (A). Tumor vascularity is seen within a mass (arrowheads) overlying and compressing the urinary bladder.

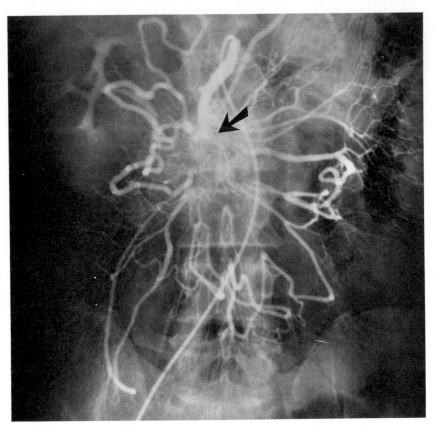

FIG. 13.17. CARCINOID TUMOR

Superior mesenteric arteriogram on a patient with rectal bleeding. The superior
mesenteric artery (arrow) and several jejunal arteries are occluded. Retraction of
mesenteric arterial branches is due to desmoplastic reaction which is characteristic
of carcinoid.

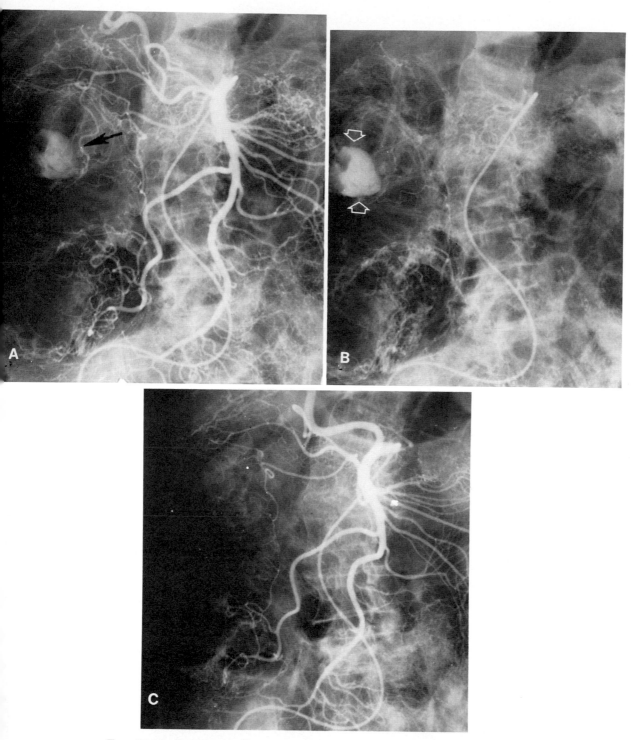

FIG. 13.18. BLEEDING DIVERTICULUM OF THE ASCENDING COLON

(A) Superior mesenteric arteriogram in a patient with massive rectal bleeding. There is contrast extravasation in the ascending colon (arrow). (B) During the late phase the extravasated contrast persists, outlining the diverticulum (arrowheads). (C) Superior mesenteric arteriogram during infusion of vasopressin, 0.2 U/min, in the superior mesenteric artery shows no extravasation. The bleeding was also clinically controlled.

It is often difficult to assess on clinical grounds whether a patient is actively bleeding or not. Radionuclide studies have been applied as a screening method prior to arteriography. The presence of radioactivity in the bowel following the intravenous administration of a blood pool agent (technetium-labeled red blood cells) implies active bleeding (Fig. 13.19). The experience with this procedure is limited. A few positive studies have been reported. It is, however, feared that a high false-positive rate will diminish the clinical importance of the procedure.

Seventy-five percent of angiographically demonstrated bleeding diverticula have been on the right side of the colon. This observation has altered the surgical approach to bleeding diverticulosis and has raised questions about differences in the origin of right-sided diverticula vs those found on the left.

Once extravasation of contrast medium has been demonstrated, the bleeding may be acutely controlled in 90–95% of these patients with infusion of vasopressin into the vessel supplying the bleeding point (Figs. 13.18 and 13.19). Infusion is at dose rates of 0.2–0.3 U/min for 24–36 hr. Acute but less massive bleeding from left-sided diverticula has been controlled with intravenous infusions of vasopressin at similar dose rates. Transcatheter embolization of the bleeding vessel with autologous blood clot has been attempted in cases of vasopressin failure, but the efficacy and safety of this method has not been established. Recurrent bleeding which occurs within hours after vasopressin therapy is discontinued requires surgery.

Following acute control of bleeding with angiographic methods a barium enema should be performed to exclude the presence of co-existing lesions. Operative resection of the colonic segment containing the diverticulum may be electively performed, although there is no evidence to suggest that if bleeding recurs it will originate from the same diverticulum.

Angiodysplasia

Current knowledge about angiodysplasia may be summarized as follows: (1) It is an acquired vascular lesion of the colon that may become the source of rectal bleeding in elderly patients. (2) It may be incidentally found in elderly nonbleeding patients undergoing angiography for other reasons. Therefore, it does not always bleed. (3) It is not associated with cutaneous vascular lesions or lesions of other viscera. (4) It is located, or at least it has been observed, only in the cecum and the ascending colon. (5) It has a specific angiographic appearance which makes the diagnosis feasible. (6) Right hemicolectomy proves to be curative in most patients with rectal bleeding and angiographic evidence of angiodysplasia. (7) In resected specimens the lesion can be best seen with special injection techniques.

The term "angiodysplasia" is used because of its consistently Greek derivation (*angos* or *angeion* = vessel; *dys* = ill or badly; *plasis* = a fashioning or molding) and its lack of a strong connotation of congenital origin. The entity has been also referred to as "vascular ectasia" which is a combination of Latin and incorrect Greek (vascular + *ectasis* = stretching not ectasia). This term should be abandoned or substituted by the etymologically correct term of "angiectasis."

Bleeding from colonic angiodysplasia may be manifested either as low grade chronic blood loss requiring iron replacement and an occasional transfusion or in the form of massive rectal hemorrhage. The lesion has been found in patients over the age of 50 and it is more frequently encountered among patients with aortic valvular disease, although an etiologic relationship has not been established.

Angiodysplasia cannot be detected by barium studies of the colon. It may be seen at colonoscopy by the experienced observer. A firm diagnosis can only be made

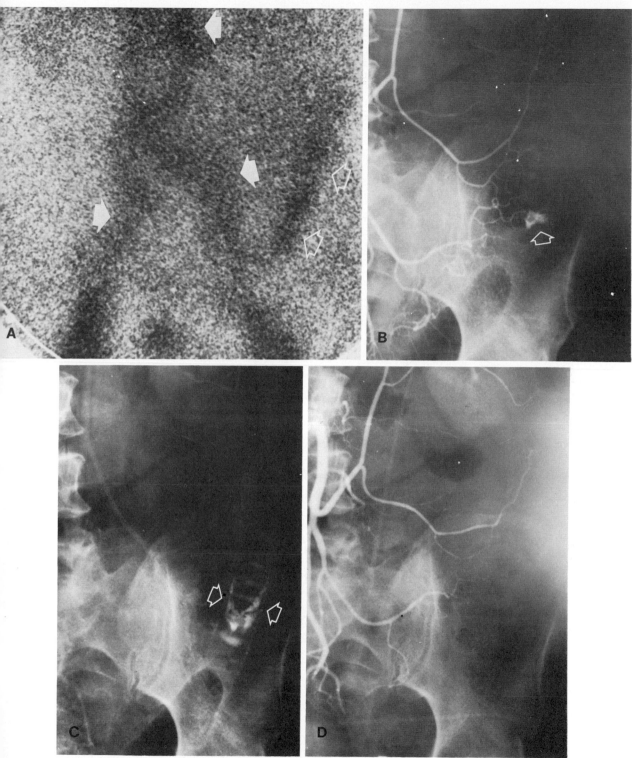

Fig. 13.19. Bleeding Diverticulum of the Descending Colon

(A) Radionuclide study with technetium-labeled red blood cells in a patient with rectal bleeding. The arrowheads point to the aorta and the iliac vessels. The open arrowheads point to radioactivity in the left colon, indicative of active bleeding at the time of the study. (B) Inferior mesenteric arteriogram shows extravasation from bleeding diverticulum of the sigmoid (open arrowhead). (C) Late phase shows persistent extravasation in the sigmoid colon (arrowheads). (D) Inferior mesenteric arteriogram during infusion of vasopressin, 0.2 U/min, shows constriction of arterial branches and no extravasation. Bleeding was also clinically controlled.

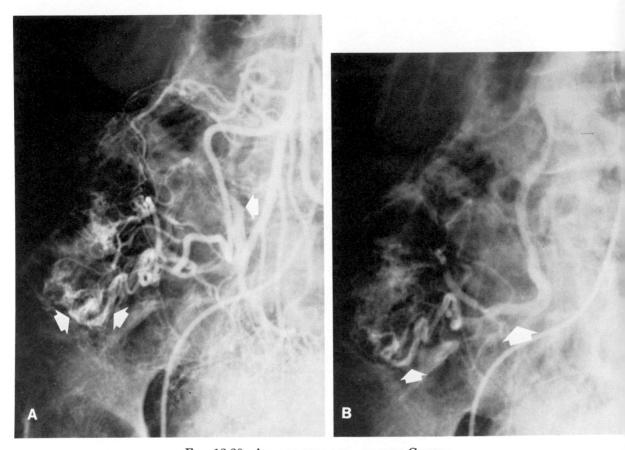

FIG. 13.20. ANGIODYSPLASIA OF THE CECUM
(A) Superior mesenteric arteriogram in a 65-year-old man with recurrent episodes
of rectal bleeding. Barium examinations and endoscopy were negative. The arrowheads point to vascular tuft and early opacified vein in the cecum. (B) During the
late phase of the arteriogram there is persistent opacification of the vein draining
the lesion in the cecum (arrowheads).

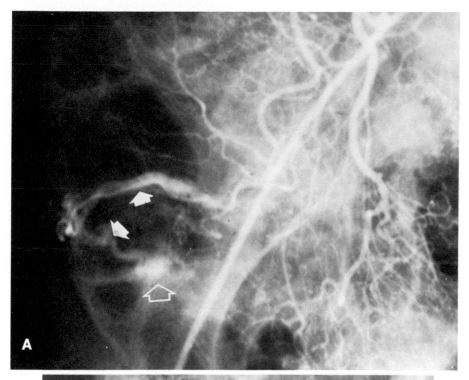

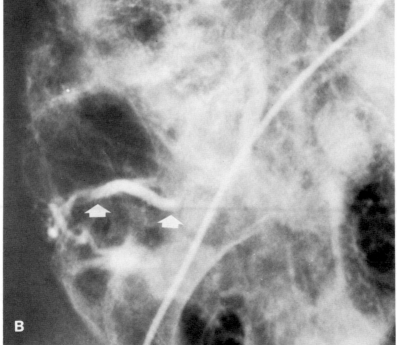

FIG. 13.21. CECAL ANGIODYSPLASIA

Coned down view from a superior mesenteric arteriogram in a 65-year-old patient with rectal bleeding. (**A**) The open arrowhead points to a vascular tuft in the cecum. The arrowheads point to simultaneous artery and vein opacification in the cecum. (**B**) Late phase of the arteriogram shows persistent opacification of the vein draining the cecum (arrowheads).

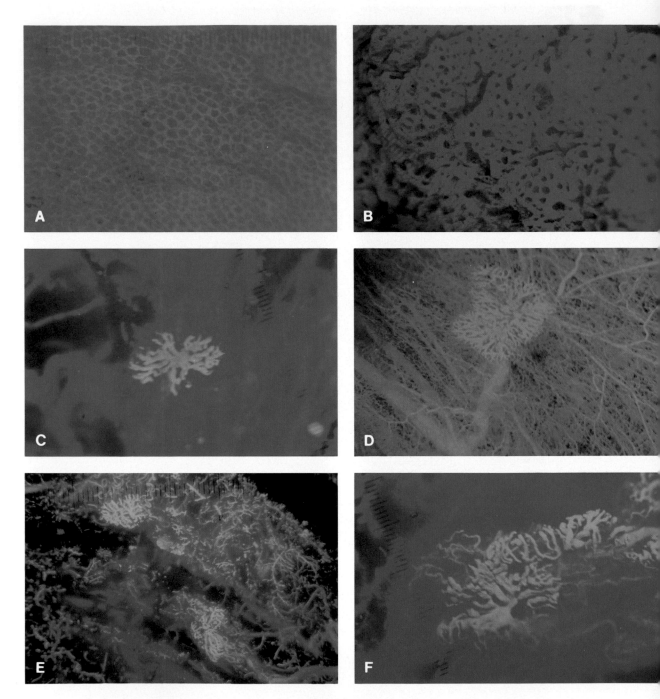

PLATE 13.1
Photomicrographs of cleared specimens, viewed under dissecting microscope.
Vessels injected with silicon rubber. (**A**) Normal colonic mucosa (×30); Honeycomb
pattern of the vascular channels surrounding the luminal openings of the Lieberkühn
crypts. (**B**) Ulcerative colitis (×30). The honeycomb pattern is deranged. (**C–F**)
Angiodysplasia (×15): flower-like (**C**); with large submucosal draining vein (**D**);
multiple (**E**); coalescent (**F**).

during angiography based on the following findings (Figs. 13.20 and 13.21): (1) Clusters of small arteries seen during the arterial phase. These clusters are frequently located along the antimesenteric border of the cecum, usually adjacent to the ileocecal valve. (2) Accumulation of contrast medium in a vascular tuft. (3) Early opacification of a draining vein usually the ileocolic. (4) Persistent opacification or late emptying of a dilated draining vein usually the ileocolic. The most important signs are the vascular tuft, the early draining vein and the persistent late opacification of the draining vein. Magnification arteriography is extremely helpful in bringing out the vascular tuft and the early draining vein when these findings are not apparent in a nonmagnified study (Fig. 13.21).

Right hemicolectomy is the definitive treatment in those patients who have bled and have an angiographic diagnosis of angiodysplasia and in whom no other lesions have been found to account for the blood loss. On the resected specimen the lesion is best seen with special injections of the blood vessels and examination under the dissecting microscope. The normal honeycomb pattern of mucosal capillaries is abruptly interrupted by congeries of enlarged, tortuous, anastomosing vessels having an organoid pattern of radial symmetry which has been described as coral-like or flower-like (Plate 13.1, C–F). Most lesions are smaller than 5 mm, ranging from 1–15 mm in size. Histologically areas of closely grouped, large thin-walled blood vessels are seen in the mucosa and submucosa with no involvement of the muscularis propria or serosa (Fig. 13.22).

The pathophysiology is not known. It has been proposed that angiodysplasia is a degenerative process caused by chronic intermittent low grade obstruction to submucosal veins, or that it is the end result of multiple chronically repeated subclinical episodes of bowel ischemia. The prevalence of the lesion in the cecum and ascending colon has been attributed to the greater wall tension developing in these segments during colonic distention.

Lower Intestinal Varices

In patients with cirrhosis and portal hypertension or in patients with prehepatic portal vein obstruction collateral flow develops mostly through gastroesophageal varices. The umbilical and inferior mesenteric veins are other potential collateral pathways and lower intestinal varices may develop as a result of the increased blood flow. Occasionally dilated hemorrhoidal veins can be distinguished as serpiginous submucosal filling defects in the barium-filled rectum (Fig. 13.23).

Another collateral pathway for the spontaneous decompression of the portal venous system is through fine venous anastomoses existing between small mesenteric venous tributaries on the parietal visceral surface and systemic venous channels in the retroperitoneum and the abdominal wall. These pathways especially develop in patients who have had previous abdominal surgery and who develop adhesions between loops of bowel and the abdominal wall (Fig. 13.24).

Postoperative Bleeding

Vasopressin has been successfully infused in either the superior or the inferior mesenteric artery to control postoperative colonic hemorrhage. Bleeding from an appendiceal stump, cecostomy, colostomy, or bleeding as the result of polypectomy through a colonoscope has been controlled with this method and re-exploration has been avoided (Figs. 13.25 and 13.26).

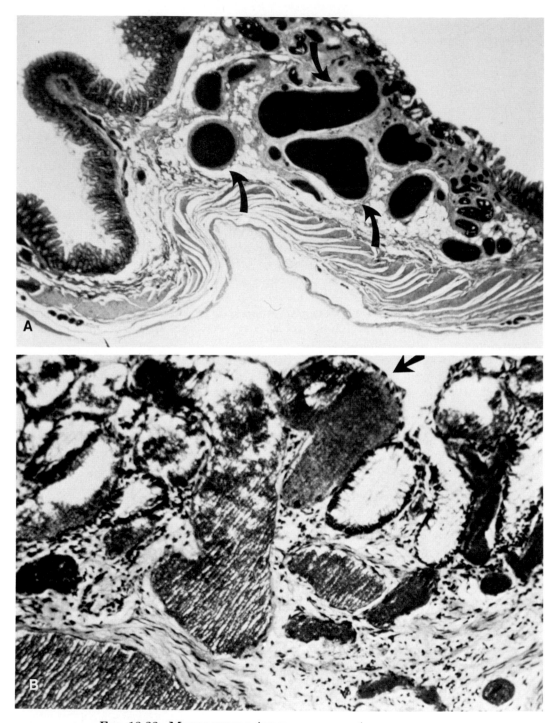

FIG. 13.22. MICROSCOPIC APPEARANCE OF ANGIODYSPLASIA
(A) Photomicrograph (×10) of area of angiodysplasia in the wall of the cecum
shows dilated submucosal vascular channels (arrows). (B) At higher magnification
(×40) the dilated vascular channels are noted to be separated from the lumen by
single layer of epithelial cells (arrow).

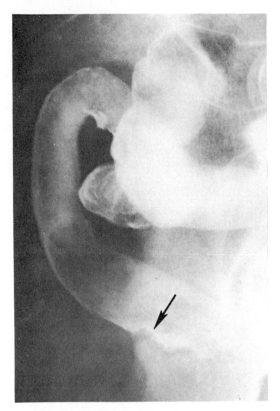

FIG. 13.23. VARICES OF RECTUM

Lateral view of the rectum showing irregular filling defects on the posterior wall due to internal hemorrhoids (arrow).

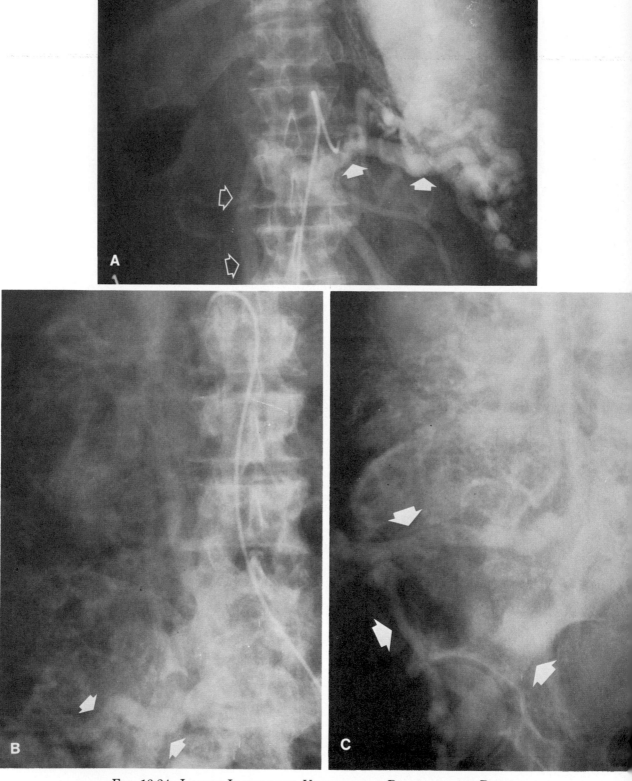

FIG. 13.24. LOWER INTESTINAL VARICES IN A PATIENT WITH PORTAL
HYPERTENSION AND PREVIOUS ABDOMINAL SURGERY

(A) Venous phase of splenic arteriogram shows enlarged spleen, patent splenic
vein (arrowheads), and retrograde flow into superior mesenteric vein (open arrowheads). (B) Venous phase of superior mesenteric arteriogram shows dilated venous
channels in right lower quadrant (arrowheads). (C) Venous phase of superior
mesenteric arteriogram. Detailed view of right lower quadrant shows opacification
of large intestinal varices and of iliac vein (arrowheads). Portosystemic communications developed through several adhesions, the result of previous oophorectomy.

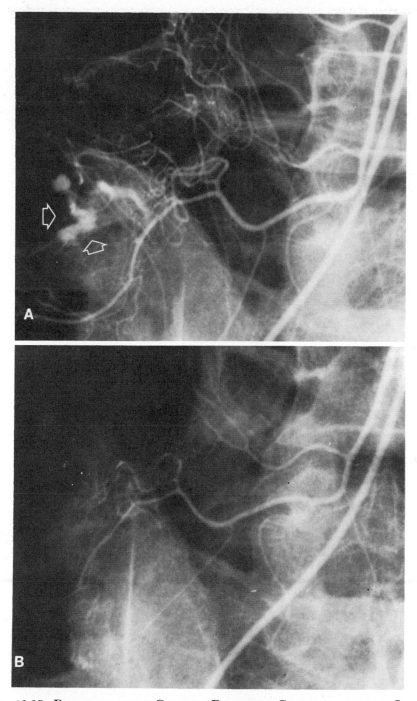

FIG. 13.25. POSTOPERATIVE COLONIC BLEEDING CONTROLLED WITH INTRA-
ARTERIAL VASOPRESSIN

(A) Superior mesenteric arteriogram in a patient with rectal bleeding 24 hr
following cecostomy. The arrowheads point to contrast medium extravasation at
the site of cecostomy. (B) Superior mesenteric arteriogram during infusion of
vasopressin at 0.2 U/min, shows arterial constriction and no extravasation. The
bleeding was also clinically controlled.

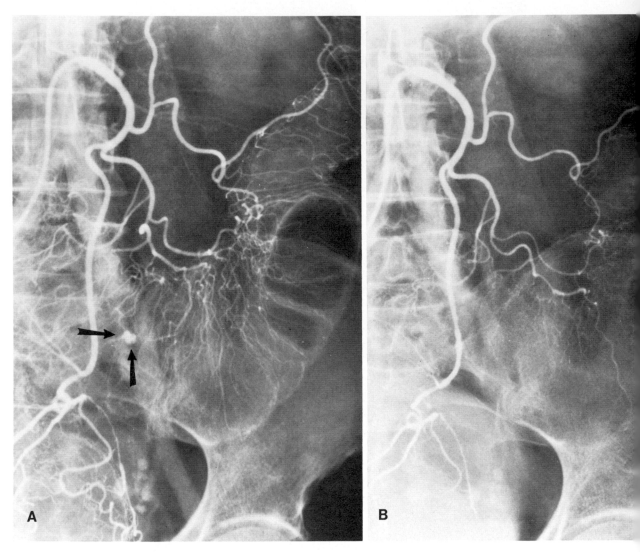

FIG. 13.26. BLEEDING FOLLOWING POLYPECTOMY VIA THE COLONOSCOPE,
CONTROLLED WITH INTRA-ARTERIAL VASOPRESSIN

(A) Inferior mesenteric arteriogram in a patient with rectal bleeding following
polypectomy via the colonoscope shows contrast medium extravasation at the
polypectomy site in the sigmoid colon (arrows). (B) Inferior mesenteric arteriogram
during infusion of vasopressin at 0.2 U/min shows no extravasation. The bleeding
was also clinically controlled. (Reproduced with permission from Athanasoulis, C.
A., Waltman, A. C., Novelline, R. A., Krudy, A. G., and Sniderman, K. W.:
Angiography: Its contribution to emergency management of gastrointestinal hemorrhage. Radiol. Clin. North Am., *14:* 2, 1976.)

BIBLIOGRAPHY

Allen, A. C.: The vascular pathogenesis of enterocolitis of varied etiology. In *Vascular Disorders of the Intestines* edited by S. J. Boley, S. S. Schwartz, and L. F. Williams, Jr. Appleton-Century-Crofts, New York, 1971.

Athanasoulis, C. A., Waltman, A. C., Novelline, R. A., Krudy, A. G., and Sniderman, K. W.: Angiography: Its contribution to emergency management of gastrointestinal hemorrhage. Radiol. Clin. North Am., *14:* 265, 1976.

Athanasoulis, C. A., and Baum, S.: Vascular disorders of the gut. Part III: Angiography. In Gastroenterology, 3rd Ed., edited by H. L. Bockus, Vol. IV, Chap. 160, pp. 329–358. W. B. Saunders, Philadelphia, 1976.

Athanasoulis, C. A., Galdabini, J. J., Waltman, A. C., *et al.*: Angiodysplasia of the colon: A cause of rectal bleeding. Cardiovasc. Radiol., *1:* 3, 1978.

Boley, S. J., Brandt, L. J., and Veith, F. J.: Ischemic disorders of the intestines. Curr. Problems Surg., *15:* 1, 1978.

Michels, W. A.: *Blood Supply and Anatomy of the Upper Abdominal Organs.* J. B. Lippincott, Philadelphia, 1955.

Ödman, P.: Percutaneous selective angiography of the superior mesenteric artery. Acta Radiol., *51:* 25, 1959.

Ottinger, L. W.: *Fundamentals of Colon Surgery.* Little, Brown and Co., Boston, 1974.

Seldinger, S. J.: Catheter replacement of the needle in percutaneous arteriography: A new technique. Acta Radiol., *39:* 368, 1953.

14

Pathology of Polypoid and Nonpolypoid Tumors of the Colon

AUSTIN L. VICKERY, JR., M.D.

POLYPOID TUMORS

Introduction

Polypoid tumors of the colon comprise one of the most common lesions in the entire gut and opinions regarding their natural history, pathologic diagnosis, and methods of clinical detection and management have historically been among the most controversial in the field of medicine. A confusing terminology has been the cause of many misconceptions. A polyp is defined as a pedunculated or sessile growth projecting into the lumen of a body cavity. Thus, "polyp," is a nonspecific, broad, generic expression embracing a variety of pathologic processes, both non-neoplastic and neoplastic, which have, as a simple common denominator, a protrusion into the bowel lumen. A classification of polyps is given in Table 14.1.

Adenomatous Polyps

Adenomatous polyps comprise over 90% of all neoplastic polypoid lesions of the

TABLE 14.1
CLASSIFICATION OF POLYPS

Neoplastic Polyps
Benign Neoplasms
    Adenomatous polyp
    Villous adenoma
    Villoglandular polyps (mixed)
    Familial adenomatous colonic polyposis
    Lipomas, leiomyomas, neurofibromas, lymphangiomas, and hemangiomas
Malignant Neoplasms
    Polypoid carcinoma
    Malignant lymphomatous polyposis
Non-Neoplastic Polyps
Inflammatory, such as the pseudopolyps in ulcerative colitis
Tumor-like lesions, including the hamartomatous growths of juvenile and Peutz-Jeghers polyps; also inflammatory polyps
Hyperplastic (metaplastic): hyperplasia of differentiated mucosal cells; the most common colonic lesion, very small (1–5 mm) and of no clinical significance

colon. These occur in probably 10% of the adult population in countries of the Western World but are very uncommon in some geographic regions. Racial groups from such areas, when transplanted to parts of the world where adenomatous polyps are common, show a tendency to develop these lesions which suggests the importance of environmental and dietary factors in addition to the genetic effect.

Adenomatous polyps may occur any place in the colon but are more common in the lower third and in the first portion of the ascending colon, particularly around the cecum. For unknown reasons, they are rarely encountered in the small intestine. Adenomatous polyps are frequently multiple with more than one occurring in about 25% or more of cases and their number increases with age.

Grossly, adenomatous polyps range in size from a few millimeters to several centimeters but most (about 75%) are less than 1 cm in diameter and relatively few are greater than 2 cm. Most are pedunculated but they may be sessile, particularly the smaller lesions (Fig. 14.1). An important aspect in the study of polyps is the formation of the stalk; its mere presence implies benign growth since it represents stretched out normal mucosa at the polyp base most likely the result of peristaltic traction. Demonstration of a definite stalk on a polypoid colonic lesion which is long enough to allow lateral mobility affords excellent assurance of clinical benignancy and cure by simple amputation (Fig. 14.2).

Microscopically, adenomatous polyps are composed of a proliferation of epithelial glands around a central fibrovascular core (Fig. 14.3). The glands are composed of normal mucous secreting and absorptive cells which are often abnormally increased in number. Varying grades of nuclear hyperchromatism and other epithelial atypicalities are common in focal areas of polyps but, in the absence of invasion, even severe atypicality (carcinoma *in situ*) poses no clinical threat to the patient and simple excision is sufficient treatment. While microscopic invasive carcinoma occurs in but a very small percent of the total number of adenomatous polyps, malignancy is closely linked to polyp size, larger lesions exhibiting a significant association with invasive carcinoma.

Villous Adenomas

Villous or papillary adenomas are much less common than adenomatous polyps constituting only about 10% of all benign neoplastic polyps. These tend to be situated in the rectosigmoid area but may appear anywhere in the colon and are usually solitary. The great majority are sessile with a broad base and a corrugated

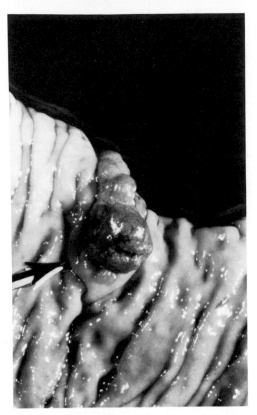

FIG. 14.1. SESSILE ADENOMATOUS POLYP
The polyp (arrow) measures 1.5 cm in diameter.

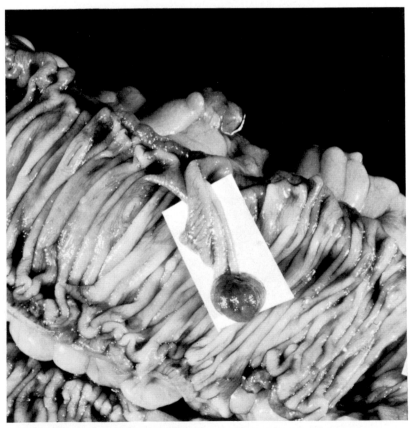

FIG. 14.2. PEDUNCULATED ADENOMATOUS POLYP
The long mucosal stalk allows great mobility of this polyp and excellent assurance that it is benign.

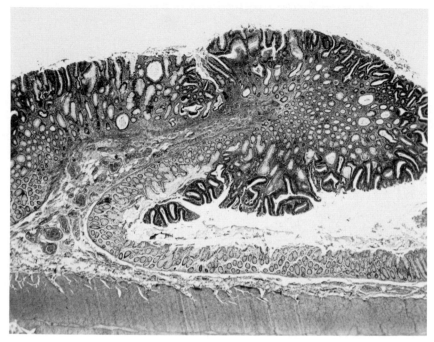

FIG. 14.3. PEDUNCULATED ADENOMATOUS POLYP

A photomicrograph reveals this small polyp to be composed of a proliferation of glands around a fibrovascular core.

surface consisting of villous fronds which often present a cauliflower-like appearance (Fig. 14.4). The average size is considerably larger than the average adenomatous polyp with about 75% exceeding 2 cm in diameter compared with only 5% of adenomatous polyps. Occasionally, villous adenomas achieve a very large diameter, 10–15 cm, and these bulky lesions may produce obstructive symptoms. An uncommon complication of these large lesions is an unusual clinical syndrome characterized by watery mucus diarrhea and a depletion of protein and electrolytes, particularly potassium.

Microscopically, although the basic cell types are the same as in adenomatous polyps, the glands in villous adenomas are arranged around thin stalks of fibrovascular stroma which tend to be perpendicular to the mucosal surface producing the characteristic frond-like surface architecture (Fig. 14.5).

In sharp contrast to adenomatous polyps, villous adenomas are often associated with malignant change with about 40% showing infiltrating carcinoma, usually at the base (Fig. 14.6). Therefore, biopsies of the surface villous adenomas may show a deceptively benign picture while the deeper portions contain infiltrating carcinoma. This is a major reason why total excision of broad based villous adenomas is advised as a general principle.

Villoglandular Polyps

These lesions represent a mixed adenomatous and villous growth pattern considered by some to represent an intermediary form suggesting that adenomatous and villous polyps are fundamentally similar lesions (Morson). They frequently have a stalk and grossly simulate adenomatous polyps (Fig. 14.7). Since villoglandular polyps have a higher incidence of invasive carcinoma than adenomatous polyps, this suggests that the mere presence of partial villous architecture in a neoplastic polyp confers a higher risk of malignancy.

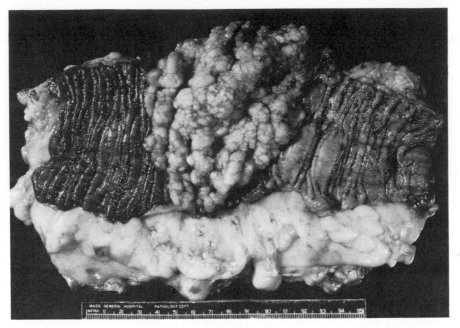

FIG. 14.4. VILLOUS ADENOMA
The surface of this bulky, broad-based tumor is characterized by a warty appearance due to numerous nodular excresences. The tumor stands out so well because the mucosa on either side is involved by melanosis coli.

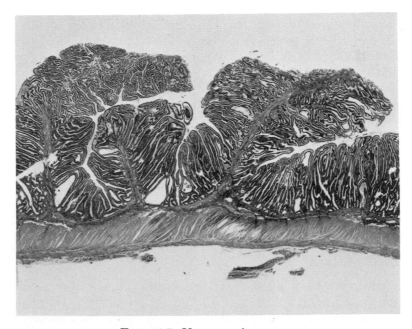

FIG. 14.5. VILLOUS ADENOMA
A microscopic section of a sessile, broad-based villous adenoma showing frond-like, glandular projections which tend to rise in a perpendicular fashion.

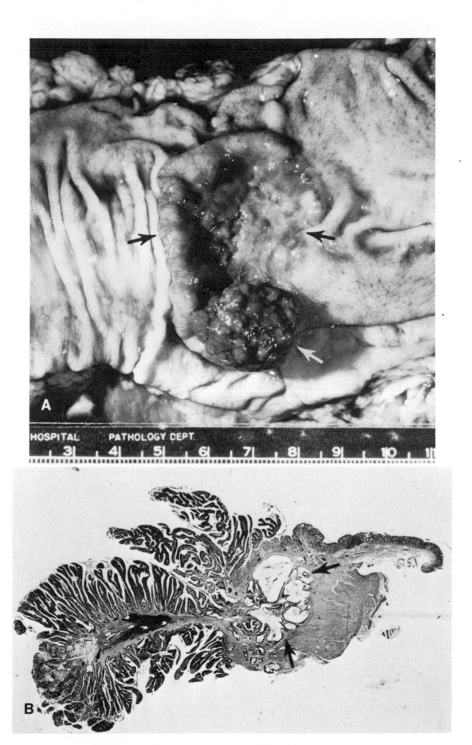

FIG. 14.6. CARCINOMA IN A VILLOUS ADENOMA

(A) An ulcerating carcinoma (black arrows) arising in a villous adenoma which is the dark polypoid mass (white arrow). (B) Microscopic section shows a typical villous pattern on the left while normal mucosa is present on the right. At the base of the villous tumor there is an invasive colloid carcinoma appearing as large clear spaces filled with mucin (arrows).

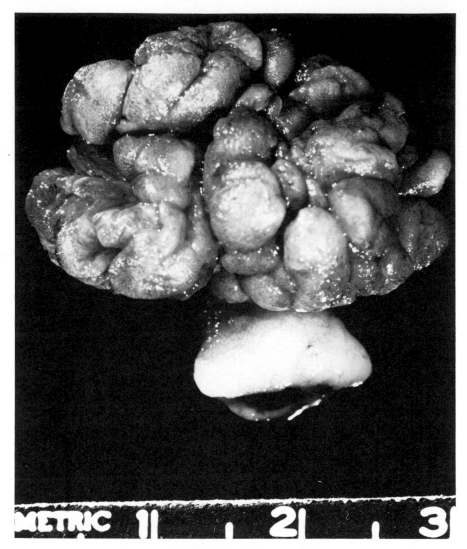

FIG. 14.7. VILLOGLANDULAR POLYP

The polyp has been amputated at the base of its short stalk. Such lesions may closely simulate an adenomatous polyp.

Familial Adenomatous Colonic Polyposis

This entity is a unique inherited disease in which the mucosal surface of the entire colon is covered with hundreds or thousands of adenomatous polyps (Fig. 14.8). The disorder is transmitted as a Mendelian autosomal dominant trait with a high degree of penetrance. The polyps usually do not appear until after 10 years of age and are not productive of symptoms. Virtually 100% of these individuals will develop invasive cancer of the colon with the average age at the time of diagnosis of cancer about 40 years which is approximately 20 years earlier than intestinal cancer observed in patients without polyposis.

With the predictable occurrence of an invasive cancer, identification of those at risk is important in the early years of life before carcinoma develops. The treatment is colectomy, usually with an ileo-rectal anastomosis.

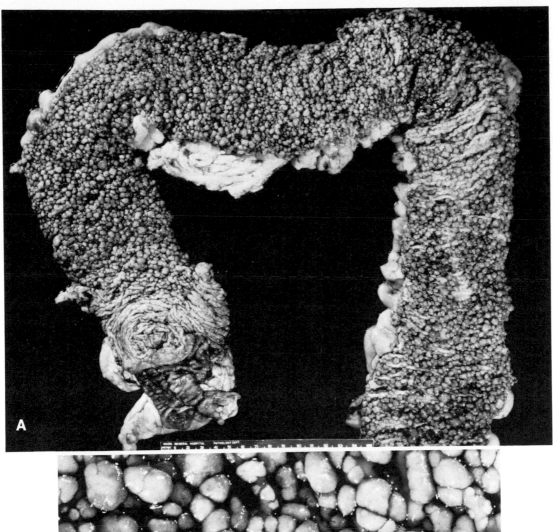

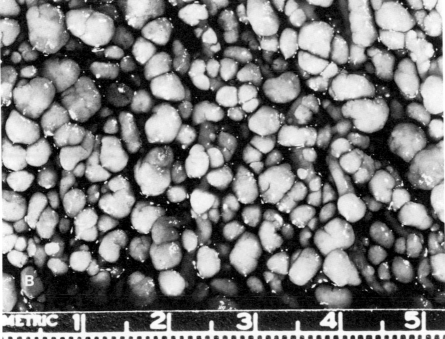

FIG. 14.8. FAMILIAL ADENOMATOUS COLONIC POLYPOSIS
(A) The colon of a teenaged youth. The mucosal surface is literally studded with polyps of relatively uniform size. Note the cessation of the process at the ileo-cecal valve, lower left. (B) Close-up of the countless adenomatous polyps.

Relationship of Benign Neoplastic Polyps to Carcinoma

Two basic schools of thought have argued this issue for many years with first one view prevailing and then the other. An old attitude that virtually all polyps were either malignant or premalignant lesions was mainly based on the frequent association of benign polyps in colons with invasive cancer and the common occurrence of atypicalities in the histology of neoplastic polyps. Excision of all polyps as a prophylaxis was generally advocated. An almost opposite conservative position followed this radical view, namely that most colon cancers arise *de novo*, unassociated with pre-existing benign lesions, with the exception of villous adenomas. The advocates of this latter viewpoint maintained that malignant conversion of benign adenomatous polyp was an exceedingly rare occurrence, a conclusion largely predicated on the lack of pathologic evidence of recognizable benign polyp tissue in invasive cancers.

More recently, the pendulum has swung back in the other direction with evidence advanced by the proponents indicating that the majority of colon cancers have their genesis in a pre-existing benign neoplastic polyp.

Points Favoring a Benign Polyp to Cancer Sequence

1. The frequent presence of cellular atypism in benign neoplastic polyps ranging from slight to carcinoma *in situ* suggests a gradual transition from benign to malignant.

2. The occurrence of invasive cancer in otherwise benign neoplastic polyps correlated with increasing size of the lesions suggests a malignant change with the passage of time (Table 14.2 and Fig. 14.9).

3. The rarity of small "early" invasive colon cancers unassociated with benign neoplastic polyps (*de novo* carcinomas) is suggestive.

4. Familial adenomatous polyposis disorders are strikingly correlated with the eventual development of carcinoma.

5. In about one-third of the colons with an invasive cancer, one or more benign neoplastic polyps are also present. These patients have a significantly higher risk of developing a second cancer than those cancer patients without associated benign neoplastic polyps.

6. The differential in average age of patients with benign polyps vs cancers (58 vs 62 years) is indirect evidence that the polyp-cancer sequence takes several years (Morson).

Management Guidelines for Colonic Polyps

1. Since only a small percent of the total have a proven malignant potential, unnecessary morbidity and mortality will result from surgical treatment of all

TABLE 14.2
INCIDENCE OF INVASIVE CARCINOMA IN COLONIC POLYPS (ST. MARK'S HOSPITAL)

Histologic Type	1 cm	1–2 cm	2 cm	Total
Adenomatous	1% (1382)*	10% (392)	35% (101)	5% (1875)
Villoglandular	4% (76)	7% (149)	46% (155)	22% (380)
Villous adenoma	10% (21)	10% (39)	53% (174)	42% (234)
Total	1% (1479)	10% (580)	46% (430)	11% (2489)

* Figures in parentheses = Total number of patients.
(Lane has presented similar findings from the New York Presbyterian Hospital citing a 1.3% incidence of cancer in 1016 lesions less than 1.5 cm in diameter vs 10% in 336 lesions larger than 1.5 cm.)

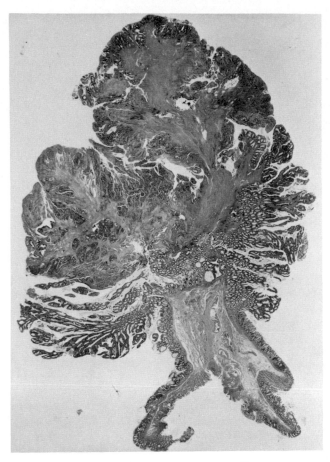

FIG. 14.9. VILLOGLANDULAR POLYP

Microscopic section of a villoglandular polyp on a pedicle. The polyp is largely replaced by carcinoma. Note the small amount of residual villous glandular tissue near the base of the tumor.

polyps. Clinical judgment is obviously very important in the management of these lesions.

2. Lesions less than 1 cm comprise the majority of *all* polyps and present no significant threat to the patient.

3. Polyps with a definite long stalk also have a low risk, even if there is microscopic invasive cancer. The mere presence of a long pedicle indicates no downward growth. Amputation is adequate treatment.

4. All polypoid lesions over 2 cm must be considered significant risks and in the absence of a long stalk should probably be excised to exclude malignancy.

5. Villous adenomas with their large size and proven malignant potential generally should be completely excised, for surface biopsies may not disclose a cancer at the base.

Polypoid Carcinoma

A polypoid carcinoma is a malignant neoplasm entirely composed of adenocarcinoma (Fig. 14.10). This is an uncommon colon cancer and has a relatively low grade of malignancy with rare distant metastatic spread.

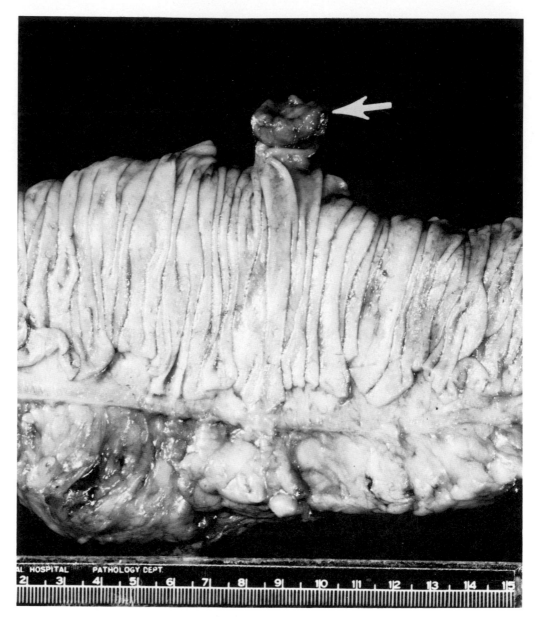

FIG. 14.10. POLYPOID CARCINOMA
This 2-cm tumor (arrow) has a short, broad stalk.

There are two basic conflicting concepts as to the pathogenesis of polypoid cancer: (1) The polyp-cancer transition school considers polypoid carcinoma as the ultimate stage of this sequence with all benign elements now replaced by carcinoma; and (2) the *de novo* proponents simply interpret the lesion as a low grade form of primary carcinoma.

HEREDITARY POLYPOSIS DISORDERS

Adenomatous Polyposis Disorders

In addition to familial adenomatous colonic polyposis, there are two other syndromes, Gardner and Turcot, characterized by multiple adenomatous polyps of the colon. The Gardner syndrome is inherited as an autosomal dominant and is associated with a curious mixture of soft tissue and osseous lesions including fibromas, skin cysts, osteomas, and dental abnormalities. The Turcot syndrome is a rarity and consists of a combination of neurogenic tumors (*e.g.,* glioblastoma or medulloblastoma) and colonic polyposis.

The relative frequency of familial adenomatous colonic polyposis has been estimated as 1 in 8,300 births compared with 1 in 14,000 births for the Gardner syndrome.

All of the familial adenomatous polyp syndromes are associated with a very high incidence of colonic carcinoma.

Non-Neoplastic (Hamartomatous) Polyposis Disorders

Peutz-Jeghers Syndrome

The Peutz-Jeghers syndrome is a rare disease characterized by multiple polypoid lesions of the gut and melanin pigmentation of buccal mucosa, lips, and digits. The mucosal tumors are most common in the small intestine. The polyps are considered developmental defects or hamartomas rather than true neoplasms. Although there are a few reports of cancer arising in these lesions, compared to the familial adenomatous polyposis disorders, the malignant potential is very low.

Juvenile Polyposis Coli

Juvenile polyposis coli is another disorder inherited as an autosomal dominant trait. The lesions are often pedunculated. They may be single or multiple and tend to be concentrated near the rectum but may occur anywhere in the colon and rarely in other portions of the gut (Fig. 14.11). Pathologically, these polyps characteristi-

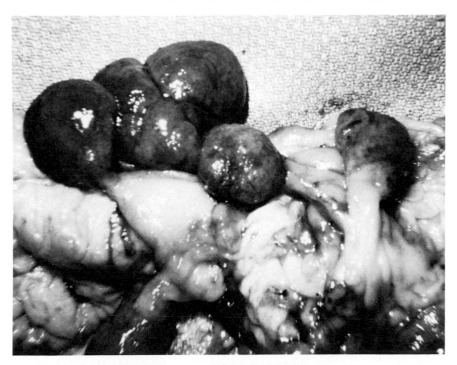

FIG. 14.11. JUVENILE POLYPOSIS COLI

Multiple juvenile or "inflammatory" polyps. The dark color of the polyps on this black and white photograph reflects their bright red appearance. Note the long pedicle on the far right polyp.

cally have a smooth surface and microscopically consist of a mixture of glands, often dilated or cystic, amid an abundant loose connective tissue stroma. Because of the cystic architecture, these lesions have been called retention polyps. The frequent presence of inflammation in juvenile pólyps caused some investigators to believe they were primary inflammatory lesions, hence the term "inflammatory" polyp. However, the prevailing viewpoint is that inflammation and local sepsis are secondary to the vulnerability of juvenile polyps to trauma. They often appear bright red on endoscopic visualization and may undergo autoamputation with passage in the stool. Juvenile polyps are considered to be hamartomas without malignant potential.

NONPOLYPOID TUMORS

Introduction

Carcinomas comprise the great majority of all large intestinal neoplasms which are not polypoid. All other nonpolypoid tumors and tumor-like lesions of clinical significance are relatively very uncommon or rare. A classification of the major nonpolypoid tumors of the large intestine is given in Table 14.3.

Carcinoma

Natural History and Epidemiology

Colon cancer is the second most frequent fatal malignancy in the western world. The incidence in the United States is about equal in the sexes and has remained relatively stable in comparison to stomach and lung cancer. The peak age incidence is 60–70 years. There are some striking variations in frequency on a worldwide basis with the highest risk in the English speaking countries. In areas of South Africa,

---

TABLE 14.3

CLASSIFICATION OF MAJOR NONPOLYPOID TUMORS OF THE LARGE INTESTINE

Epithelial Tumors
    Adenocarcinoma
    Mucinous (colloid) adenocarcinoma
    Signet cell carcinoma
    Undifferentiated carcinoma
Carcinoid Tumors
Nonepithelial Tumors
    Benign
        Leiomyoma and Leiomyoblastoma
        Neurilemoma (schwannoma)
        Lipoma
        Hemangioma and lymphangioma
    Malignant
        Leiomyosarcoma
        Malignant lymphoma
Tumor-like Lesions
    Endometriosis

Asia and South America, the incidence is as low as 1/10 that of western world countries. Migrant populations from these areas have shown increased rates of colon cancers similar to their adopted western world cultures (*e.g.,* colon cancer rate is low in Japan but Japanese living in Hawaii have rates similar to Caucasians). Another unusual geographic feature is that countries tending to have a higher rate of stomach cancer have low colon cancer rates. Such interesting epidemiologic observations have suggested that a difference in diet may be an important factor in the development of colon cancer. Populations ingesting natural foods with a high fiber content have bulkier stools and a faster fecal transit time. Burkitt believes this may alter the effects of intestinal carcinogens and bacterial flora on colonic mucosa.

Other Etiologic Factors

Familial adenomatous colonic polyposis and ulcerative colitis are both diseases with a known predilection for secondary cancer development.

Growth Rate

Carcinoma of the colon appears to have the same wide variation in rate of growth as observed in many other neoplasms. Collins measured the doubling time of metastatic colon cancer to lung and calculated a 34–210 day range with a mean of 116 days. Allowing for 30 doubling times for 1 tumor cell to grow to a 1 cm mass (1 billion cells), the extrapolated ages for these metastases would be from 3–17 years with a mean of 9½ years. Such studies document the long silent period of growth of most colonic cancers, *i.e.,* before the tumor achieves a size allowing clinical detection. It is thus ironic that the so-called "early" clinical cancer is actually several years old. Another feature relating to tumor growth is that size of the primary tumor may have no relation to the lethal potential of the neoplasm. In contrast to some carcinomas of other organs, there is no correlation between size of a colonic carcinoma and the stage of disease. Regardless of size at the time of clinical discovery, colonic cancers may have equivalent malignant potentials, and the obvious implication is that some tumors metastasize when they are very small, even microscopic and clinically undetectable. Furthermore, there is poor correlation between duration of symptoms and disease stage. Small cancers with long histories and large ones with short histories are not uncommon.

Such data relating to tumor growth document the inappropriateness of the terms "early," "late," and "advanced" in describing colon cancers. Small lesions with a high lethal potential may be of recent origin and already have metastasized. Conversely, a large tumor may have a low growth rate and not have metastasized. A depressing conclusion from this evidence is that present methods of detecting colon cancer in a truly early phase are very inadequate.

Gross and Microscopic Pathology

About 75% of colon carcinomas occur in the rectum and sigmoid areas with the cecum the second most common site. Carcinomas of the colon are extremely variable in gross appearance, ranging from small infiltrating lesions to large bulky masses with extensive ulceration (Fig. 14.12). Some tumors tend to grow in a circumferential fashion with a tendency for obstructive symptoms (Fig. 14.13). Microscopically, the great majority of carcinomas are gland-forming adenocarcinomas but about 10% are of an undifferentiated type. A distinctive form of adenocarcinoma is the mucinous or colloid cancer. A rare type is the signet-cell variant of mucinous carcinoma which provokes a scirrhous response and a radiographic picture similar to linitis plastica of the stomach or an inflammatory stricture of the colon.

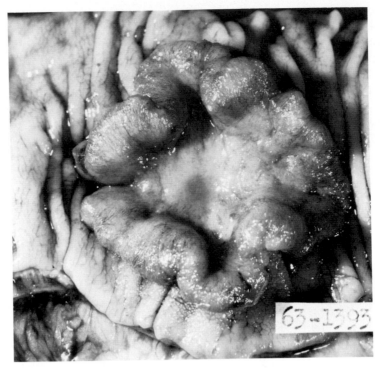

FIG. 14.12. ADENOCARCINOMA
Close-up of a colonic cancer with raised margins and central ulceration.

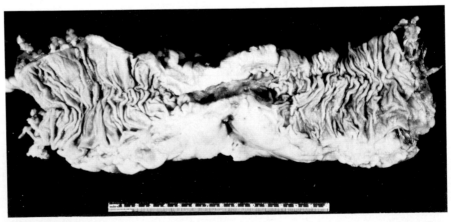

**FIG. 14.13. OBSTRUCTING, ELONGATED ANNULAR CARCINOMA OF THE LEFT
COLON**
Note the smooth ulceration of the mucosa, the extensive tumor infiltration in the
wall, and the sharp demarcation between the tumor and adjacent mucosa (tumor
shelf).

Etiology

As stated previously in the section on polypoid adenomas, there is considerable evidence to suggest that many, if not most, carcinomas of the large intestine arise in pre-existing villous or adenomatous polyps. *De novo* cancers remain controversial as to their contribution to the total number of cases of colon carcinoma. The very infrequent finding of a truly small carcinoma unassociated with a benign polypoid tumor is offered as proof that carcinoma arising in normal mucosa must be a rare phenomenon. Mention has been made previously regarding a higher risk of carcinoma in ulcerative colitis and also familial adenomatous colonic polyposis.

Patterns of Tumor Spread, Staging and Prognosis

Colon carcinomas extend by direct invasion of the bowel wall and by invasion of lymphatics and blood vessels. The Dukes method of tumor staging is based on the extent of local tumor infiltration of the bowel wall and the status of regional lymph nodes.

Stage A—Tumor limited to the bowel wall without lymph node metastases.

Stage B—Extension through bowel wall without lymph node metastases.

Stage C—Extension through bowel wall with lymph node metastases.

In patients operated for curative resection, tumor stage is closely related to survival. Lesions confined to the bowel wall (Stage A) are the most favorable with an 80–90% 5-year survival. Stage B tumors, with extension through the bowel wall but without lymph node metastases, have a 5-year survival of about 70%. Stage C carcinomas, which comprise approximately half of all colon cancers resected for cure, have the worst prognosis with only about 1 patient in 3 still alive after 5 years.

Although the average patient with colon cancer (all stages) has about a 50% chance of being alive (and probably cured) at the end of 5 years, the statistics relate only to the more favorable cases and exclude the approximately 30% of all patients with disease who are either inoperable or have palliative procedures. The 5-year survival of *all* patients with colon carcinoma is only about 35%.

Other factors which tend to worsen the prognosis of patients with colonic adenocarcinoma include undifferentiated carcinomas, ulcerative colitis, mucinous (colloid) carcinomas, venous invasion and metastases to multiple (more than 5) lymph nodes.

Complications

Bowel obstruction is the most frequent complication of colonic cancer but frank perforation is quite uncommon. Intussusception may occur, particularly with bulky tumors.

Recurrences and Mortality Causes

Most patients who develop recurrent or metastatic tumor do so within the first 3 years, and, if the patient is still free of disease after 5 years, chances of complete cure are very good. Local recurrences in the pelvis or suture line account for only about 20% of those dying after surgery. Most postoperative deaths (70%) are due to hematogenous spread with liver the most frequent site of distant metastasis, being involved in about 75% of all fatal cases while the lungs are second in frequency (15% of cases).

Carcinoid Tumors

Carcinoid tumors are rare, comprising only about 0.5% of all malignant tumors of the large intestine. The rectum is by far the most common site, being second only to the ileum in the frequency of intestinal carcinoids (exclusive of appendix). They are situated in the submucosa and present as an elevated nodule of mucosa.

Most rectal carcinoids are asymptomatic, discovered incidentally at sigmoidoscopy, are less than 1 cm in size and without clinical significance being adequately treated by local excision. Rectal carcinoids greater than 1 cm occur very infrequently, may be symptomatic and are associated with a higher risk of malignant growth behavior. Although carcinoids elsewhere in the colon are very rare, when present they tend to be relatively large and have a poorer prognosis than rectal carcinoids. The "carcinoid syndrome" is an exceedingly rare occurrence with carcinoid tumors of either the rectum or colon.

Benign Nonepithelial Tumors

Smooth muscle tumors, leiomyomas and leiomyoblastomas are relatively rare in the colon and rectum compared to the small intestine. These tumors, as in the small intestine, are usually intramural but may both project into the lumen and also bulge the serosa outward in a dumbbell fashion.

Other benign mesenchymal neoplasms include those of neurogenic origin—neurofibromas and neurilemomas—and also lipomas and vascular lesions such as hemangiomas and lymphangiomas.

Malignant Nonepithelial Tumors

Malignant tumors of smooth muscle, leiomyosarcomas, are uncommon. They may be bulky lesions and often metastasize to the liver and disseminate in the peritoneal cavity.

Malignant Lymphoma

Although the gastrointestinal tract is the most common location of primary extranodal lymphoma, the colon is the least often affected gut segment. Of 117 patients with gastrointestinal lymphoma reported by Lewin *et al.* from Stanford,

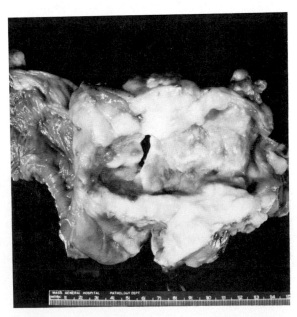

FIG. 14.14. RETICULUM CELL SARCOMA
A large, bulky tumor with central ulceration.

the location of the tumor was: stomach 41%; small intestine 32%; ileo-cecal region 11%; and colon 9%. The presentation of lymphoma in the large intestine is usually as a single, relatively large lesion (Fig. 14.14). Rarely, there may be multiple tumors. Lymphomas are frequently infiltrative and may be obstructive, simulating carcinoma.

Tumor-like Lesions

Endometriosis

Endometriosis, usually of the rectosigmoid area, may simulate primary neoplasia of the intestine for the endometrial implants provoke a hyperplasia of both smooth muscle and stroma within the affected bowel segment with resultant narrowing of the lumen.

BIBLIOGRAPHY

Bartholomew, L. G., and Schutt, A. J.: Systemic syndromes associated with neoplastic disease including cancer of the colon. Cancer, *28:* 170, 1971.

Buckwalter, J. A., Jr., and Kent, T. H.: Prognosis of surgical pathology of carcinoma of the colon. Surg. Gynecol. Obstet., *136:* 465, 1973.

Collins, V. P.: Time of occurrence of pulmonary metastasis from carcinoma of colon and rectum. Cancer, *15:* 387, 1962.

Cornes, J. S.: Multiple lymphomatous polyposis of the gastrointestinal tract. Cancer, *14:* 249, 1961.

Donaldson, G.: The management of perforative carcinoma of the colon. N. Engl. J. Med., *258:* 201, 1958.

Dukes, C. E., and Bussey, H. J. R.: The spread of rectal cancer and its effect on prognosis. Br. J. Cancer, *7:* 309, 1958.

Falterman, K. W., Hill, C. B., Markey, J. C., Fox, J. W., and Cohn, I., Jr.: Cancer of the colon, rectum and anus: A review of 2313 cases. Cancer, *34:* 951, 1974.

Fenoglio, C. M., and Lane, N.: The anatomical precursor of colorectal carcinoma. Cancer, *34:* 819, 1974.

Gilbertsen, V. A.: The earlier diagnosis of adenocarcinoma of the large intestine. Cancer, *27:* 143, 1971.

Haenszel, W., and Correa, P.: Cancer of the colon and rectum and adenomatous polyps. A review of epidemiologic findings. Cancer, *28:* 14, 1971.

Lewin, K. J., Ranchod, M., and Dorfman, R. F.: Lymphomas of the gastrointestinal tract. A study of 117 cases presenting with gastrointestinal disease. Cancer, *42:* 693, 1978.

MacLeod, J. H., Chipman, M. L., Gordon, P. C., and Graham, C. H.: Survivorship following treatment for cancer of the colon and rectum. Cancer, *26:* 1225, 1970.

Morson, B. C.: Evolution of cancer of the colon and rectum. Cancer, *34:* 845, 1974.

Morson, B. C., and Dawson, I. M. P.: *Gastrointestinal Pathology,* 1st Ed. F. A. Davis, Philadelphia, 1972.

Morson, B. C., and Sobin, L. H.: *Histological Typing of Intestinal Tumours.* World Health Organization, Switzerland, 1976.

Sheahan, D. G., Martin, F., Baginsky, S., Mallory, G. K., and Zamcheck, N.: Multiple lymphomatous polyposis of the gastrointestinal tract. Cancer, *28:* 408, 1971.

Sizer, J. S., Frederick, P. L., and Osborne, M. P.: Primary linitis plastica of the colon: Report of a case and review of the literature. Dis. Colon Rectum, *10:* 339, 1967.

Spratt, J. S., Jr., and Ackerman, L. V.: Small primary adenocarcinoma of the colon and rectum. J.A.M.A., *179:* 125, 1962.

Spratt, J. S., Jr., and Spjut, H. J.: Prevalence and prognosis of individual clinical and pathologic variables associated with colorectal carcinoma. Cancer, *20:* 1976, 1967.

Stewart, H. L.: Geographic pathology of cancer of the colon and rectum. Cancer, *28:* 25, 1971.

Symonds, D. A., and Vickery, A. L., Jr.: Mucinous carcinoma of the colon and rectum. Cancer, *37:* 1891, 1976.

Welch, C. E., and Burke, J. F.: Carcinoma of the colon and rectum. N. Engl. J. Med., *266:* 211, 1962.

Wynder, E. L., Kajitani, T., Ishikawa, W., Dodo, H., and Takano, A.: Environmental factors of cancer of the colon and rectum. II. Japanese epidemiological data. Cancer, *23:* 1210, 1969.

Wynder, E. L., Kajitani, T., Ishikawa, S., Dodo, H., and Takano, A.: Epidemiology of cancer of the colon and rectum. Cancer, *28:* 3, 1971.

15

Polyps

JACK R. DREYFUSS, M.D.

BACKGROUND

Few topics in medicine have swirled in more controversy, been the subject of wider swings in dogma, or precipitated the writing of more papers than colonic polyps. Efforts to find and categorize these tumors, to elucidate their relationship to cancer, and to devise more effective methods of diagnosis and treatment have highlighted an age of confusion and discovery. Only recently has there begun to develop a rational multidisciplinary approach with which most authorities agree.

In 1958, Dockerty made the flat statement that eventually 100% of polyps will become malignant, while in the same year Spratt and Ackerman were saying that the theory of origin of adenocarcinomas of the colon within adenomatous polyps had little to support it.

In 1962, Castleman and Krickstein defused the significance of focal atypia in adenomatous polyps and stressed the benign implication of a long, thin stalk in these tumors. However, they believed the overwhelming majority of colon cancers arose *de novo* or in villous adenomas and not in adenomatous polyps, which they said were lesions of negligible malignant potential.

In the 1970's the accumulated evidence caused a swing back toward the older concepts. It is now believed that the majority of colonic cancers arise in pre-existing benign neoplastic polyps. The adenomatous polyp has been shown to have a definite, if low, malignant potential. There has been further confirmation of the marked malignant potential of villous adenomas and the more recently described villoglandular polyps. Morson, Lane, Fenoglio, among others, have been strong advocates of the newer concepts of malignant transformation in benign neoplastic polyps.

Although polyps of the colon have been reported since the very beginning of radiology, no attempt was made until recently to define them in terms of their growth potential or actual threat to the patient's life. In addition, the inability to clean a colon for adequate radiography was an excuse for not being able to find small polyps. To further confuse the issue, statistics from sigmoidoscopy were given an inordinate emphasis since so many more polyps were found by direct visualization than by x-ray examination, including 0.2–0.5 mm mammillations of no clinical significance.

The incidence of malignancy in a polyp under 1 cm in size is now estimated to be 1%. However, size alone should not be used either radiologically or grossly to predict histology. Metastases have been reported from carcinomas of only 2 or 3 mm in size, hardly more than mammillations to the naked eye. Therefore, such terms as "early" or "minimal" cancers should not be used if meant to imply that a small malignant lesion has been found and that its removal guarantees safety from eventual metastatic disease. The determinant of critical importance for survival is whether the cancer is invasive and has extended from epithelial elements beyond the muscularis mucosa at the time of resection.

The challenge to be met by radiologists can be precisely stated: to find and categorize polyps of the colon with an accuracy that equals the data obtained from expert colonoscopy, surgical specimens, and autopsy material. In order to do this, the colon must be cleansed of all particulate debris, the x-ray examination must be individualized for each patient and designed to find small lesions, and the radiologist must express an opinion on the growth potential of each lesion he finds.

DEFINITIONS

Polyp

When the word "polyp" is used without qualification, its medical meaning must be restricted to the simple clinical entity of a small mass of tissue, with or without a stalk, arising from the mucous membrane and projecting into the lumen of the gut. Similarly, the term "polypoid lesion" must not connote a more ominous tumor than the word polyp. The two are synonymous terms, descriptive but not definitive; in no way does use of either term carry the implication of benignancy or malignancy. By common usage, polyp has become the term of choice.

Sessile Polyp

A polyp which appears attached to the mucosa by a broad base is termed sessile (Fig. 15.1). It has a central fibrovascular core, arising from the submucosa, not detectable by x-ray. All polyps of the colon are sessile in the early stages of their growth (Fig. 15.2). It is impossible to differentiate by x-ray a tiny benign sessile polyp from one that is malignant.

Pedunculated Polyp

A polyp which is attached to the mucosa by a pedicle or stalk is termed pedunculated (Fig. 15.3). The stalk is actually an elongated central fibrovascular core covered by normal colonic mucosa.

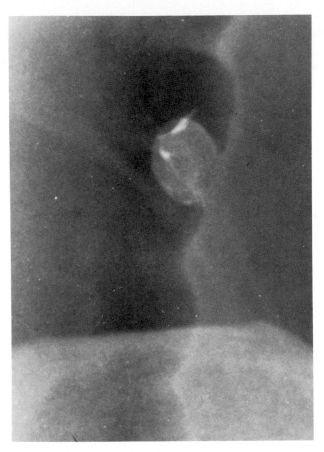

FIG. 15.1. SESSILE POLYP
A 1 cm sessile polyp is attached to the wall of the descending colon by a broad
base (double-contrast enema).

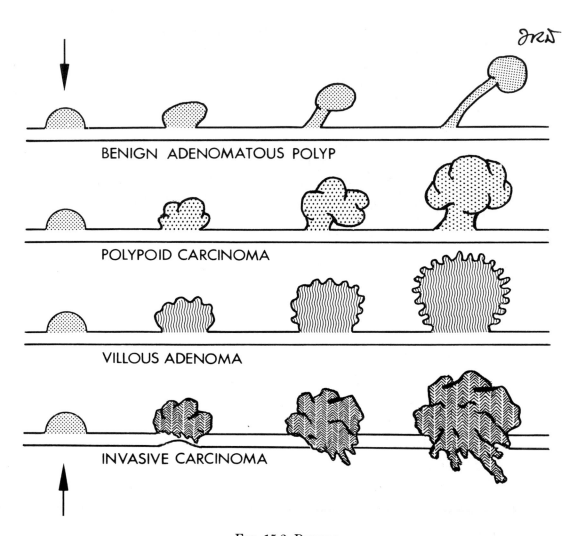

BENIGN ADENOMATOUS POLYP

POLYPOID CARCINOMA

VILLOUS ADENOMA

INVASIVE CARCINOMA

FIG. 15.2. POLYPS

The tiny polyp—which way will it grow? In the early stages of their growth, all polyps appear small and sessile (arrows). It is only with increase in size and evolution of form that the morphologic characteristics of each lesion may become apparent. This gradual change in appearance is demonstrated in schematic form as the above polyps progress in growth from left to right.

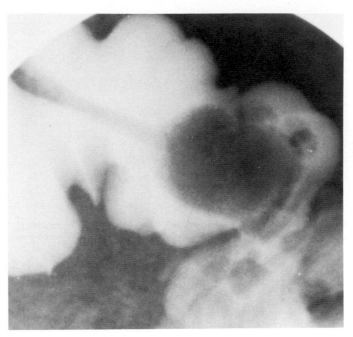

FIG. 15.3. PEDUNCULATED POLYP
The polyp is attached to the wall of the sigmoid colon by a long, thin stalk.

The presence of a long, thin pedicle is virtually always a sign of a benign polyp. The absence of malignant infiltration allows a long mucosal stalk to develop, most likely secondary to the constant tugging of peristalsis and the fecal stream.

A malignant sessile polyp which very early in its growth has invaded deep to the mucosa will not develop a long stalk. A polypoid carcinoma, or a polyp with malignant degeneration, may have a stalk, but it is likely to be short and thick.

Neoplastic Polyps

Because of their malignant potential, there are four polyps of particular interest to the radiologist.

Adenomatous Polyp

Basically this is a benign epithelial tumor, with a very low malignant potential.

Villous Adenoma (Papillary Adenoma)

This is a benign tumor characterized by papillary fronds which has a significant malignant potential.

Villoglandular Polyp (Mixed Polyp)

This tumor is intermediate in histology between the adenomatous polyp and villous adenoma; it also has an intermediate malignant potential.

Polypoid Carcinoma

This is a totally malignant polyp.

PATHOLOGY

The pathology of colonic polyps is presented in Chapter 14.

INCIDENCE AND LOCATION

What are the incidence and location of colonic polyps in the general population? These seem to be two easily answered questions, but consistent and therefore reliable statistics are hard to come by. In surveying over 50 papers for the incidence of colonic polyps, it is frustrating to find so many different sets of figures. How can this be?

The incidence of polyps in published autopsy series of the general population ranges from 2–39%, while in similar large clinical series the reported incidence varies between 3–15%. The explanation for such a spread has to be differences in methods of compilation and in the techniques used to examine the patients. For example, some autopsy series of colon polyps are based only on older patients in institutions, or on patients who have died of cancer of the colon. Similarly, some clinical reports are based on sigmoidoscopic findings alone, while others are based on conventional barium enema study only. Still other series are based on combinations of endoscopic and x-ray findings, but the radiology may have been the single-contrast enema or the double-contrast examination or even a combination of both. Two other variables affecting the results are the type of bowel preparation and whether the examined group was asymptomatic or symptomatic, or a mixture of the two. It is thus easy to see why such divergent statistical reports abound.

Perhaps the closest approach to the truth is the series from Malmo, Sweden. For many years, the meticulous preparation and double-contrast examination technique of Welin and his group have produced extraordinarily rewarding colon studies. Many thousands of patients are now included in their series. In one adult series of over 3,000 double-contrast studies, the incidence of polyps of all sizes found by the Welin method was 12.5%. In a similar general population series of over 3,000 cases, the Malmo autopsy incidence is also reported at 12.5%. This is the most impressive correlation currently available in the world literature.

As might be expected, the incidence of polyps increases with the age of the patient. Also, a patient with one polyp has a greater risk of having two or more polyps than a person in the general population has of having even one polyp (Fig. 15.4). Similarly, there is an increased incidence of the coexistence of colon cancer in patients with one or more polyps over the incidence of cancer alone in the general population (Fig. 15.5). In the Malmo series of double-contrast enemas, 76% of the patients with polyps had only one polyp, while 17% had two, and 7% had three or more polyps. The Malmo surgeons and pathologists found polyps in 20% of patients operated for carcinoma of the colon.

The distribution of polyps in the colon is also subject to the same wide divergence in reported statistics, and for the identical reasons of variables in the patient pool, the techniques of examination, and the combinations of technique used to obtain mappings of polyp location. For example, the reported percentage of polyps within sigmoidoscopic range varies from 52–93%. In the older literature, the usually stated figures are 80% of polyps in the rectum and sigmoid, and 20% in the remainder of the colon. From various autopsy series the reported distribution of polyps ranges from 27–37% in the rectum and sigmoid, 12–20% in the left colon, and 40–50% in the right and transverse colon segments.

Again, from the Malmo series of over 3,000 cases using the double contrast x-ray method of colon examination, the location of polyps is stated to be: rectum, 42.3%; sigmoid, 25.5%; left colon, 15.2%; transverse colon, 12.6%; and right colon, 4.4%.

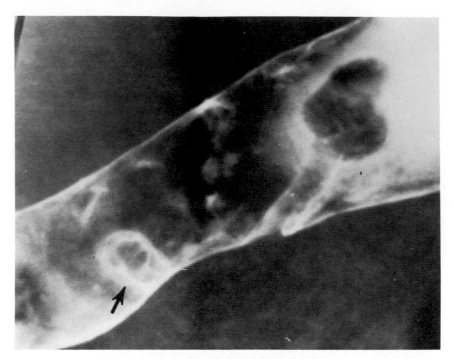

FIG. 15.4. TWO SIGMOID POLYPS

A 0.8 × 1.2 cm sessile polyp (arrow) arises from the sigmoid colon adjacent to a 1.5 × 1.8 cm stalked polyp. Both were benign adenomas.

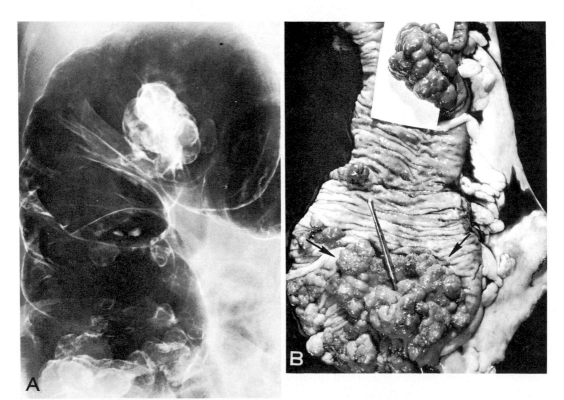

FIG. 15.5 MULTIPLE POLYPS OF COLON

(A) Detail from an air-contrast film of right colon showing multiple polyps of varying sizes and shapes. (B) Detail of the resected right colon showing the polyps which were identified on the air-contrast enema. The large tumor at the bottom of the specimen (arrows) was a villous adenoma in the cecum which had undergone malignant degeneration.

DEVELOPMENT AND GROWTH OF COLONIC POLYPS AND THEIR RELATIONSHIP TO CARCINOMA

Morson in England and Lane in the United States have championed "the polyp-cancer sequence" or "the adenoma-carcinoma sequence" to explain the relationship of colonic polyps to carcinoma. Their theories state that the majority of adenocarcinomas of the colon arise in pre-existing, benign neoplastic adenomas.

As Lane and his colleagues have stressed, if there has been one consistent observation during the period in which colonic polyps have been carefully studied, it is that intramucosal cancer (carcinoma *in situ*) has not been found in normal colonic mucosa or in nonadenomatous mucosal polyps under 5 mm in size, whereas it is frequently found in adenomas in the size range from 0.5–1.5 cm or larger. It is this fact which has been used to deny the concept of cancer arising *de novo* in cells of the normal, tubular shaped mucosal glands of the colon, the crypts of Lieberkühn.

To understand the current theory on the origin of adenocarcinoma of the colon, it must be appreciated that there are two key types of colonic polyps: hyperplastic polyps and adenomas (Fig. 15.6). *Hyperplastic polyps,* which comprise over 90% of all polyps of the colon, are benign mammillations, under 5 mm in size (Fig. 15.7). They arise from excessive cellular proliferation in the crypts of Lieberkühn, but with maintenance of their cellular differentiation. These polyps are thus formed by benign hyperplasia of normal mucosa and are of no consequence; they are not neoplastic and they are totally unrelated to adenomas or carcinomas. *Adenomas,* however, although only 1/10 as common as hyperplastic polyps are true neoplasms and may contain foci of intramucosal carcinoma with or without evidence of microinvasion. It is the adenoma with invasive cancer, capable of metastasizing, that is the true villain in the new concept of colonic carcinogenesis.

Invasive cancer is present when cells from malignant foci in adenomatous mucosa have penetrated the muscularis mucosa and entered the submucosa (Fig. 15.8). Such invasion is more ominous if present in a sessile polyp than in a polyp with a long stalk. Where microscopic invasion is limited to the submucosa of the head of a polyp and has not extended into the stalk, the chance of local or distant spread is negligible.

While rare, an adenomatous polyp may measure only a few millimeters or a fraction of a millimeter in size and already contain a microcancer. Similar minute foci of cancer have not been detected *de novo* in hyperplastic polyps even though countless thousands of them have now been examined. It is estimated that of 1,000 polyps, 900 will be totally benign hyperplastic polyps, 90 will be small adenomas in which focal carcinoma may be present but is rare and 10 will be larger adenomas (over 1.5 cm) of which one will show invasive carcinoma. This gives a 0.1% incidence of invasive carcinoma in all polyps, but a 10% incidence in larger adenomas. Therefore, the likelihood of invasive cancer increases with the size of the adenoma, particularly if sessile or villous elements are also present in the adenomatous epithelium. These lesions are the true precursors of colorectal carcinoma.

Morson has used the term polyp-cancer sequence to describe the evolution of colorectal carcinoma from adenomatous polyps and villous adenomas. He has stressed the significance of finding both benign and malignant tissue in a polyp as evidence that the cancer arose from a previously benign tumor.

In the St. Mark's Hospital study, it has been found that when a series of tumors which are both part benign and part malignant is examined, the relative frequency of cancer in the benign component of each of the 3 main histologic types is similar. Therefore, the adenomatous polyp, villoglandular polyp, and the villous adenoma are each responsible for one-third of colon cancers. Although adenomatous polyps are more common, it would thus appear that the less common villoglandular polyps and villous adenomas have the greater malignant potential.

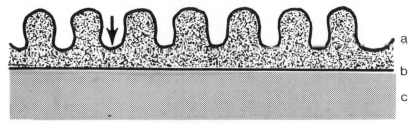

Normal mucosa

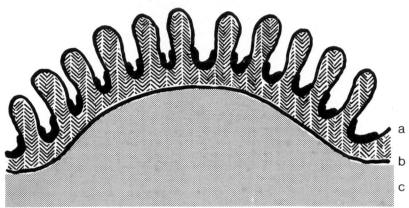

Hyperplastic polyp

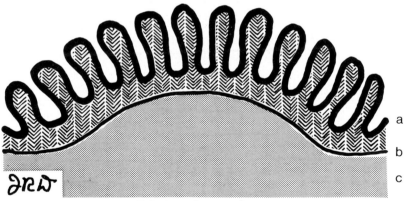

Adenomatous polyp

FIG. 15.6. SCHEMATIC PRESENTATION OF NORMAL MUCOSA AND OF HYPERPLASTIC
AND ADENOMATOUS POLYPS

a, mucosa; b, muscularis mucosa; c, submucosa. *Normal mucosa*: There are no
villi, only simple glands with normal cell division occurring in the lower part of the
crypts of Lieberkühn (arrow). *Hyperplastic polyp*: There is excessive cell proliferation in the crypts of Lieberkühn (heavy black portion of the mucosal line, a).
Although cellular differentiation is maintained, this benign hyperplasia results in
the formation of villi, a crowding together of the glands and the tiny mound of tissue
which is a non-neoplastic polyp. *Adenomatous polyp*: There is unrestricted cell
division throughout the mucosa (heavy black line, a). Cell differentiation is also
incomplete, the total result being the formation of a neoplastic polyp.

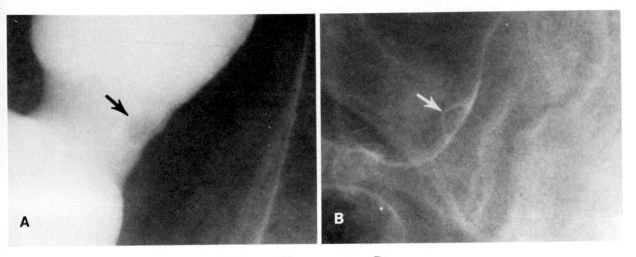

FIG. 15.7. HYPERPLASTIC POLYP

A 3 mm benign mammillation of the sigmoid colon demonstrated on (**A**) barium enema, and (**B**) double-contrast enema (arrows). The patient also had a 1.5 cm adenomatous polyp in the rectosigmoid. Both were resected through a colonoscope.

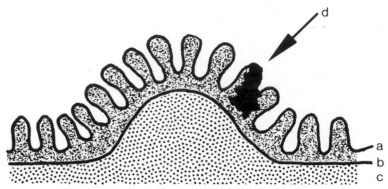

A. Sessile adenoma with intramucosal carcinoma
(carcinoma *in situ*)

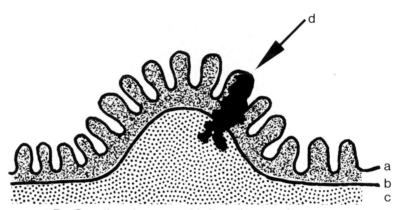

B. Sessile adenoma with invasive carcinoma

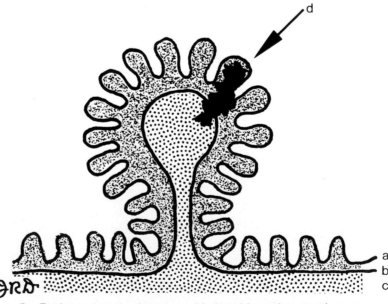

C. Pedunculated adenoma with focal invasive carcinoma

It is estimated that the evolution of cancer of the colon from adenomatous and villous polyps takes at least 5 years and may take as much as 20 years, with an average between 10–15 years. The overall malignancy rate for adenomatous polyps is given at 5%, for villous adenomas at 40%, and for villoglandular polyps at 22%. This means that most adenomatous polyps never evolve into cancer (Fig. 15.9), although the risk increases with increasing size of the polyp. The risk of cancer is also increased when an adenomatous polyp contains evidence of a villous growth pattern or when a polyp is a pure villous adenoma.

DIAGNOSTIC METHODS

Laboratory Tests

Tests for Blood Loss

The detection of occult intestinal bleeding has been the single most rewarding test in alerting the clinician to the possibility of colonic neoplasia. While it does not make the diagnosis, a positive test, especially in an otherwise asymptomatic patient, leads to the performance of other diagnostic methods of study such as endoscopy and radiology. As a screening procedure, however, the guaiac test is not as reliable as the Hemoccult Slide Test.* These subjects are covered in Chapter 17.

Carcinoembryonic Antigen (CEA)

While the CEA assay will occasionally show an elevated titer in patients with colonic polyps, it has no value as a screening test for such lesions. Once thought specific for detecting colon cancers, the CEA assay has not proven to be a consistently rewarding diagnostic method. The subject is discussed in more detail in Chapter 17.

Barium Enema and Air-Contrast Enema

Conventional barium enema and air-contrast studies of the large bowel remain the most utilized and least expensive methods of examining the large bowel. However, as with any medical procedure, the final degree of accuracy and value will depend totally on meticulous preparation and technique.

The details of performing the various radiologic studies of the colon are described in Chapter 3. There are, however, certain points which should be stressed when evaluating the colon for tumors.

During filling of the colon the head of the barium column should be followed at fluoroscopy as the patient's position is controlled so as to uncoil overlapping loops of bowel. Radiolucent filling defects in the barium column should be checked carefully and compression spot-films taken of any that are suspicious in addition to routine spot-films of areas that may be difficult to visualize on the overhead films.

---

* SmithKline Diagnostics

FIG. 15.8 A–C. SCHEMA OF THREE DEGREES OF CARCINOMA INVOLVING ADENOMATOUS POLYPS

a, mucosa; b, muscularis mucosa; c, submucosa; d, carcinoma. Note that in the sessile adenoma (**B**) invasive carcinoma has crossed the muscularis mucosa and involved the submucosa. The risk of later spread to pericolic fat, local nodes, and distant organs is great. Although the same situation obtains with focal invasive carcinoma in the pedunculated polyp (**C**), the risk of local or distant spread is less because the tumor is confined to the submucosa of the head of the polyp and does not extend into the stalk.

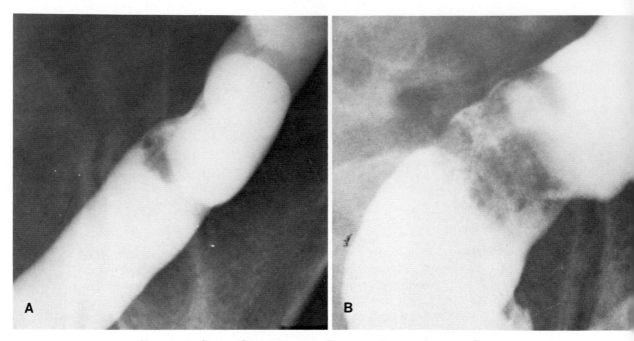

FIG. 15.9. SLOW GROWTH OF A BENIGN ADENOMATOUS POLYP
(**A**) The polyp was first demonstrated in the mid-descending colon when it was 1
cm in size. (**B**) Seventeen years later it measured 3 cm in diameter and was resected.
Multiple sections showed no evidence of malignancy.

Fecal material, air or castor oil bubbles, diverticula, and, occasionally, undissolved
tablets or undigested food may be confused with polyps (Fig. 15.10). Fortunately, all
of these objects, except the diverticula, move with the flow of barium or usually can
be dislodged by palpation with the gloved hand. Fecal material tends to be shapeless
and irregularly coated with barium, especially on an air-contrast study. Air and oil
bubbles tend to cluster together and have flattened contiguous surfaces. The
differentiation of diverticula from polyps may present a more difficult problem. One
simple maneuver to help distinguish the two is turning the patient 90°. If the area
of suspicion then projects in profile beyond the bowel wall it can readily be identified
as a diverticulum (Fig. 15.11). When it is impossible to see a suspected lesion in
profile, evaluation of its *en face* appearance must suffice. On a regular barium enema
a dependent diverticulum (not filled with feces) will appear as a dense white spot,
or, when in a superior position, it may be filled with air and appear relatively lucent.
When a double-contrast study is done, a diverticulum seen *en face* has a sharply
defined rim of barium against the mucosal surface of the sac and, when distended
with air, may appear more lucent than adjacent bowel (Fig. 15.12). A polyp, on the
other hand, always appears slightly more dense than adjacent bowel when thinly
coated with barium on a double-contrast study (Fig. 15.13).

Endoscopy

For many decades, sigmoidoscopy and the single-contrast barium enema examination were the sole methods available for detecting colonic polyps. Each had
limitations, which still exist.

The rigid sigmoidoscope is a poorly named instrument; the sigmoid colon is never
visualized. By placing surgical clips in the mucosa at the limit of sigmoidoscopic
visualization, then obtaining x-ray films of the pelvis and a barium enema, it can be
shown that the endoscopist does not see beyond the rectosigmoid junction or curve,

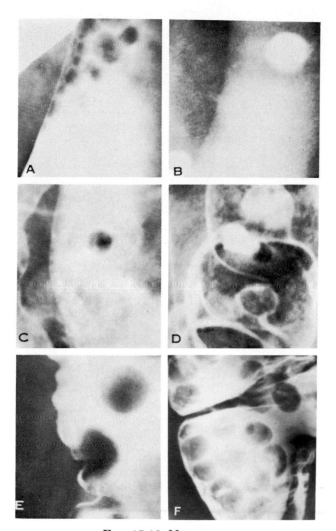

FIG. 15.10. NONPOLYPS

(A) Air bubbles clustered against the colon wall. (B) Diverticulum filled with barium *en face*. (C) A diverticulum pointing superiorly and filled with air. (D) Diverticula filled with air and barium. (E) Undissolved tablets in the colon. (F) Uncooked green peas in cecum.

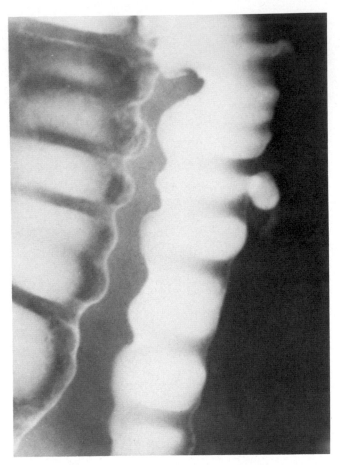

FIG. 15.11. DIVERTICULUM IN PROFILE

By turning the patient 90°, a diverticulum can be projected in profile and not be confused with an intraluminal density.

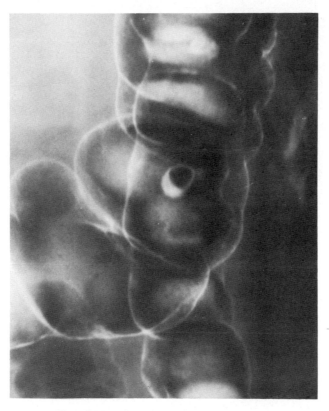

FIG. 15.12. DIVERTICULUM, EN FACE

On a double-contrast enema, a diverticulum seen *en face* has a sharp rim of barium against its mucosal surface and, because it is also distended with air, appears more lucent than adjacent bowel.

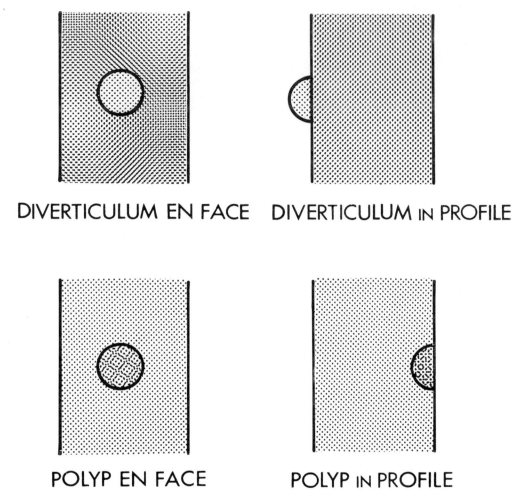

DIVERTICULUM EN FACE   DIVERTICULUM ɪɴ PROFILE

POLYP EN FACE   POLYP ɪɴ PROFILE

Fɪɢ. 15.13. Dɪᴠᴇʀᴛɪᴄᴜʟᴜᴍ ᴀɴᴅ Pᴏʟʏᴘ

Schematic appearance of a diverticulum and a polyp on double-contrast study. A diverticulum filled with air and seen *en face* appears slightly less dense than adjacent bowel and projects beyond the bowel wall when viewed in profile. A polyp *en face* appears slightly more dense than adjacent bowel and projects within the lumen when seen in profile.

even with maximum penetration. The single-contrast barium enema examination has its faults too. Although its province has long been to evaluate the colon above reach of a sigmoidoscope, with less than optimal bowel preparation and incomplete visualization of the interior of the colon, it has failed to find the number of colonic polyps which autopsy figures suggest are present in the general population.

When only these two methods were used, undue emphasis was accorded the statistics from sigmoidoscopy and too much reliance placed on the results of the single-contrast barium enema. These failures of technique and interpretation of results have now largely been corrected by both endoscopists and radiologists.

With the development of a flexible fiberoptic colonoscope, the diagnostic capability of endoscopy has been significantly advanced. The early reports from colonoscopists suggested that radiology was missing nearly 50% of all colonic polyps. This was a dismal record considering that just over 12% of the general population has colonic polyps.

Study of these early reports, however, shows that colonoscopists were comparing their results after exceptionally meticulous bowel preparation and examinations done with great expertise against radiologic studies performed after less than optimal preparation, by examiners of widely divergent experience who did not always utilize the best of currently available double-contrast techniques. As might be expected, colonoscopy found many more polyps than did radiology.

More recent reports suggest that although colonoscopy is indeed more accurate than x-ray in detecting lesions in the 2–5 mm range, there is little difference in accuracy of the two methods with lesions over 5 mm in size—assuming comparable bowel preparation, examination technique, and expertise of the endoscopist and radiologist. Radiology is least accurate when only a conventional single-contrast barium enema is performed and most accurate using the double-contrast technique. A polyp is more likely to be missed by x-ray in a redundant sigmoid, redundant flexures, or in a redundant transverse colon. Colonoscopy is most vulnerable to error where there is a redundant sigmoid, in redundant flexures, behind interhaustral folds or when the right colon and cecum cannot be reached for technical reasons.

Because of these vulnerabilities, colonoscopy must not be used as the yardstick to measure its own accuracy or that of the double-contrast barium enema. Actually, there is presently no adequate way to equate the accuracy of either method generally or in a given patient. The closest approximation is to compare the find rate of polyps over 5 mm in size by both methods against large autopsy series. Allowing for the difficulties of establishing a proper basis for comparison, current studies suggest that the error rate for detecting polyps by various techniques is: single-contrast barium enema, 45%; double-contrast barium enema, 12%; and colonoscopy, 11%.

Although the incidence of complications with expert colonoscopy is very low, there have been cases of bowel perforation during diagnostic colonoscopy as well as cases of uncontrollable hemorrhage during endoscopic polypectomy. The procedure is also costly and time-consuming. The charge approaches the surgical fee for a laparotomy in many centers, and complete colonoscopy can take from 10–60 min or up to 4 hr if polypectomy is also performed.

Certainly, colonoscopy is not to be considered as a routine screening procedure for polyps. However, its use in cases of obscure intestinal bleeding in patients at high risk for colon cancer, in patients at high risk for laparotomy, or where the double-contrast enema has not provided acceptable reassurance is invaluable and a real contribution to polyp detection and management.

SYMPTOMS

The most frequent symptom of a colonic polyp is bleeding, although it may occur in less than 50% of patients. A malignant polyp is more likely to bleed than a benign polyp. The blood is more likely to be bright red and to streak the surface or be mixed with the stool if the lesion is in the left or lower colon. A right-sided polyp is more likely to cause repeated guaiac-positive stools than to cause visible blood on the stool. Other symptoms that may be associated with colonic polyps are intermittent or alternating constipation and diarrhea, crampy abdominal pain, decreased caliber of the stools, and mucous discharge.

Except for bleeding, most polyps are asymptomatic, especially those below 1 cm in size. Symptoms tend to increase as the lesion becomes larger or if carcinoma is present. Larger benign polyps or carcinomas are the ones most likely to cause hemorrhage, pain, and change in bowel habits.

CLASSIFICATION AND CHARACTERISTICS

Colonic polyps can be separated into two major groups: non-neoplastic and neoplastic. The latter group can be further subdivided into benign and malignant neoplasms.

Non-Neoplastic Polyps

Juvenile Polyp

Most polyps in children are hamartomas, sometimes called retention or inflammatory polyps, and occur in the distal colon. They are first suspected because of bleeding, and have no malignant potential. By x-ray examination they may have a smooth or lobulated surface and are usually pedunculated. They are thought to represent errors in the formation of colonic mucosa and colonoscopic or surgical removal is only indicated to alleviate symptoms, most often bleeding.

When numerous such polyps are present in the colon, or in the colon, small bowel, and stomach, one of the juvenile polyposis disorders must be suspected; they are discussed in Chapter 16.

Hamartoma

This is considered to be identical to the juvenile polyp in appearance and significance.

Pseudopolyp

Pseudopolyps are discussed in Chapters 8, 9, and 10. Although they may resemble benign adenomas, pseudopolyps are not true polyps and the term is a poor one; they are localized areas of hyperplastic or regenerated colonic mucosa.

Hyperplastic Polyp

These mammillations, 1–5 mm in size, represent localized hyperplasia of differentiated mucosal cells. They are rarely identified by radiologic methods and are of no clinical significance.

Neoplastic Polyps

Benign Neoplasms

Adenomatous polyp

At least 75% of benign neoplastic polyps of the colon are adenomatous. They range in size from a few millimeters to several centimeters and are either sessile

(Figs. 15.14 and 15.15) or have a stalk which may be short and thick, or, more often, long and thin (Fig. 15.16). When seen on end and behind a polyp, a long thin stalk may appear as a bull's-eye within a target (Fig. 15.17). The head of the polyp is usually smooth but may be lobulated.

It is not possible by x-ray to distinguish a benign adenomatous polyp on a short stalk from a polypoid carcinoma. If the stalk is long and thin, however, then a benign lesion is much more likely (Fig. 15.18). For added reassurance, the stalk of a benign polyp should be freely movable through a 90° arc to either side (Fig. 15.19). For these reasons, and because there is no significant danger in following an asymptomatic, long stalked polyp in a patient for whom the operative risk might be greater than the risk of malignancy, it is important to establish its presence or absence. This can best be done by fluoroscopic spot-films made during inflow of barium, or by air-contrast films (Fig. 15.20).

There have been isolated case reports of carcinoma arising in stalked adenomatous polyps as well as metastases from such lesions. However, review of the x-ray films has almost invariably shown the stalk to have been short and broad with relation to

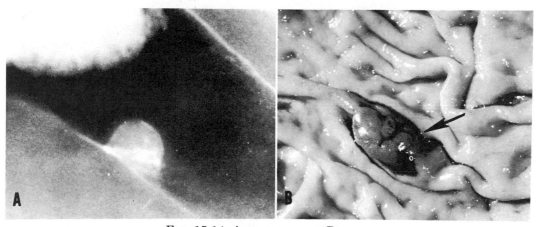

FIG. 15.14. ADENOMATOUS POLYP

(**A**) Detail from an air-contrast examination. (**B**) Detail of the specimen from a similar case in which the polyp measured 1 cm in size.

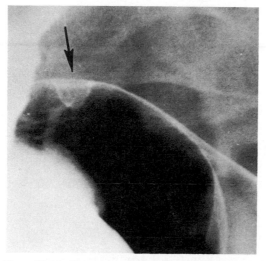

FIG. 15.15. BENIGN ADENOMATOUS POLYP

A 4 mm sessile polyp (arrow) demonstrated by double-contrast examination.

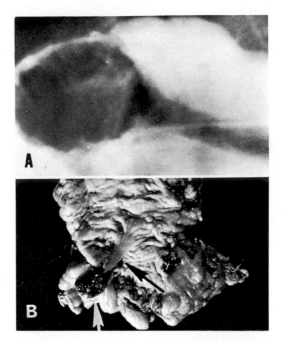

FIG. 15.16. ADENOMATOUS POLYP ON LONG, THIN STALK

(**A**) Spot-film from barium enema examination. (**B**) Photograph of resected polyp. The long, thin stalk is marked by a black arrow and the head by a white arrow. A segmental resection was done because of multiple polyps.

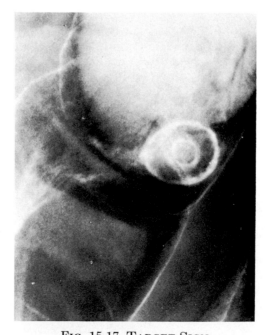

FIG. 15.17. TARGET SIGN

The stalk, on end, appears as a circle within the outer circle of the head of the polyp.

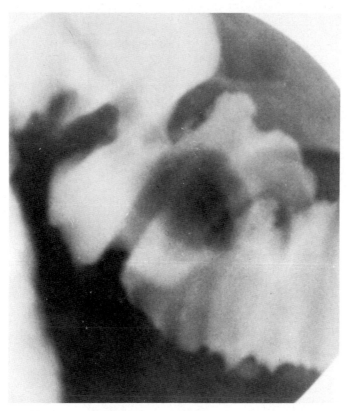

Fig. 15.18. Benign Adenomatous Polyp with a Long, Thin Stalk
Note the length and thinness of the stalk in relation to the size of the head of the polyp.

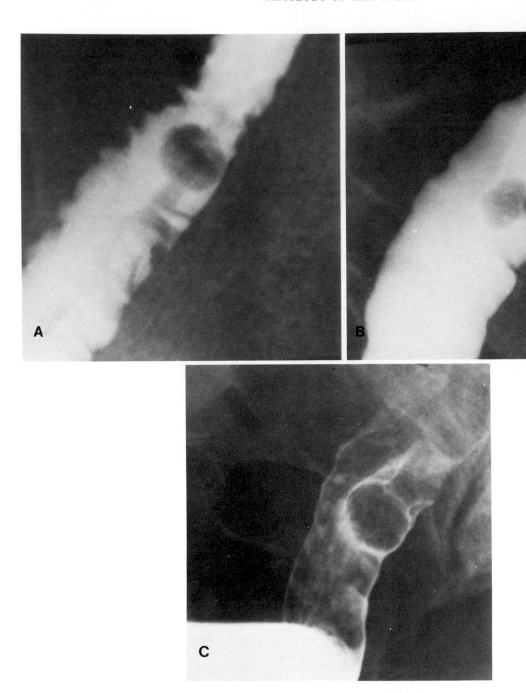

Fig. 15.19. A "Swinging Polyp"

A 1.5 cm polyp in the proximal sigmoid colon is freely movable through a 90° arc
to either side. (**A**) During inflow of barium the head of the polyp points in a cephalad
direction. (**B**) On a filled-colon film the polyp lies perpendicular to the axis of the
bowel. (**C**) On a double-contrast film the head of the polyp points caudally. This
free movement of the stalk is strongly in favor of its being a simple mucosal pedicle
without the rigidity often associated with malignant invasion.

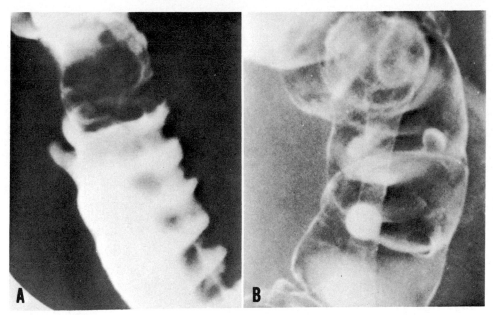

FIG. 15.20. BENIGN ADENOMATOUS POLYP ON LONG STALK
(**A**) Outlined by barium and (**B**) by air.

the size of the head of the polyp, and therefore, *not* violating the generally accepted rule that a polyp on a long, thin, freely movable stalk is benign.

The overall incidence of malignancy in adenomatous polyps is about 5%, but less than 1% for tumors under 1 cm in size.

Villous adenoma (papillary adenoma)

Villous adenomas are benign tumors, about 40% of which will eventually undergo malignant degeneration. They are usually sessile, but may have a stalk and are often over 2 cm in size when first discovered. Although nearly 70% of all villous tumors occur in the rectum and rectosigmoid (Fig. 15.21), they may be found anywhere in the colon particularly the cecum.

The villous adenoma accounts for about 10% of benign neoplastic polyps of the large bowel. Most often, it is a soft, bulky tumor covered with velvety fronds and may attain great size (10–15 cm) before causing the passage of blood and mucus by rectum, the most frequent symptoms. Diarrhea and obstruction may also occur, and very rarely there may be a copious, mucous diarrhea resulting in severe electrolyte depletion.

Many villous adenomas, particularly the larger ones, have an almost diagnostic appearance on x-ray examination; they resemble a barium-soaked sponge due to barium filling of the deep clefts between the multiple fronds (Fig. 15.22). The size and shape of such a villous adenoma may appear to change slightly from film to film, a reflection of its soft nature, and may easily be mistaken for fecal material if the colon is not clean. Some villous adenomas, however, and particularly those in the proximal colon, do not have this so-called "classic" appearance and may be indistinguishable from any other smooth or lobulated polyp (Fig. 15.23). Carcinoma in a villous adenoma is rarely diagnosed on x-ray examination. Malignancy may be suspected at surgery when areas of ulceration or induration are found.

The villous adenoma most frequently occurs in the elderly, and although local invasion or metastasis from a malignant villous adenoma may occur, a conservative

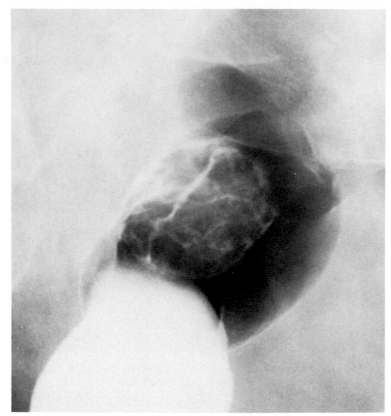

FIG. 15.21. VILLOUS ADENOMA

A 3.5 cm villous adenoma of the proximal rectum. The barium-filled clefts, which are so often typical of this tumor in the distal colon, are clearly demonstrated.

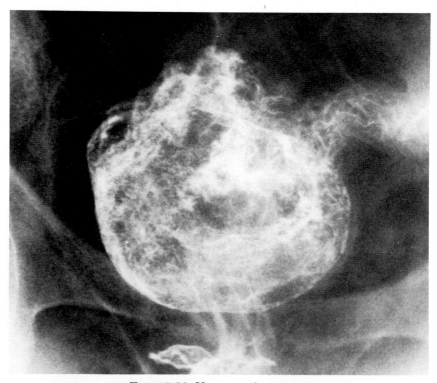

FIG. 15.22. VILLOUS ADENOMA

Detail from a postevacuation film of the rectum demonstrating a large tumor, the surface of which is patterned by innumerable barium-filled clefts.

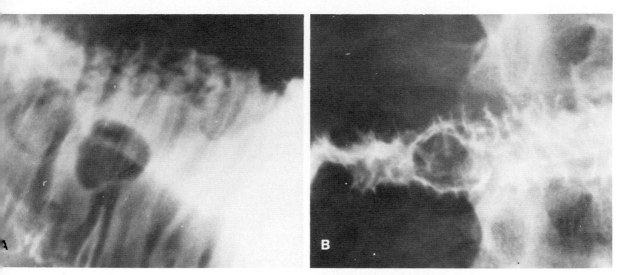

FIG. 15.23. VILLOUS ADENOMA

A smooth 1.3 cm villous adenoma in the proximal transverse colon which does not show the so-called "classic" mucosal surface of a villous tumor. (**A**) Spot-film from a single column examination. (**B**) Spot-film after evacuation of the barium.

resection is usually indicated. Frequent follow-up examination is recommended because local recurrence is common, although the recurrence is almost invariably benign, even when the original lesion showed malignant degeneration.

Villoglandular polyp (mixed polyp)

Composed of both adenomatous and villous elements, this mixed tumor more closely resembles an adenomatous polyp both by x-ray and grossly. It often has a stalk and rarely shows a barium-filled crevice pattern even on compression spot-films. Villoglandular polyps comprise about 15% of benign neoplastic polyps and range in size from under 1 cm to 3 cm, rarely growing as large as a pure villous adenoma. The incidence of malignancy is about 20%, higher than in adenomatous polyps but less than in villous adenomas.

Malignant Neoplasm

Polypoid carcinoma

At x-ray examination and grossly, a polypoid carcinoma may resemble a benign adenoma although it is more likely to have an irregular or lobulated contour (Fig. 15.24).

A polypoid carcinoma is usually sessile but may have a short stalk (Fig. 15.25). The great danger in evaluating a polypoid tumor on a stalk is to place too much reliance on the mere presence of a stalk, especially when it is poorly visualized (Fig. 15.26). A short, thick stalk is more often associated with a polypoid carcinoma, whereas the long, thin stalk is more typical of a benign adenoma. Even when cancer is found in the head of a polyp on a long stalk, invasion of the stalk is so rare that local excision is considered to be the operation of choice.

When the tumor is sessile, "puckering" of the bowel wall may be seen, and this is considered to be a highly suspicious sign of malignancy (Fig. 15.27). Puckering refers to a slight concavity of the bowel wall at the base of a sessile polyp and is probably caused by invasion deep to the mucosal layer with subsequent retraction of these layers toward the base of the tumor (Fig. 15.28). A similar retraction of the bowel

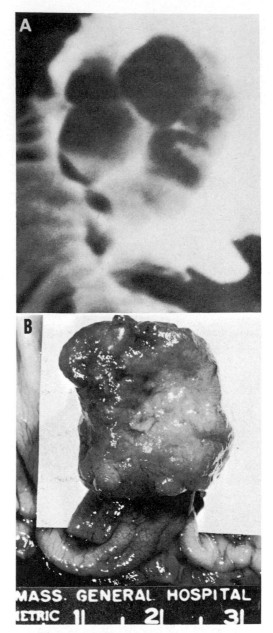

FIG. 15.24. POLYPOID CARCINOMA
A 2-cm lobulated tumor with a short, broad stalk. (A) Spot-film from barium enema examination. (B) The resected tumor.

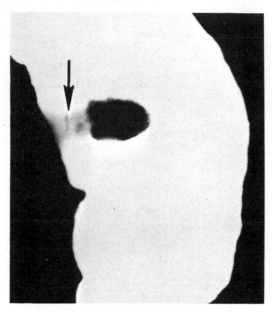

Fig. 15.25. Small Polypoid Carcinoma
Note the short, broad stalk (arrow).

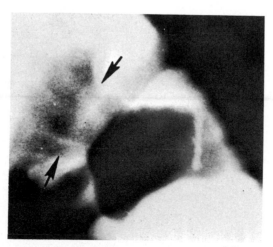

Fig. 15.26. Polypoid Carcinoma
A 2-cm irregular polypoid filling defect on an apparent "broad stalk" (arrows)
which is actually due to "tugging" of the mucosa.

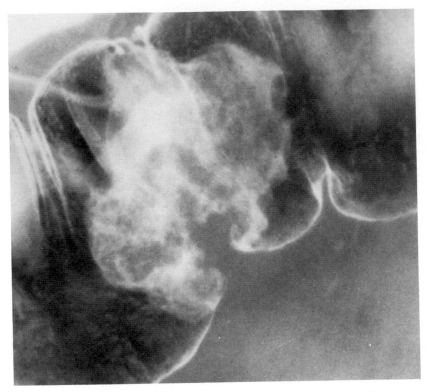

Fig. 15.27. Polypoid Carcinoma with "Puckering"
The bowel wall at the site of attachment of this 4 × 6 cm tumor appears retracted toward the tumor, a highly suspicious radiographic sign of malignancy.

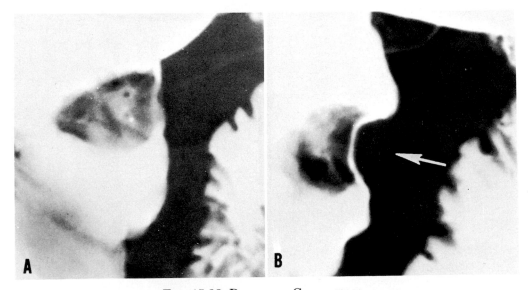

Fig. 15.28. Polypoid Carcinoma
(A) A 1.5-cm irregular, sessile polyp. (B) On turning the patient, "puckering" at the base of the tumor is demonstrated (arrow), a sign of malignancy.

wall may be seen at the base of a short, broad stalk and has the same significance (Fig. 15.29). When present at the point of origin of a long, thin stalk, it is due to tugging of the stalk and the observation is thus of no value in suspecting malignancy (Fig. 15.30).

X-RAY CRITERIA: BENIGN VS MALIGNANT POLYP

A number of diagnostic features have with great consistency been observed by those who follow polyps. While no one of them alone is necessarily critical, the presence of several may make the presumptive x-ray diagnosis of benignancy or malignancy in a polyp much easier and more likely to be correct.

These helpful features are listed in Tables 15.1 and 15.2 with the understanding that they are guides and not absolute rules.

CURRENT CONCEPTS OF POLYP MANAGEMENT

Now that improved techniques for cleansing and examining the colon are available, the radiologist and endoscopist can find polyps with greater accuracy, demonstrate a stalk, if one is present, and look for the signs of malignancy described earlier in this chapter. In addition, the pathologist has downgraded the significance of focal atypicality and has more accurately assessed the malignant potential of adenomatous, villous, and mixed polyps. With all of these advances in the ability to find and define them, how should polyps of the colon be managed?

Before discussing management, one must recognize that these very advances have posed their own problem: How far should one go in removing polyps? Since the incidence rate is about 12% in the general population, a large number of polyps are available for detection. As Behringer has so clearly stated the dilemma, "To consider all such lesions innocent will result in the tragic neglect of some malignancy, and yet to treat all as malignant will result in unnecessary morbidity and mortality. Each of these cases demands of the clinician the ultimate in judgment, based on a knowledge of the changing concepts of the histopathology of polypoid lesions of the colon."†

As a general principle of management, and if for no other reason than good housekeeping, any polyp found during sigmoidoscopy or colonoscopy should be removed if possible. If a polyp is first found by radiology, the decision as to whether or not it should be removed must be based on the size and characteristics of the polyp and the clinical setting. It is, therefore, essential to have knowledge of these characteristics as well as the behavioral pattern of polyps, in order to exercise enlightened judgment in their management.

Sessile Polyp

If the polyp is first detected by radiology and is less than 1 cm in size, smooth in outline and without symptoms or signs of bleeding, it can be watched with reasonable reassurance that it is benign.

Follow-up barium enema examination should be done in 6 months, or sooner if there are interval symptoms or if bleeding occurs. If there is no interval growth or change in contour of the polyp or the adjacent bowel wall at 6 months, the barium enema should then be repeated each year. The incidence of malignancy in such a tumor is extremely low, in the range of 0.5–1.0%. Even if malignant cells should be found after total excisional biopsy, the likelihood of infiltrating carcinoma or distant metastases are nil if the muscularis mucosa has not been breached.

---

† Reprinted with permission from Behringer, G. E.: Changing concepts in the histopathologic diagnosis of polypoid lesions of the colon. Dis. Colon Rectum, *13:* 116, 1970.

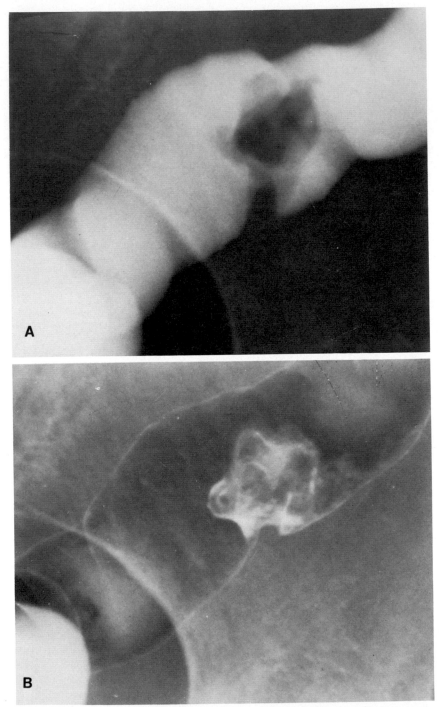

FIG. 15.29. POLYPOID CARCINOMA WITH A SHORT, BROAD STALK AND
"PUCKERING" OF THE BOWEL WALL

A 1.6 × 2.0 cm lobulated polyp in the sigmoid colon also has an ominous short,
broad stalk. The retraction of the wall at the point of attachment of the stalk is
consistent with "puckering" and therefore is another observation in favor of malignancy. (A) Spot-film from barium enema. (B) Spot-film from double-contrast
enema.

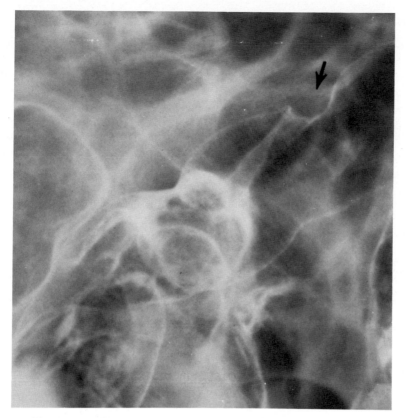

FIG. 15.30. TUGGING OF THE STALK IN A BENIGN POLYP
On double-contrast study, the point of attachment of this long, thin stalk to the wall of the bowel appears puckered (arrow). However, with this type of benign appearing stalk, the retraction of the wall is due to tugging of the stalk and not malignant invasion of the bowel wall.

TABLE 15.1
BENIGN POLYP

1. Sessile, 1 cm or less in size
2. Smooth surface
3. Smooth colon wall at site of origin (when seen in profile)
4. Pedunculated, with head 2.0 cm or less in size
5. If pedunculated, stalk should be long and thin in relation to head
6. If pedunculated, stalk should move freely through a 90° arc to either side
7. Very slow or no interval growth on serial examination
8. No sign of intestinal bleeding

TABLE 15.2
MALIGNANT POLYP

1. Sessile, over 1 cm in size
2. Irregular or lobulated surface
3. Base of sessile polyp measures greater than its height
4. Pedunculated, but stalk is short and broad in relation to size of head
5. Retraction of colon wall at site of origin of a sessile polyp or of a short, broad stalk when seen in profile ("puckering")
6. Stalk relatively rigid to inflow of barium or air, and to palpation
7. Evidence of sudden or steady growth on interval examination
8. Gross or occult intestinal bleeding

Long-Stalked Polyp

If a polyp is first found by radiology above sigmoidoscopic range, on a long, thin stalk, and if the head of the polyp is less than 2.0 cm in size, it too may be watched. The first follow-up barium enema should be done in 6 months and at yearly intervals thereafter. With this type of stalk, the head of the polyp should be freely movable on its stalk through a 90° arc in all directions. If the polyp presents a problem because of bleeding or if it shows change in size or shape of the head or stalk on interval barium examination, it should be resected. A simple polypectomy done through a colonoscope is all that is required. Local invasion or distant metastasis from a polyp on a long, thin stalk is rare and does not warrant segmental bowel resection, regardless of the histologic diagnosis of the polyp. If within reach of the sigmoidoscope, it can easily be amputated when first demonstrated.

Short-Stalked Polyp

If a polyp on a relatively short stalk in relation to the size of the head is first found by radiology, it should be resected through a sigmoidoscope or colonoscope. If there is no microscopic evidence of invasion of the stalk, no further treatment is indicated. If not resected when first found, it should be followed by barium enema study at 6 months, and yearly thereafter. Any evidence of change in size or shape of the head of the polyp, or shortening of the stalk, is a sufficient reason for prompt resection.

BIBLIOGRAPHY

Amberg, J. R., Berk, R. N., Burhenne, H. J., *et al.:* Colonic polyp detection: Role of roentgenography and colonoscopy. Radiology, *125:* 255, 1977.

Behringer, G. E.: Changing concepts in the histopathologic diagnosis of polypoid lesions of the colon. Dis. Colon Rectum, *13:* 116, 1970.

Castleman, B., and Krickstein, H. I.: Do adenomatous polyps of the colon become malignant? N. Engl. J. Med., *267:* 469, 1962.

Dockerty, M. B.: Pathologic aspects in the control of spread of colonic carcinoma. Mayo Clin. Proc. *33:* 157, 1958.

Ekelund, G., Lindström, C., and Rosengren, J. E.: Appearance and growth of early carcinomas of the colon-rectum. Acta Radiol. [Diagn.] *15:* 670, 1974.

Enterline, H. T.: Management of polypoid lesions. J.A.M.A., *231:* 967, 1975.

Fenlon, J. W., and Margulis, A. R.: Current concepts in cancer. Cancer of the G.I. tract: Colon, rectum, anus. The radiologic diagnosis. J.A.M.A., *231:* 752, 1975.

Fenoglio, C. M., and Lane, N.: The anatomic precursor of colorectal carcinoma. J.A.M.A., *231:* 640, 1975.

Finkelstein, A. K., Stein, G. N., and Roy, R. H.: Colonic polyps: A radiologist's viewpoint. Radiol. Clin. North Am., *1:* 175, 1963.

Figiel, L. S., Figiel, S. J., and Wietersen, F. K.: Is surgical removal of every colonic polyp necessary? Am. J. Roentgenol., *88:* 721, 1962.

Kaye, J. J., and Bragg, D. G.: Unusual roentgenologic and clinicopathologic features of villous adenomas of the colon. Radiology, *91:* 799, 1968.

Lane, N., and Fenoglio, C. M.: Observations on the adenoma as precursor to ordinary large bowel carcinoma. Gastrointest. Radiol., *1:* 111, 1976.

Lane, N., Kaplan, H., and Pascal, R.: Minute adenomatous and hyperplastic polyps of the colon: Divergent patterns of epithelial growth with specific associated mesenchymal changes. Gastroenterology, *60:* 537, 1971.

Laufer, I.: *Double Contrast Gastrointestinal Radiology with Endoscopic Correlation.* W. B. Saunders, Philadelphia, 1979.

McCabe, J. C., McSherry, C. K., Sussman, E. B., *et al.:* Villous tumors of the large bowel. Am. J. Surg., *126:* 336, 1973.

McDivitt, R. W.: "Early" large bowel cancer. A morphologist's dilemma. Cancer, *34:* 904, 1974.

Malt, R. A., and Ottinger, L. W.: Carcinoma of the colon and rectum. N. Engl. J. Med., *288:* 772, 1973.

Marshak, R. H., Lindner, A. E., and Maklansky, D.: Adenomatous polyps of the colon. A rational approach. J.A.M.A., *235:* 2856, 1976.

Miller, R. E., and Lehman, G.: Polypoid colonic lesions undetected by endoscopy. Radiology, *129:* 295, 1978.

Morson, B.: The polyp-cancer sequence in the large bowel. Proc. R. Soc. Med., *67:* 451, 1974.

Sleisenger, M. H., and Fordtran, J. S.: *Gastrointestinal Disease,* pp. 1432–1444. W. B. Saunders, Philadelphia, 1973.

Spratt, J. S., Jr., Ackerman, L. V., and Moyer, C. A.: Relationship of polyps of the colon to colonic cancer. Ann. Surg., *148:* 682, 1958.

Spratt, J. S., Jr., and Ackerman, L. V.: Small primary adenocarcinomas of the colon and rectum. J.A.M.A., *179:* 337, 1962.

Thoeni, R. F., and Menuck, L.: Comparison of barium enema and colonoscopy in the detection of small colonic polyps. Radiology, *124:* 631, 1977.

Turek, R. E., Davis, W. C., Wilson, W. J., *et al.:* The roentgenographic diagnosis of villous tumors of the colon. Am. J. Roentgenol., *113:* 349, 1971.

Welin, S., and Welin, G.: *The Double Contrast Examination of the Colon. Experiences with the Welin Modification.* Georg Thieme Verlag, Stuttgart, 1976.

Wolff, W. I., and Shinya, H.: A new approach to colonic polyps. Ann. Surg., *178:* 367, 1973.

16

The Polyposis Disorders

JACK R. DREYFUSS, M.D.

BACKGROUND

Several hereditary and nonhereditary disorders have been described in which there is gastrointestinal polyposis alone or accompanied by manifestations outside of the gastrointestinal tract (Table 16.1). Since some of these well-known entities are not true syndromes, "polyposis disorders" is a better generic term and will be used in this chapter.

Each of the genetic polyposis disorders is inherited in an autosomal dominant pattern except the Turcot syndrome in which the pedigrees are consistent with an autosomal recessive inheritance. The Cronkhite-Canada syndrome has never been identified in more than one family member. The malignant potential of the various disorders ranges from low in generalized juvenile gastrointestinal polyposis to 100% in such devastating entities as familial adenomatous colonic polyposis and the Gardner syndrome. With regard to these latter two disorders, some have suggested that they are both part of the spectrum of a single genetic disorder, while others have proposed that they differ in both clinical manifestations and natural history so that their distinction in any given patient is important. Although further information is needed to finally resolve the controversy, the evidence to date favors the concept that familial adenomatous colonic polyposis and the Gardner syndrome are distinct genetic disorders.

The importance of recognizing these polyposis disorders is not only to identify the individual patient who may be at risk of having or developing colonic cancer, but also to investigate the relatives and offspring of such an individual to determine whether or not they have inherited the gene for the disorder, a point that is all too often overlooked. A *proband* is the term used to denote the individual with a genetic disorder whose diagnosis brings a family to medical attention. The proband, therefore, may lead the physician to other similarly affected family members. Genetic counseling should be provided to such individuals who may plan to have children

TABLE 16.1

The Polyposis Disorders

Disorder	True Syndrome	Inheritance	Age Group	Type of Polyp	Location of Polyps	Extragastrointestinal Manifestations	Malignant Potential	Treatment
Familial adenomatous colonic polyposis	No	Autosomal Dominant	Polyps, at puberty Diagnosis, age 30–40 Death, age 45	Adenomatous	Rectum and colon	None	100%	Colectomy
Gardner syndrome	Yes	Autosomal Dominant	Polyps, late childhood or early adult life Diagnosis, age 30 Death, age 41	Adenomatous	Rectum and colon	Osteomas, fibromas, sebaceous cysts, dental abnormalities, keloid formation	100%	Colectomy
Peutz-Jeghers syndrome	Yes	Autosomal Dominant	Pigmented lesions, infancy or childhood Polyps, at puberty Diagnosis, age 22	Hamartomatous	Entire gastrointestinal tract, but principally in jejunum	Melanin mucocutaneous pigmentation: buccal mucosa, lips, face, hands, feet, genitalia	2–3% predisposition to gastrointestinal cancer, involving stomach, duodenal region, and colon	Surgical for: bleeding; anemia; intussusception or obstruction
Juvenile polyps	No	Not genetic	First decade	Hamartomatous	Rectum and colon	None	None	Polypectomy for bleeding
Juvenile polyposis coli	No	Autosomal Dominant	First decade	Hamartomatous	Rectum and colon	None	To date, colon cancer reported only in relatives of some patients	Polypectomy for bleeding
Generalized juvenile gastrointestinal polyposis	No	Autosomal Dominant	Infancy or first decade	Hamartomatous	Rectum and colon (but may involve stomach and small bowel)	None	Increased incidence of malignant tumors of stomach, duodenum, pancreas, and colon	Surgical for: intussusception and obstruction
Cronkhite-Canada syndrome	Yes	Probably not genetic	Fifth decade or over	Hamartomatous	Stomach, small bowel, and colon	Brownish skin pigmentation, alopecia, loss of nails	Rare reported coexistence with carcinoma of colon	Supportive: fluids; electrolytes and antibiotics
Turcot syndrome	Yes	Autosomal Recessive	Second decade	Adenomatous	Colon	Central nervous system tumors (most are glioblastomas)	3 of 8 reported cases have had carcinoma of colon	Probably colectomy, if early diagnosis could be made, but central nervous system tumors likely to cause symptoms and death before colon cancer can develop

since each potential offspring has a 50% chance of inheriting the autosomal dominant gene responsible for the disorder. Early diagnosis and treatment may be critically important.

GENERAL CONSIDERATIONS

A polyposis disorder should be suspected whenever a polyp is demonstrated in a young person, when 2 or more polyps are found in any individual, or when carcinoma of the colon is found in a patient under 40 years of age. A careful search should then be made for any of the extraintestinal manifestations of the several syndromes and, if indicated, a survey of the patient's immediate family, *i.e.*, parents, siblings, offspring. To miss the opportunity of diagnosing a potentially fatal disease in its premalignant phase is indeed a tragedy.

If there are any presenting intestinal symptoms, they are likely to be bleeding and diarrhea. Abdominal pain is a less frequent complaint. The various extragastrointestinal manifestations of these disorders (*e.g.*, the mucocutaneous pigmentations in Peutz-Jeghers syndrome) may, however, be the only presenting clue. It is, therefore, imperative to recognize them in order to suspect a disorder and initiate the appropriate serial radiologic studies, perhaps even before the appearance of gastrointestinal polyps and, hopefully, before the occurrence of a malignant bowel tumor. Patients who are at risk, but initially without polyps, should thereafter be studied periodically.

While a particularly virulent form of colon cancer may occur at an early age in several of these polyposis disorders, it should be stressed there is no convincing evidence that formation of a polyp is a necessary intermediate step. The colonic cancer may well be a separate effect of the gene itself, or the occurrence of carcinoma may be entirely analogous to the development of colonic cancer in patients with isolated colonic polyps who do not have a polyposis disorder.

As more effective methods of bowel preparation have evolved over the years and as improved techniques for examining the large bowel by x-ray have been described, there has been a significant advance in ability to detect and define colonic polyps. The advent of expertise in colonoscopy has also added immeasurably to the accuracy of diagnosing the polyposis disorders.

The specific clinical features, radiologic findings, and pertinent statistics of these disorders are presented in the following sections.

FAMILIAL ADENOMATOUS COLONIC POLYPOSIS

In 1882, Cripps, in England, described 2 cases of disseminated polyps of the colon. This was the first documentation of what is the best known, most frequent, and deadliest of the polyposis disorders. Inherited as a simple autosomal dominant, the incidence in the general population is estimated at about 1 in 8,000, with each offspring of an affected patient having a 50% risk of inheriting the causative gene.

On the average, symptoms due to the polyps appear at about age 30, and the diagnosis of polyposis is made at age 40—by which time two-thirds of the patients will already have colonic cancer and half of those will have multiple primary lesions. If untreated, the average patient will be dead at age 45 from metastatic colon carcinoma.

Unlike some of the other inherited polyposis disorders, there are no extraintestinal manifestations in familial adenomatous colonic polyposis and the polyps are limited to the colon and rectum. However, there have been scattered reports of patients who also had adenomas of the stomach and duodenum.

Since the penetrance of the familial polyposis gene is high, although not complete, two-thirds of affected patients will have other family members with colonic polyps or cancers. (Occasionally a skipped generation is observed with an affected individual related through an apparently unaffected parent to an affected grandparent. This may be the result of what geneticists term *incomplete penetrance*, but it is perhaps more likely due to incomplete diagnostic evaluation of the relevant family members, here the parent.) The inheritance pattern and the relentless progression of the disorder demand early suspicion, detection, and prompt treatment. A careful screening of all at-risk relatives (parents, siblings, and offspring) as well as genetic counseling becomes as mandatory as dedicated follow-up studies for both surgically treated and asymptomatic at-risk individuals.

Clinical Features

The presenting symptoms of familial adenomatous colonic polyposis are intermittent rectal bleeding and diarrhea, with less than half of the patients complaining of abdominal pain or mucous discharge. Because the polyps are relatively small and limited to the colon, intussusception is not a problem.

The polyps may begin to develop by puberty and increase steadily in size and number during the teens and twenties until hundreds or thousands are present throughout the colon. This blanketing by polyposis may be so extensive that normal colonic mucosa cannot be recognized. The polyps range in size from a few millimeters to 1–3 cm but tend to be rather uniform in the 0.5 cm range. The overwhelming majority of the polyps are adenomas, although there may be a rare inflammatory polyp or villous adenoma. Lymphoid hyperplasia of the terminal ileum may be noted, but true polyps are not present in the small bowel.

Colectomy is the only available treatment. It should be carried out both for demonstrated carcinoma, or as a prophylactic procedure in symptomatic or asymptomatic individuals when the diagnosis of familial adenomatous colonic polyposis is first made. Total colectomy is favored by some, while others recommend subtotal colectomy and ileorectal anastomosis. However, if the subtotal procedure has been done, frequent inspection of the rectum by proctoscopy is required to detect and remove remaining polyps or new polyps if they develop, and to look for malignancy. If the disease is first detected in early adolescence, it is considered safe to wait until the late teens to perform surgery, particularly if total colectomy is to be done. The young person is then better able, physically and emotionally, to tolerate such drastic treatment, or to understand the importance of life-long medical follow-ups if the rectum is to be spared.

Roentgen Findings

The x-ray study of patients with familial adenomatous colonic polyposis is usually requested because they have complained of rectal bleeding or diarrhea, often with mucus. Polyps may have been observed at sigmoidoscopic examination done for the same symptoms, or the patient may be related to a proband.

Depending on the age of the patient, the polyps may appear as scattered lesions of about 0.5–1 cm in size in one or more areas of the colon—or there may be hundreds of polyps throughout the colon (Fig. 16.1). If polyposis is diffuse, the colon may appear to be "poorly prepared." However, with true polyps, the filling defects do not scatter with palpation, but remain fixed in position. In profile, they clearly arise from the wall of the bowel and resemble the pseudopolyps of ulcerative colitis although smaller and more uniform in size.

Compression spot-films will easily confirm the constancy of the polyps. Perhaps

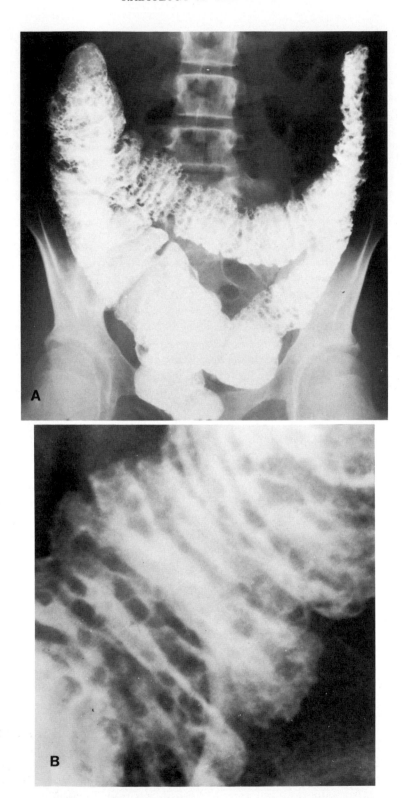

FIG. 16.1. FAMILIAL ADENOMATOUS COLONIC POLYPOSIS
(A) Countless polyps are present throughout the colon in this 13-year-old male.
The boy's mother was found to have an adenocarcinoma of the colon 10 years earlier
at the time of colectomy for "polyps of the colon." (B) Spot-film of the colon
showing the 0.5–1 cm polyps.

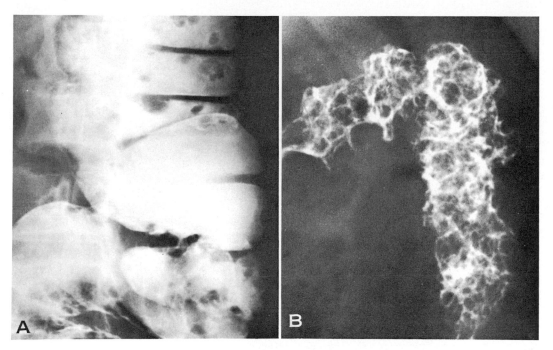

FIG. 16.2. FAMILIAL ADENOMATOUS COLONIC POLYPOSIS
(A) Multiple, round filling defects are seen in the barium-filled descending colon.
(B) The postevacuation film demonstrates the true extent of the polyps as well as
failure of the colon to contract completely due to the bulk of the polyps.

the most striking confirmation is obtained on the postevacuation films, where a light
coating of retained barium outlines the filling defects with clarity. Another important
observation is that with countless polyps, the colon will not clamp down to its usual
postevacuation diameter of 1.5–2.0 cm, but will appear wider than normal due to the
bulk of the mucosal polyps (Fig. 16.2). If doubt still persists, an immediate repeat
barium enema should be done.

Air-contrast studies of a clean colon will also provide dramatic demonstration of
the distribution and size of the polyps. Colonoscopy is yet another diagnostic
procedure of value, especially when biopsy confirmation of the nature of the polyps
or of a lesion suspicious of cancer is required.

When cancer of the colon develops in patients with familial adenomatous colonic
polyposis, its morphologic appearance is not different from colonic malignancy in a
patient without the genetic disorder. The cancer will either be lobulated and larger
than surrounding polyps, or it will have a plaque-like or annular configuration,
depending on its stage of development. It is, however, much more likely to be
multifocal than in the non-genetic types.

GARDNER SYNDROME

In articles starting in 1950, Gardner and his co-workers described a syndrome
characterized by osteomatosis, cutaneous and subcutaneous lesions in association
with an hereditary form of polyposis similar to familial polyposis. Since then, over
300 additional cases have been reported, but the actual incidence is estimated to be
as high as 1 in 14,000 births. Because of the wide variety of extraintestinal presentations, many cases are overlooked until the intestinal manifestations demand
attention. The syndrome is inherited as a simple autosomal dominant produced by

a single pleiotropic gene. Skipped generations have also been described but again may present incomplete penetrance or inadequate diagnosis. This is a lethal disease. If colectomy is not performed when the diffuse colorectal polyposis is first discovered, 100% of the patients will die of metastatic colon cancer before the end of their fourth decade. The mean age at diagnosis is 31, and in one series of 29 symptomatic patients, 19 developed colon cancer within 2 years of diagnosis of the polyps. The average age at death is 41 years.

Clinical Features

The extraintestinal signs of the Gardner syndrome generally develop earlier than the intestinal polyposis. For this reason, the clinician may have the opportunity to suspect the syndrome when prepubertal patients seek advice because of their distressing cosmetic appearance. Among these early manifestations are single or multiple sebaceous cysts of the face, scalp and back, together with subcutaneous fibromas, lipomas, and leiomyomas. The fibrous tissue tumors tend to progress in number and size regardless of whether colon polyps are present or the colon has been resected for polyposis. In addition, there may be one or more osteomas or exostoses of the skeleton, particularly of the skull (Fig. 16.3) and also areas of cortical thickening in the long bones and ribs. The patients may also have dental abnormalities such as odontomas, extra teeth, unerupted teeth, and numerous caries. Further, they tend to form dense scars or keloids following surgery. This propensity to proliferation of fibrous tissue may also be manifested in the abdomen

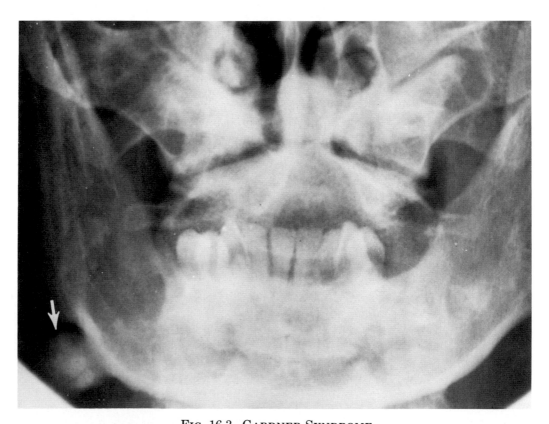

FIG. 16.3. GARDNER SYNDROME
Osteoma of the mandible (arrow). (Reprinted by permission from Case Records of the Massachusetts General Hospital (Case No. 53-1976, Gardner's Syndrome). N. Engl. J. Med., *295:* 1526, 1976.)

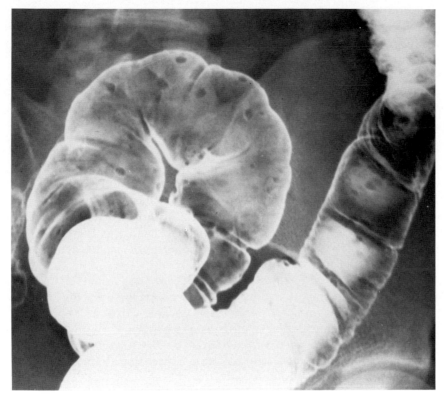

FIG. 16.4. COLONIC POLYPS IN A PATIENT WITH GARDNER SYNDROME
Resembling the polyps of familial adenomatous colonic polyposis, these polyps also measure from 0.5–1 cm in diameter. (Reprinted by permission from Case Records of the Massachusetts General Hospital (Case No. 53-1976, Gardner's Syndrome). N. Engl. J. Med., *295:* 1526, 1976.)

as adhesions or mesenteric and retroperitoneal fibrosis. If severe enough, small bowel or intra-abdominal vascular obstruction may occur.

While any one patient may not have the entire triad of soft tissue abnormalities, bone lesions, and polyposis, recognition of the pleiotropic signs is critical for early diagnosis of the syndrome. At this point, a careful radiologic study of the entire intestinal tract becomes mandatory.

Roentgen Findings

The adenomatous polyps found in patients with Gardner syndrome are almost invariably limited to the rectum and colon. Rarely, they may also occur in the stomach and small bowel. Whereas the extraintestinal components of the disorder tend to appear early, the polyps develop later, usually in late childhood or early adult life. In all ways they resemble the polyps found in familial adenomatous colonic polyposis, varying in size from mammillations to sessile lesions of about 1 cm (Fig. 16.4). Pedunculated polyps also occur but are less common than the sessile variety. The colon will eventually be blanketed with polyps. Compression spot-films or air-contrast studies are the best roentgen methods for detecting the polyps. Colonoscopy and biopsy should be done as well.

When cancer develops, it is of the plaque-like form, later becoming annular. Because of the almost certain development of colon cancer in mid-life, all patients who have the polyposis part of the syndrome are usually advised to have a prophylactic total colectomy when the polyps are first demonstrated. Recently, colectomy with ileorectal anastomosis has been performed in some patients, even though polyps have been present in the retained rectum. Frequent follow-up proctoscopy has often shown regression in the number and size of the remaining polyps. In a few cases, they have completely disappeared.

Further careful clinical and roentgen monitoring of these patients is indicated, even after total or subtotal colectomy, for they seem to have a higher than normal risk of developing malignant lesions of the thyroid, pancreas, and periampullary areas of the duodenum.

PEUTZ-JEGHERS SYNDROME

The Peutz-Jeghers syndrome is inherited by an autosomal dominant gene responsible for both gastrointestinal polyposis and mucocutaneous pigmentation. First described by Peutz in 1921, and expanded and clarified by Jeghers, McKusick, and Katz in 1949, over 300 patients have been reported in the literature. The true incidence, however, is unknown; isolated cases are not reported nor are family studies always carried out.

Because the polyps are hamartomas, the syndrome was originally thought to be unassociated with malignancy. However, recent studies have suggested a predisposition to the development of gastrointestinal cancer, a risk of about 2–3% with predilection for the stomach, duodenal region and colon.

The hamartomatous polyps of this syndrome occur throughout the gastrointestinal tract, predominantly in the jejunum, with decreasing frequency in the ileum, colon and rectum, stomach, and duodenum.

Clinical Features

The hallmark of this syndrome is the mucocutaneous pigmentation which occurs in nearly all cases, and usually develops in infancy or early childhood. These brownish-black lesions are flat and 1–5 mm in size. They appear predominantly on the lips and buccal mucosa (Fig. 16.5) but may also occur on the face, abdomen, genitalia, hands, and feet. The cutaneous melanotic spots may fade in adult life but the buccal pigmentation generally persists.

The presenting intestinal symptoms are bleeding and intermittent colicky pain, often severe and due to small bowel intussusception led by one of the polyps. While the pigmented lesions develop early, the gastrointestinal symptoms due to polyps appear later—in puberty or adolescence. Even so, the mean age at actual diagnosis of the syndrome is 22 years (Fig. 16.6).

The attacks of pain are recurring, consistent with the usual transient nature of the intussusception. However, some patients have required surgical intervention on more than one occasion for relief of small bowel obstruction (Fig. 16.7). There may, conversely, be long periods of total lack of intestinal symptoms (Fig. 16.8).

The relatively rare colonic hamartoma of the Peutz-Jeghers syndrome is often found only when rectal bleeding or anemia indicate the necessity of a barium enema or colonoscopy. Even though the incidence of colonic polyps in Peutz-Jeghers patients is low, these diagnostic procedures should be part of the work-up of patients suspected of having the syndrome.

Surgery is indicated in the presence of acute or repeated intestinal bleeding, chronic anemia, or frank obstruction due to an intussusception. All demonstrated or palpable polyps should be removed when possible, preferably by multiple enterostomies. This is important to preserve as much absorptive small bowel surface as possible, since further surgery may be necessary as new polyps occur and the cycle of bleeding and intussusception is repeated. When symptomatic and demonstrated,

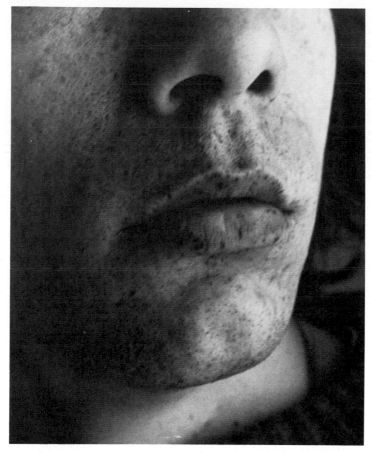

FIG. 16.5. PEUTZ-JEGHERS SYNDROME

A 22-year-old male showing the typical melanotic pigmentation of the lips and face. He also has similar pigmentation on his buccal mucosa, genitalia, and knees.

colon polyps should be removed by colonoscopy or colotomy. Only one case of colo-colic intussusception has been reported.

Roentgen Findings

Although Peutz-Jeghers polyps are less difficult to demonstrate in the stomach and colon, they are relatively uncommon in these locations. The polyps occur more frequently in the small bowel, especially the jejunum and may be extremely difficult to demonstrate, even when suspected clinically. A careful study of the small bowel by serial films and fluoroscopy, however, may reveal single or multiple tumors, often pedunculated.

When one or two small bowel polyps are found on x-ray examination, it can be assumed with certainty that there are more present which defy current methods of detection. While serial films of the small bowel are mandatory, they are apt to be confusing because of overlapping loops and spurious filling defects which represent merely pockets of gas or normal bowel content. Intestinal enemas and air-contrast examinations of the small bowel may be helpful if meticulously performed. However, conventional, intermittent fluoroscopy with spot-filming is apt to be the most rewarding type of study. During fluoroscopy, transient intussusceptions may draw the fluoroscopist's eye to the polyps.

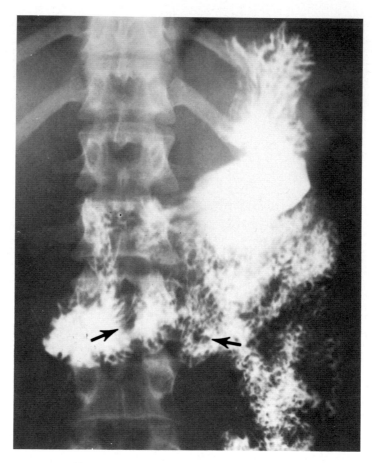

FIG. 16.6. PEUTZ-JEGHERS SYNDROME

Examined because of repeated guaiac-positive stools, the patient was found to have multiple jejunal polyps, two of which are demonstrated (arrows). This is the young man shown in Fig. 16.5.

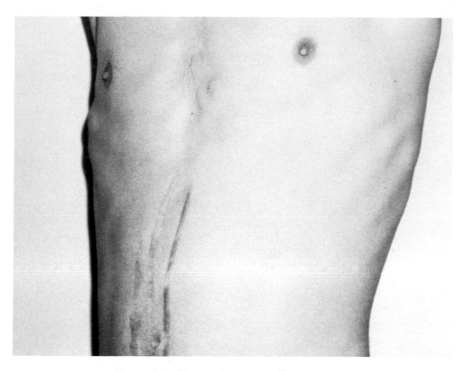

FIG. 16.7. PEUTZ-JEGHERS SYNDROME

Photograph of the abdomen of the patient shown in Figs. 16.5 and 16.6. This 22-year-old male has undergone 5 abdominal operations for bleeding, intussusception, or obstruction. In the course of these procedures polyps have been removed from his stomach, duodenum, small bowel, and colon, all hamartomas. He has also undergone 24 sigmoidoscopies or colonoscopies because of rectal bleeding, with resection of numerous colonic polyps.

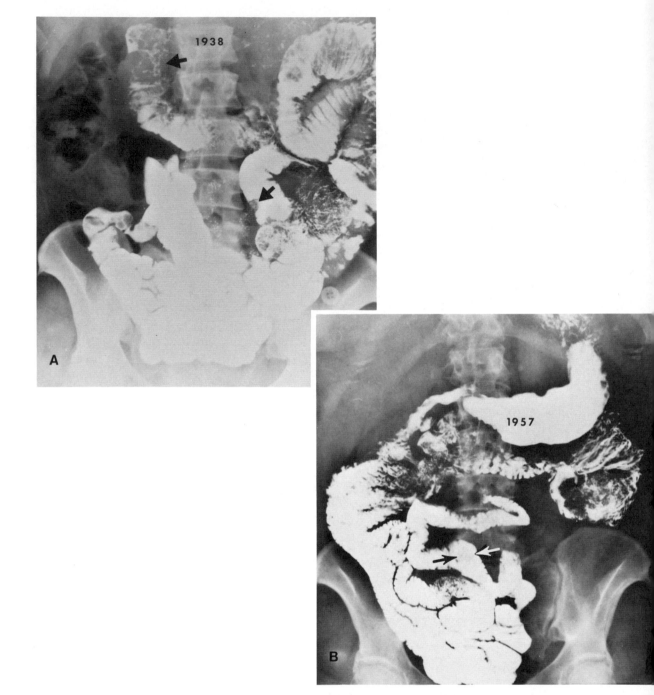

FIG. 16.8. PEUTZ-JEGHERS SYNDROME

Four films from the many small bowel examinations done on a 72-year-old female between 1935 and 1975. This woman was one of the patients described by Jeghers, McKusick, and Katz in their 1949 article in the *New England Journal of Medicine*, and has been followed at the Massachusetts General Hospital since 1938. The patient has required 7 abdominal operations for bleeding or intussusception. The multiple polyps resected over the years have all been hamartomas, and there has been no sign of gastrointestinal malignancy to date. (**A**) Duodenal and jejunal polyps in 1938 (arrows). (**B**) Transient jejunal intussusception with polyps, in the left upper quadrant, and a large ileal polyp (arrows) in 1957. (**C**) Jejunal polyps in 1969 (arrows). (**D**) Multiple small and one large jejunal polyp (arrow) in 1975.

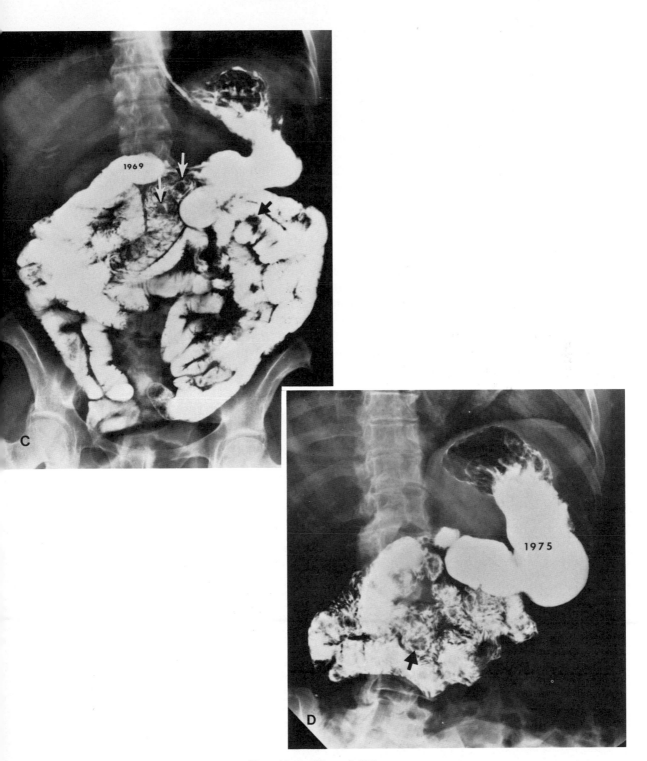

FIG. 16.8. (C) and (D)

JUVENILE POLYPS

The presence of one or several juvenile polyps in the colon of a young child is not uncommon in the absence of a heritable disorder and without any extraintestinal manifestations or evidence of associated intestinal malignancy. As the name suggests, these polyps occur in children, usually as isolated tumors, developing during the first decade of life.

The juvenile polyp is a hamartoma and is sometimes referred to as a retention or inflammatory polyp. A juvenile polyp contains multiple cysts filled with mucin and there is an abundant connective tissue stroma. Inflammatory cells are numerous, the thin surface epithelium bleeds easily, and the polyps may ulcerate at the base and undergo autoamputation. The juvenile or inflammatory polyp is identical in type to that seen in adults with the Cronkhite-Canada syndrome.

Clinical Features

With a peak incidence between 2 and 5 years of age, the young patients present with symptoms of rectal bleeding, a mucous discharge or diarrhea, and occasionally abdominal pain. The bleeding is bright red if a polyp is in the distal colon or rectum whereas the blood will be mixed with the stool if the lesion is more proximal in the colon. When detected at sigmoidoscopy, the juvenile polyp usually shows a hemorrhagic surface; the isolated stalk of a sloughed-off polyp may be seen as well. If located in the rectum, the polyp may prolapse. Rarely, autoamputation may cause the polyp to be deposited in the toilet bowl, where it may be detected by a startled parent as a red, fleshy mass.

In nearly all cases, the polyp is solitary. When multiple polyps are found, there are rarely more than several in the rectum or colon. Since juvenile polyps are benign when discovered and without malignant potential, conservative treatment is indicated. Surgical removal is reserved for those cases where significant or repeated rectal bleeding is a problem.

Roentgen Findings

On barium enema examination, the juvenile polyp appears round, 1–3 cm in size and may show a smooth or slightly lobulated surface. The lesion is usually sessile. In the more distal colon and rectum, pedunculation is more common.

A vigorous bowel preparation and purge is rarely warranted in children, and the barium enema itself is the best preparation followed by a repeat barium enema if necessary for a clearer view of the cleansed bowel. Overfilling of the colon with subsequent small bowel reflux should be avoided; the barium inflow is best stopped when the hepatic flexure is reached. The postevacuation mucosal relief film is likely to be the most rewarding one for the detection of polyps in children. There is no contraindication to an air-contrast examination as an additional procedure and the detection of small polyps can be as easily accomplished in children as in adults.

The subject of polyps in children is also covered in Chapter 5.

JUVENILE POLYPOSIS COLI AND GENERALIZED JUVENILE GASTROINTESTINAL POLYPOSIS

Two probable familial juvenile polyposis disorders have been reported which may involve children, teenagers, and adults. Since the data are still incomplete with regard to prognosis and treatment, it will be important to observe such patients frequently and carefully. There has been no change, however, in the belief that the isolated juvenile polyp of the colon is itself a benign hamartoma without malignant potential.

In 1966, Veale and colleagues described juvenile polyposis coli, an entity which appeared to be distinct from simple juvenile polyposis. Their 11 patients, from 4 families, had multiple juvenile polyps of the colon. In addition, there was a history of colon cancer in relatives of 4 of the patients, although none had occurred in the 11 patients themselves. There have been no extraintestinal manifestations.

Kindreds have also been reported by Sachatello, Stemper, and others, in which some family members have single or multiple juvenile polyps in the stomach and small intestine, as well as the colon. In this entity, known as generalized juvenile gastrointestinal polyposis, there appears to be an increased incidence of malignant tumors in the stomach, duodenum, pancreas, and colon. Blood loss and intussusception are the usual presenting symptoms. The disorder is thought to be heritable by a single autosomal dominant gene with a high degree of penetrance. No extraintestinal manifestations have been reported.

CRONKHITE-CANADA SYNDROME

A bizarre combination of brownish pigmentation of the skin, alopecia, atrophy and subsequent loss of fingernails and toenails together with gastrointestinal polyposis was reported in 2 patients by Cronkhite and Canada in 1955. Since then, 48 additional cases have been reported, bringing the total number of recorded cases to 50. There has been no evidence to date that this syndrome is heritable.

Although originally there was no suggestion that the polyps were associated with colonic malignancy, 2 cases have now been reported in which coexisting cancer of the colon occurred. Whether this is a chance occurrence or indicative of a true malignant potential will have to be tested by time.

The disorder presents later in life than the other polyposis disorders and syndromes, the average age of onset being over 50 (range 42–85 years). The presenting symptoms are usually those of intestinal malabsorption and include diarrhea, abdominal pain, anorexia, nausea, vomiting, weight loss, peripheral edema, and marked weakness. In some patients, the ectodermal changes may precede the more gross intestinal symptoms by months or years. The diffuse intestinal polyposis is probably responsible for the defect in absorption and the resultant deficiency state.

The degree of gastrointestinal polyposis is striking. Although it was originally suggested that these polyps were adenomatous, subsequent reports have shown that they are actually inflammatory polyps with cystic glandular dilatation, similar to juvenile polyps. In 1971, Diner (née Canada) reported that a retrospective analysis of the original case material also showed the polyps to be inflammatory rather than adenomatous. Roentgen and gross examination of the gastrointestinal tracts of patients with this syndrome show the stomach and colon to be blanketed by polyps, which also occur in the small bowel, more numerous in the distal half. The polyps vary in size from mammillations to over 1 cm. Because of the usual difficulty of demonstrating small bowel polyps, the roentgen examination of the stomach and colon is always more striking. Compression spot-films and air-contrast examination are the most rewarding methods of finding the polyps.

Since the cause of the disorder is unknown, treatment is largely supportive and designed to combat the extraordinary deficiency state—which is probably responsible for the ectodermal changes as it is for the degree of inanition. Spontaneous remissions have been reported, but the disease is likely to be relentlessly progressive and death within 1 year of diagnosis has been the rule, especially in females.

TURCOT SYNDROME

A combination of multiple adenomatous polyps of the colon and tumors of the central nervous system are the features of this syndrome. First reported in 1959 by Turcot and colleagues, in a brother and sister, the offspring of unaffected parents (who were third cousins), the syndrome is considered to be on the basis of autosomal recessive inheritance rather than the autosomal dominance pattern of the other major polyposis disorders.

Of the total of 8 patients with Turcot syndrome reported thus far, 6 have been from only 2 families. It is, therefore, the newest and "smallest" of the heritable polyposis disorders and there is less known about it than the others. The presenting symptoms have occurred in the second decade of life and have been either neurologic due to brain or spinal cord tumors or intestinal—diarrhea possibly related to the colonic polyps. Three of the patients had carcinoma of the colon in addition to adenomatous polyps of the colon.

Since death at an early age, in the teens or twenties, has been the usual outcome due to the central nervous system tumors, of which glioblastoma of the brain is most common, the actual potential for fatal outcome due to metastatic colon cancer is unknown. It is probable that if these patients survived long enough, they would show the same high incidence of death from colon cancer as do patients with the Gardner syndrome and familial adenomatous colonic polyposis.

BIBLIOGRAPHY

Case Records of the Massachusetts General Hospital (Case No. 53-1976, Gardner's Syndrome). N. Engl. J. Med., *295:* 1526, 1976.

Cripps, H.: Two cases of disseminated polyps of the colon. Trans. Pathol. Soc. Lond., *33:* 165, 1882.

Cronkhite, L. W., Jr., and Canada, W. J.: Generalized gastrointestinal polyposis. An unusual syndrome of polyposis, pigmentation, alopecia, and onychotrophia. N. Engl. J. Med., *252:* 1011, 1955.

Diner, W. C.: The Cronkhite-Canada syndrome. Radiology, *105:* 715, 1971.

Dodd, G. D.: Genetics and cancer of the gastrointestinal system. Radiology, *123:* 263, 1977.

Dodds, W. J.: Clinical and roentgen features of the intestinal polyposis syndromes. Gastrointest. Radiol., *1:* 127, 1976.

Erbe, R. W.: Inherited gastrointestinal-polyposis syndromes. N. Engl. J. Med., *294:* 1101, 1976.

Gardner, E. J., and Richards, R. C.: Multiple cutaneous and subcutaneous lesions occurring simultaneously with hereditary polyposis and osteomatosis. Am. J. Hum. Genet., *5:* 139, 1953.

Gardner, E. J., and Stephens, F. E.: Cancer of the lower digestive tract in one family group. Am. J. Hum. Genet., *2:* 41, 1950.

Itai, Y., Kogure, T., *et al.:* Radiographic features of gastric polyps in familial adenomatous coli. Am. J. Roentgenol., *128:* 73, 1977.

Jeghers, H., McKusick, V. A., and Katz, K. H.: Generalized intestinal polyposis and melanin spots of the oral mucosa, lips and digits. A syndrome of diagnostic significance. N. Engl. J. Med., *241:* 993, 1949.

Long, J. A., Jr., and Dreyfuss, J. R.: The Peutz-Jeghers syndrome: A 39-year clinical and radiographic follow-up report. N. Engl. J. Med., *297:* 1070, 1977.

McAllister, A. J., and Richards, K. F.: Peutz-Jeghers syndrome. Experience with twenty patients in five generations. Am. J. Surg., *134:* 717, 1977.

Murashima, Y., *et al.:* Cronkhite-Canada syndrome. Report of 26 cases. Stomach Intestine, *12:* 495, 1977.

Peutz, J. L.: Ober eeen zeer merkwaardige, geocombineerde familiare polyposis van de slijmvliezen van den tractus intestinalis met die van de neuskeelholte en gepaard met eigen aardige pigmentaties van huiden slijmvliezen. Nederl Maandschr Geneesk *10:* 134, 1921.

Sachatello, C. R., Pickren, J. W., and Grace, J. T. Jr.: Generalized juvenile gastrointestinal polyposis. A hereditary syndrome. Gastroenterology, *58:* 699, 1970.

Stauffer, J. Q.: Hereditable multiple polyposis syndromes of the gastrointestinal tract. In *Gastrointestinal Disease,* edited by M. H. Sleisenger and J. S. Fordtran, p. 1051. W. B. Saunders, Philadelphia, 1973.

Stemper, T. J., Kent, T. H., and Summers, R. W.: Juvenile polyposis and gastrointestinal carcinoma. A study of the kindred. Ann. Intern. Med., *83:* 639, 1975.

Turcot, J., Despres, J., and St. Pierre, F.: Malignant tumors of the central nervous system associated with familial polyposis of the colon: Report of two cases. Dis. Colon Rectum, *2:* 465, 1959.

Veale, A. M. O., McColl, I., Bussey, H. J. R., and Morson, B. C.: Juvenile polyposis coli. J. Med. Genet., *3:* 5, 1966.

Wayne, A. L., Core, S. K., and Carrier, J. M.: Gardner's syndrome. Surg. Gynecol. Obstet., *141:* 53, 1975.

17

Malignant Tumors and Other Colonic Neoplasms

JACK R. DREYFUSS, M.D.

BACKGROUND

Among malignant tumors, cancer of the colon and rectum is the number two killer of both sexes, second only to cancer of the lung in males and cancer of the breast in females. Despite all efforts to alert the public to the early symptoms of colonic carcinoma, and despite steady improvement in methods for diagnosis and treatment, the 5-year survival rate has not changed significantly since 1960.

A disease which predominantly afflicts those in the fifth to seventh decades, colon cancer is now being seen with increasing frequency not only in this group but also in younger individuals. There continues to be no appreciable difference in the death rate between males and females; there has, however, been a gradually increasing incidence and death rate for both sexes in western cultures.

From 1945 to 1960, there was a slight decrease in colon cancer deaths, attributed to earlier detection, more radical surgical procedures, and a decrease in operative

TABLE 17.1
CARCINOMA OF COLON AND RECTUM: MASSACHUSETTS GENERAL HOSPITAL, 1937–1970*

	1937–48	1949–60	1961–70
Total patients treated	1,940	1,886	1,566
Five year survival			
Available for 5-year follow-up study	1,088	1,205	1,162
Total survival	26%	39%	41%
After resection for cure	45%	57%	54%

* Adapted from: Welch, J. P., and Donaldson, G. A.: Am. J. Surg. *127*: 258, 1974.

mortality. Even though these laudable factors continue, the death rate has leveled off and remains unassailable even to better understanding of the malignant potential of certain polyps, improved endoscopic and radiologic techniques and to the advent of aggressive chemotherapy.

The American Cancer Society estimated that in 1978 there would be 49,000 new cases of cancer of the colon and rectum in males and 53,000 new cases in females. The Society also estimated that there would be 25,000 deaths from this disease among males and 27,000 among females.

The overall 5-year survival rate remains in the 35–45% range, as it has since 1960. It is estimated that the best obtainable figure is 55%, assuming that primary physicians and radiologists detect all colon cancers on initial presentation of patients with symptoms and that curative rather than palliative resections can be carried out (Table 17.1).

Analysis of current statistics on colonic cancer suggests that an age has been entered where no further improvement will be achieved until we discover and are able to control the factors responsible for this disease whether they be genetic, environmental, hormonal, enzymatic, immunologic, diet-related or a combination of them.

PATHOLOGY

The pathology of malignant tumors and other neoplasms of the colon is presented in Chapter 14.

DIAGNOSTIC METHODS

The methods available to evaluate the possibility of colonic neoplasia are history, physical examination, laboratory tests, radiology, and endoscopy. Although any one of these may provide the information needed to make a presumptive diagnosis, it is more likely that a combination of two or more methods will lead from suspicion to final histologic diagnosis.

History

In its earliest stages of growth a colonic cancer may be totally asymptomatic. Patients with right-sided tumors are more likely to complain of dull abdominal pain, or present with symptoms due to bleeding or anemia. The symptoms most frequently reported by patients with left-sided colonic tumors are rectal bleeding, change in bowel habits, and crampy abdominal pain. The symptoms which cause patients to seek medical attention according to the specific location of the tumor are given in Table 17.2.

A left-sided tumor will usually cause earlier symptoms than one on the right side of the colon. Severe changes in bowel habits, anemia, weight loss, and obstruction occur late in the disease. Occult bleeding, an early sign of colonic neoplasia, is not

TABLE 17.2
Symptoms by Location: Massachusetts General Hospital, 1937–1970*

	Percent with Symptoms	Percent with Rectal Bleeding	Percent with Change in Bowel Habits	Percent with Abdominal Pain	Percent with Obstruction	Percent with Weight Loss	Percent with Mass	Percent with Anemia
Right colon	92.3	20.0	24.5	44.7	7.9	19.4	6.3	13.8
Transverse colon	88.8	21.1	23.2	40.1	16.2	18.3	3.5	8.4
Descending colon	89.4	27.6	26.3	35.5	23.7	11.8	1.3	3.9
Sigmoid colon	94.8	43.1	39.7	26.6	15.1	12.8	1.7	2.3
Rectum	96.3	60.0	50.8	19.2	6.9	17.7	0.7	0.0

* Adapted from: Welch, J. P., and Donaldson, G. A.: Am. J. Surg., *127:* 258, 1974.

evident to the patient. As more bleeding occurs, the stool may be reported as dark or maroon colored. With fresh bleeding, particularly from a left-sided lesion, the blood is often reported as mixed with the stool, rather than at the end of defecation, as often seen with hemorrhoidal bleeding. Alternating diarrhea and constipation and then progressive constipation are often noted by patients with left-sided tumors who then resort to the use of cathartics.

Physical Examination

Digital examination of the rectum is still the quickest and surest method to detect a cancer in that location. It is an essential part of every physical examination, even in asymptomatic individuals; three-fourths of all rectal cancers are within reach of the examining finger.

Lesions in other locations are more difficult to detect by palpation. The bulky right-sided tumors, or tumors of 4 cm or more in size in the transverse and left colon segments may be palpable depending on the patient's build.

The physical appearance of the patient is notoriously deceptive. Depending on the duration and stage of a colonic tumor, the patient may appear in excellent health, or pale, anemic and fatigued, or may show frank cachexia.

Laboratory Tests

Tests for Blood Loss

Patients with chronic blood loss may show a hypochromic, microcytic anemia typical of iron deficiency. Leukocytosis is not usually seen in patients with colonic cancer unless there is associated necrosis, inflammation, or metastatic disease. An elevated alkaline phosphatase may indicate hepatic metastasis.

Many colon cancers are first suspected because of a single, random guaiac-positive test of the stool, or repeated positive tests. The guaiac test is, nevertheless, an unreliable screening procedure; a negative test does not provide reassurance and positive tests may result from a variety of other conditions, including a diet high in meat content.

The Hemoccult Slide Test,* however, has been shown to be very effective in detecting occult bleeding. The ease of performance, the low rate of false-positives, even when the patient is not on a meat-free diet, and its high rate of accuracy in detecting small asymptomatic cancers (Fig. 17.1) has resulted in its endorsement by the American Cancer Society. It should be a part of every patient work-up, whether or not colon cancer is suspected.

---

* SmithKline Diagnostics

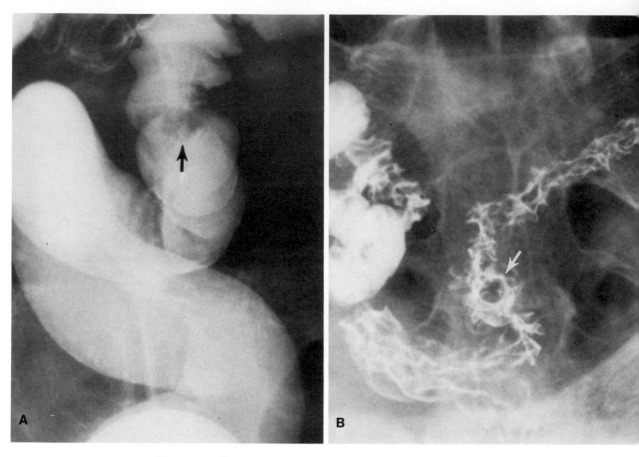

FIG. 17.1. SEVEN MILLIMETER ASYMPTOMATIC CARCINOMA
Two positive tests for occult blood at the time of a yearly physical examination
prompted this barium enema in a 63-year-old man. A 7 mm sessile polyp (arrow)
was found which proved to be adenocarcinoma. (**A**) Posteroanterior angled view of
the barium-filled sigmoid. (**B**)Postevacuation film.

Cytology

In contrast to its success in detecting cervical cancer, cytology has not thus far
played a significant role in colonic cancer. The low yield of identifiable cells from
the surface of a colon tumor, the time and cost of the procedure, and the lack of well
trained cytologists have combined to make this a screening test of limited value.
Recently, colonoscopic brushings have yielded better results, but still not as sensitive
as endoscopic biopsy.

Carcinoembryonic Antigen (CEA)

CEA was originally isolated from specimens of human colon cancer in 1965. Later,
when radioimmunoassay methods were devised for detecting CEA in human serum,
it was hoped that the test would be specific and, therefore, invaluable for the
diagnosis of colonic neoplasia. Such has not been the case. While there is a high
incidence of elevated CEA levels in patients with carcinoma of the colon, elevated
levels may also be demonstrated concurrent with malignancies of the pancreas,
breast, lung, genitourinary tract, and bone. To further dampen its hoped for
specificity, the CEA titer may also be elevated in patients with inflammatory bowel
disease, cirrhosis, chronic renal disease, diverticular disease and even in patients

who are heavy smokers, or who have no evidence of organic disease. Numerous false-negative results have also marred testing accuracy—normal CEA's in the presence of demonstrable colon cancers by x-ray and subsequent surgery.

When colon cancer is resected in a patient in whom the CEA was positive, there seems to be a relation between the level of titer elevation and size of the tumor, as well as the recurrence rate. The CEA assay also has some limited value in following patients under chemotherapy. However, as a test to pick up early localized recurrent cancer, the CEA method is of little value. Elevated titers more often are associated with disseminated metastases. At this stage the disease is usually clinically apparent and not amenable to any current therapy.

When the serum CEA titers are utilized in conjunction with radiologic studies of the colon, the overall accuracy of cancer detection is slightly improved over either method alone. However, if only one test is to be done, the x-ray examination remains more rewarding than CEA assay in detecting new colonic cancer.

Radiology

Radiologic study of the colon remains the least invasive, least expensive, and most rewarding method for the detection of carcinoma. When a meticulously performed double-contrast examination is done, the accuracy approaches or equals the statistics of surgery or autopsy material in the detection of colonic lesions of 5 mm or larger in size.

The details of performing single- and double-contrast examinations of the large bowel are covered in Chapter 3 on Technique. The role of radiology in the detection of polyps is covered in Chapter 15. The radiographic characteristics of the larger, more obvious colonic malignancies are described in this chapter under Roentgen Findings.

Endoscopy

The sigmoidoscope has a real place in the diagnosis of colonic cancer, provided one realizes that the instrument does *not* reach into the sigmoid colon.

Although colonoscopy should not be used as a screening procedure for the initial detection of either colonic polyps or carcinoma, it does have great value in the work-up of patients with obscure intestinal bleeding. This is particularly true in those patients where a double-contrast enema has not provided acceptable reassurance that there is no lesion present. Colonoscopy is the method of choice to biopsy or remove a radiologically demonstrated lesion above reach of a sigmoidoscope.

Both sigmoidoscopy and fiberoptic colonoscopy are covered in detail in Chapter 15.

CLINICAL FEATURES

Colonic tumors which are small and limited to the mucosa are usually asymptomatic. Extension of growth and increasing size will result in the clinical signs of cancer of the colon which are change in bowel habits, pain, blood in the stool, anemia, weight loss, and obstruction. The highest frequency of colon cancer is in the 50 to 70 year age group and there is no significant sex predilection. A lesion in the left colon is more likely to be flat and ulcerated or annular and to cause symptoms earlier because of bleeding and obstruction. Tumors can grow to a larger size in the wider, more distensible right colon where the contents are semiliquid; obstructive symptoms are less likely, or occur late, and blood loss is usually occult. There is an average 2 to 3 months delay in seeking medical attention after the onset of symptoms. This represents an improvement over the average 6 months delay of the 1960's.

Carcinoma of the colon in patients under 30 years of age is rare (Fig. 17.2). The reported incidence ranges from 1–5%, but is probably under 3%. In contrast with older age groups, colloid carcinoma is more common than adenocarcinoma, and males are afflicted slightly more often than females. The sites of predilection, however, are similar to those of the older population. The most frequent symptom is abdominal pain of such a diffuse, crampy, and nonspecific nature that a variety of abdominal conditions are considered before the actual diagnosis is made. Consequently, in this age group there is a 3 to 6 months delay from onset of symptoms to surgery. Colon cancer tends to be more aggressive in the young and the 5-year survival is under 20%.

The patient with a carcinoma of the colon has a 1% risk of having multiple synchronous colon cancers (Fig. 17.3) and a 3% risk of developing additional metachronous cancers at a later date (Fig. 17.4). The Malmo series of double-contrast enemas has shown a 20% incidence of the coexistence of carcinoma in the colons of patients with polyps (Fig. 17.5). With regard to growth rate, there are no constant figures for benign or malignant tumors. In general, a malignant tumor increases more rapidly in size than does a benign one. Sudden or rapid growth of a tumor beyond 1 cm, when followed by serial radiography, is an ominous finding (Fig. 17.6). Further data on the growth rate of carcinoma of the colon are presented in Chapter 14.

ROENTGEN FINDINGS

Adenocarcinoma of the colon may have varying features depending on its age, rate of growth, and size. The problems associated with the detection and differential diagnosis of a small polypoid carcinoma of the colon have been presented in detail

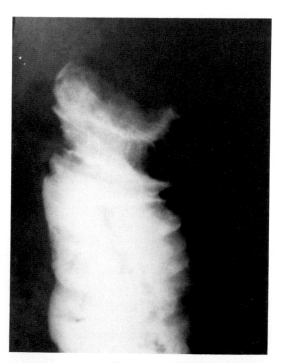

Fig. 17.2. Adenocarcinoma of the Descending Colon in a 17-Year-Old-Male
An obstructing cancer was found after the patient complained of vague abdominal pain, alternating diarrhea and constipation, weight loss and, finally, rectal bleeding and distention. The total duration of symptoms was 4 months.

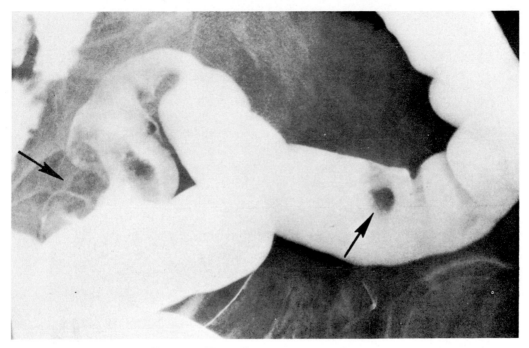

FIG.17.3. TWO CARCINOMAS OF COLON
There is a large ulcerated carcinoma of the rectosigmoid and a small polypoid carcinoma of the mid-sigmoid (*arrows*).

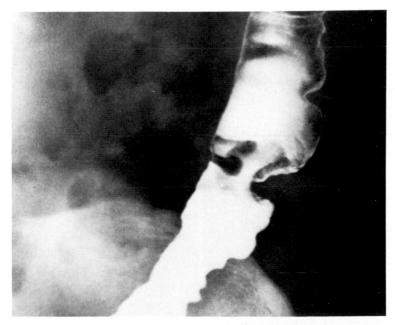

FIG. 17.4. METACHRONOUS CARCINOMA
The same patient whose synchronous cancers are shown in Fig. 17.3. Four years later, at age 67, he was found to have this third cancer in the proximal descending colon.

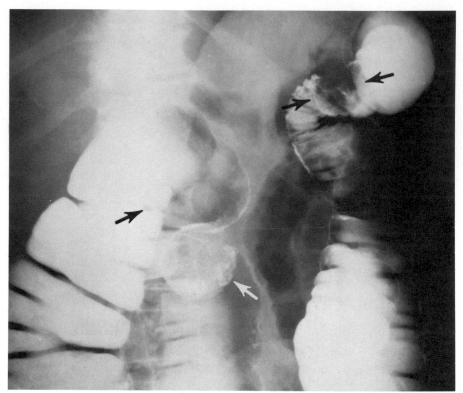

FIG. 17.5. COEXISTENCE OF CARCINOMA AND COLONIC POLYPS

A 65-year-old man with 3 colon tumors. At surgery they proved to be an adenomatous polyp (black arrow), a villous adenoma (white arrow), and an adenocarcinoma (2 black arrows).

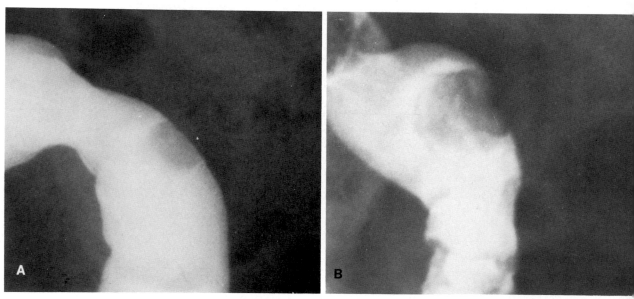

FIG. 17.6. RAPID GROWTH OF A SESSILE POLYP

When first demonstrated, this sessile polyp measured 10 mm in size (**A**). One year later it measured 18 mm (**B**) and was resected. It was adenocarcinoma.

in Chapter 15. This chapter is concerned with the less controversial and more obvious colon cancers, identifiable and named according to features of their gross and roentgen morphology. The descriptive terms for these adenocarcinomas of the colon are: flat, annular, polypoid, and scirrhous.

Flat Carcinoma (Saddle)

The flat carcinoma with a rolled-up margin and often an ulcerated center (Fig. 17.7) is among the most lethal of gastrointestinal cancers. Although it is rarely mentioned in the literature, except in passing, the small flat carcinoma may be the earliest form of colonic malignancy detectable by radiology. These flat, malignant tumors have been variously referred to as plaque-like, contour defect or medallion-shaped cancers and also as ulcerated carcinomas and carcinomas en plaque. Such a lesion might more descriptively be termed a saddle cancer for it appears to sit on the column of barium in the colon like a saddle sits on the back of a horse (Fig. 17.8).

In the early and middle stages of its growth, the flat or saddle cancer may be most difficult to detect if not seen tangentially (Fig. 17.9). In the final stages of growth a flat cancer becomes an annular carcinoma.

The saddle cancer apparently begins as a flat plaque of tissue which early in its growth becomes anchored in position. Spreading axially and circumferentially, it does not develop a significant luminal mass until it begins to encircle the bowel (Fig. 17.10). When first detected the cancer may measure only a few millimeters in size; in the late stages of its growth it may reach 5–8 cm in size before completely encircling the bowel or causing obstruction (Fig. 17.11).

The saddle cancer is in all ways analogous to a malignant Carman ulcer of the stomach, also a centrally ulcerated lesion with heaped-up edges (Fig. 17.12). In fact, in areas of the colon such as the sigmoid where compression spot-films can be taken, it is possible to trap barium in the ulcer by flattening one edge of the tumor against the opposite edge and thus producing a true Carman meniscus sign. This term refers to the crescent shape of the ulcer, when the tumor is folded over on itself. The flat base of the folded ulcer crater will always appear to sit on the margin of the bowel wall and the peripheral curving line of the ulcer will always be convex toward the colonic lumen.

These flat, ulcerating cancers seem to have a virulent biologic behavior and every effort should be made to look for them, particularly in a patient with rectal bleeding. Because of early ulceration, bleeding precedes all other bowel symptoms by months or years and may be the only symptom. The most rewarding films of the barium-filled colon have been the anteroposterior, both supine obliques, the posteroanterior angled view of the rectum and sigmoid, a lateral film of the rectum and the Chassard-Lapiné view. Careful scrutiny of the entire margin of the bowel must be made on each film, looking for a subtle, unnatural appearing area of straightening or a contour defect. Such a small and subtle lesion may be seen on only one of the many views when the tumor is caught tangentially; on the other films it may be totally obscured by the full column of barium (Fig. 17.13).

Study of the progression of these saddle tumors lends strong support to the current belief that if a cancer is found within 2 or 3 years of what was considered to be a previously negative barium enema, it can be assumed that the cancer was missed on the previous study (Figs. 17.14 and 17.15).

Annular Carcinoma

The predominant characteristic of an annular carcinoma is extensive infiltration and rigidity of the bowel wall, rather than formation of an intraluminal polypoid

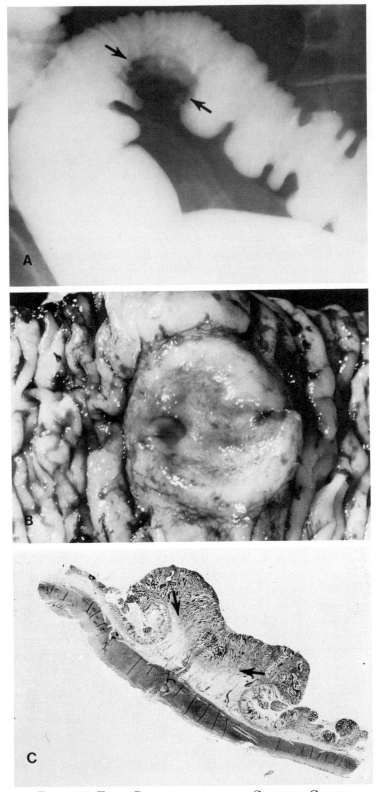

FIG. 17.7. FLAT CARCINOMA OF THE SIGMOID COLON

(A) Radiographic appearance of a 2.75 cm flat carcinoma (arrows) with a rolled-up edge and central ulceration. The tumor involved 120° of the circumference of the colon. (B) Gross specimen. (C) Histologic section of a similar (1.4 cm) flat carcinoma. Note that the mucosal surface has been destroyed by tumor as has the muscularis mucosa along the base (arrows). (A and B reproduced with permission from Radiology, *129:* 289, 1978.)

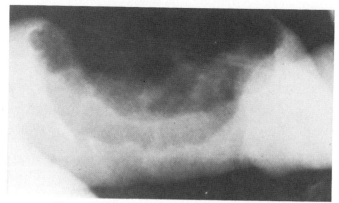

FIG. 17.8. FLAT OR SADDLE CARCINOMA

The tumor appears to sit on top of the bowel like a saddle on a horse. At surgery it involved 180° of the circumference of the sigmoid colon and was an adenocarcinoma. (Reproduced with permission from Radiology, *129:* 289, 1978.)

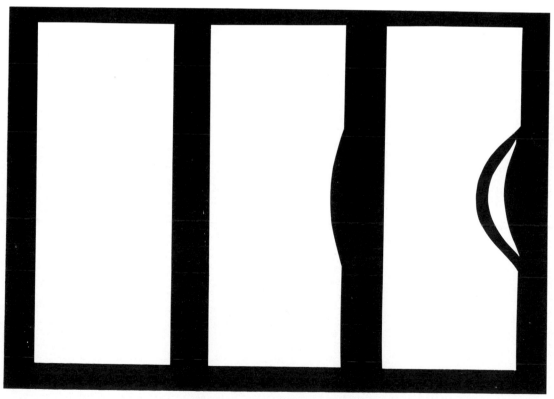

FIG. 17.9. SADDLE CANCER

Schematic presentation of a segment of barium-filled colon. On the left, the tumor is not seen. By turning the patient slightly (center) a contour defect is first suspected. On the right, with further turning, the saddle cancer is seen tangentially and becomes diagnosable.

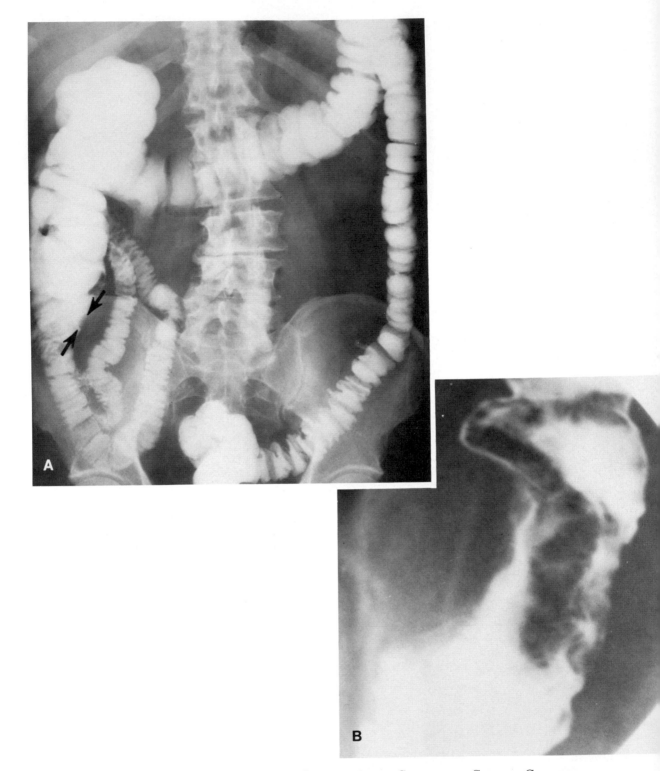

FIG. 17.10. EARLY AND LATE STAGES IN THE GROWTH OF SADDLE CANCERS
(A) A 2 cm flat cancer on the medial wall of the cecum (arrows). (B) A 5.5 cm,
ulcerated saddle cancer that had encircled 300° of the circumference of the sigmoid
colon.

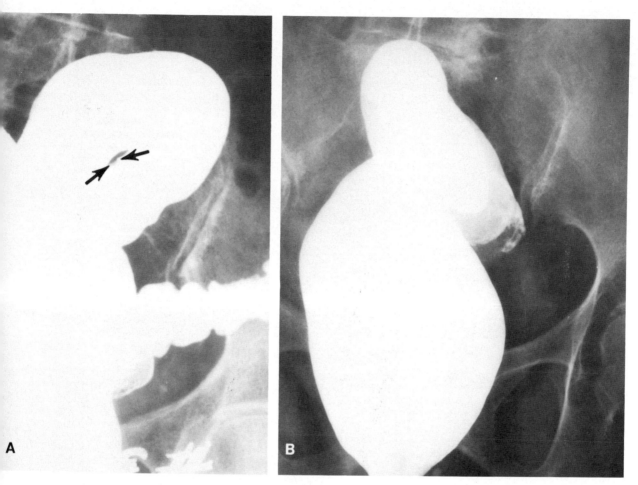

FIG. 17.11. SEVEN-YEAR GROWTH OF A CARCINOMA

(**A**) Although interpreted as negative, in retrospect there is a 7 mm contour defect in the distal sigmoid colon (arrows). (**B**) Seven years later, the patient, now age 85, presents with a 6-month history of constipation and abdominal pain. There is complete obstruction to the retrograde passage of barium by what proved to be a 6.0 cm annular carcinoma in the same location as the contour defect on the original barium examination.

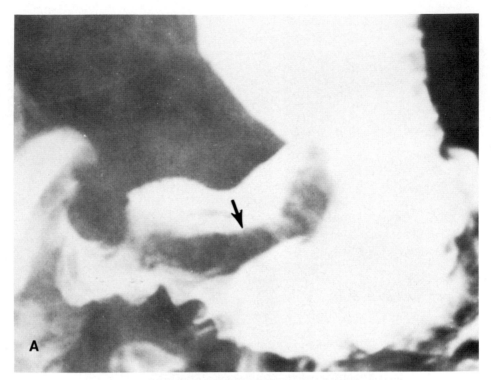

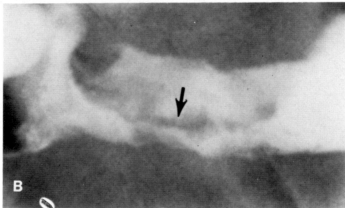

FIG. 17.12. SIMILARITY IN APPEARANCE OF A CARMAN ULCER OF THE STOMACH TO
A SADDLE CANCER OF THE COLON

These two malignant tumors are both shown with barium trapped in the ulcer
crater as one side of the rolled-up edge of the tumor is apposed to the other. The
Carman meniscus sign refers to the crescent shape of the ulcer which is convex
towards the lumen (arrow) when the tumor is folded on itself. (**A**) Malignant
Carman ulcer of the stomach. (**B**) Saddle cancer of the sigmoid colon. (Reproduced
with permission from Radiology, *129:* 289, 1978.)

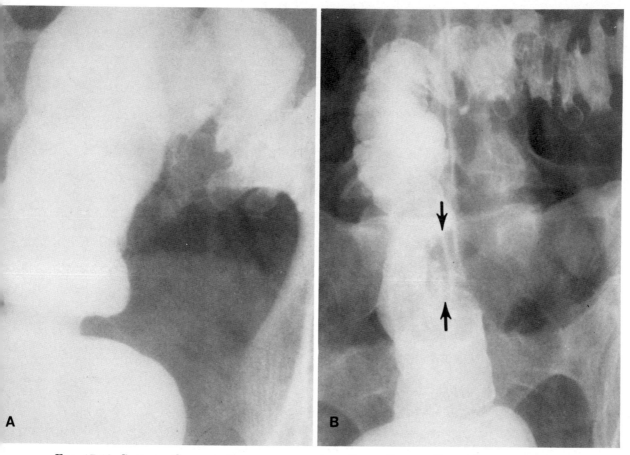

FIG. 17.13. SADDLE CANCER DEMONSTRATED ON ONLY ONE OF TWO VIEWS OF THE
SAME AREA

Because of foreshortening of the bowel, a 3 cm flat, saddle cancer is not seen on
the posteroanterior view of the high rectum (**A**) but is seen (arrows) on a posteroanterior angled view (**B**). (Reproduced with permission from Radiology, *129:* 289,
1978.)

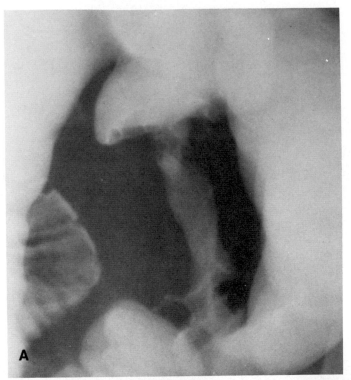

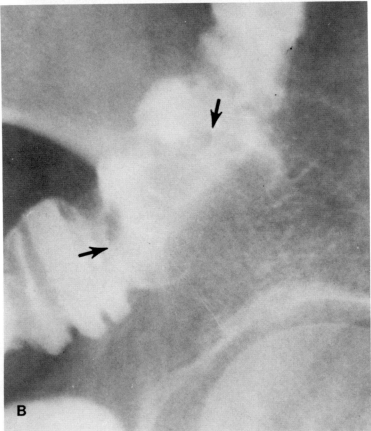

FIG. 17.14. PROGRESSION OF SADDLE CANCER TO ANNULAR CARCINOMA IN 9 MONTHS

(A) An annular carcinoma in the sigmoid colon of a 50-year-old woman. (B) In retrospect, a saddle lesion (arrows) can be seen in the same location on barium enema done 9 months earlier for rectal bleeding. (Reproduced with permission from Radiology, *129:* 289, 1978.)

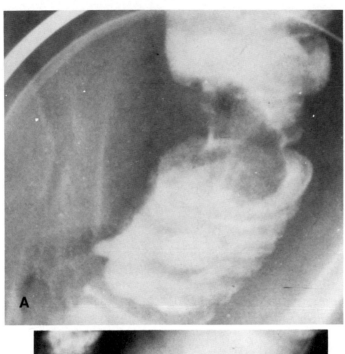

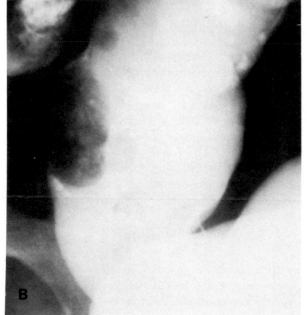

FIG. 17.15. GROWTH OF A SADDLE CANCER IN 18 MONTHS
(A) A nearly annular cancer of the sigmoid in a 55-year-old woman examined because of rectal bleeding. (B) A saddle tumor is seen in retrospect on only this one film from a barium enema performed 18 months earlier, also for rectal bleeding.

filling defect. It is more common on the left side (Fig. 17.16) but may occur anywhere in the colon (Figs. 17.17 and 17.18). The bowel lumen is narrowed by an annular carcinoma, and the abrupt change from normal bowel to tumor results in a so-called "tumor shelf" at the proximal and distal ends of the mass.

An annular carcinoma appears to develop most commonly from a flat or saddle type of lesion, as described in the previous section. However, retrospective studies have shown that an annular cancer may on occasion evolve from a polypoid tumor (Fig. 17.19).

In contrast with diverticulitis, the annular carcinoma extends over a relatively short segment of bowel and the mucosa through the narrowed central core is ulcerated. The terms "napkin ring" and "apple core" have been used to describe these centrally ulcerated, encircling tumors.

Either annular or polypoid tumors may cause total obstruction or, more commonly, there will be apparent retrograde obstruction to the flow of barium. When there is retrograde obstruction, the chance of defining the true nature and extent of the lesion may be lost.

Sustained Spasm vs Obstruction

Apparent complete retrograde obstruction may not be absolute, but rather on the basis of sustained local spasm, which can often be overcome by intravenous administration of an antispasmotic agent such as glucagon (Fig. 17.20). If successful, one may then be able to differentiate a stenotic, ulcerated carcinoma from a segment of colon involved by acute diverticulitis. If relaxation does not occur, it is unwise to force further filling. Liquid barium should not be given from above in cases of suspected obstruction.

Colon Sphincter vs Annular Carcinoma

An annular carcinoma may be simulated by an area of transient, localized spasm at any point, but particularly in the transverse, descending, and sigmoid colon (Fig. 17.21). These areas of spasm, not due to organic disease, are most likely to occur at one of the so-called "colon sphincters," many of which are disfavored with eponyms and which are probably due to localized nerve and muscle imbalance (Fig. 17.22). Features which differentiate this entity from an annular carcinoma are that with a colon sphincter the contour of the leading edge changes from film to film, the mucosa through the area of apparent narrowing is intact without ulceration, and the area of constriction does not persist or may shift slightly along the colon even during the same examination (Fig. 17.23). Intravenous glucagon or air insufflation will usually result in distention of the area in question (Fig. 17.24).

Polypoid Carcinoma

As mentioned in the chapter on polyps, the overwhelming majority of polypoid lesions less than 1 cm in size are benign; however, the incidence of malignancy increases rapidly with increase in size. A fungating or large polypoid carcinoma of the colon is characterized by its irregular or nodular contour. It appears to begin as a small sessile lesion arising in an otherwise normal segment of bowel; except at its point of attachment, the adjacent bowel wall appears pliable. Fungating carcinomas are more likely to occur in the cecum, right colon, and proximal transverse colon (Figs. 17.25 and 17.26). They may range in size from 1–10 cm and except for blood loss, are unlikely to cause symptoms until quite large (Fig. 17.27). Rarely, an intussusception may be caused by a polypoid carcinoma of the right colon.

This type of lesion is well demonstrated by compression spot-films and will coat well on double-contrast study of the colon. On the postevacuation films, a polypoid

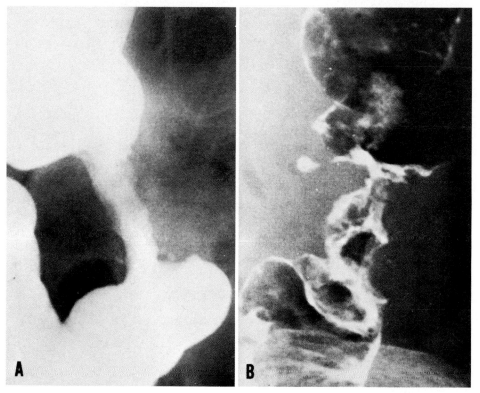

FIG. 17.16. ANNULAR CARCINOMA OF THE DESCENDING COLON
(A) Detail film of the left colon showing narrowing of the lumen due to an encircling carcinoma. The proximal and distal tumor shelves are clearly defined. (B) A similar lesion defined by air-contrast technique.

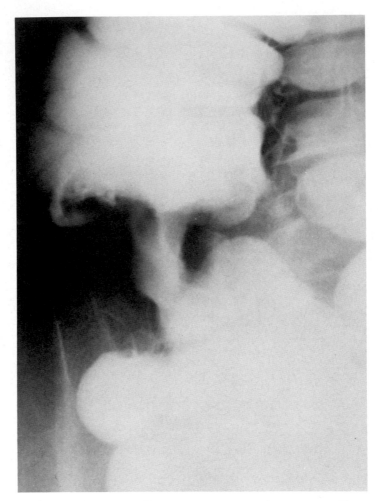

FIG. 17.17. ANNULAR CARCINOMA OF THE ASCENDING COLON

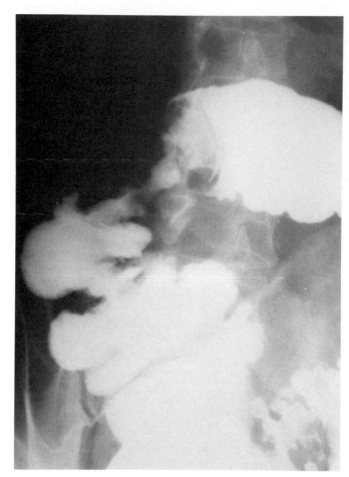

FIG. 17.18. ANNULAR CARCINOMA OF THE HEPATIC FLEXURE

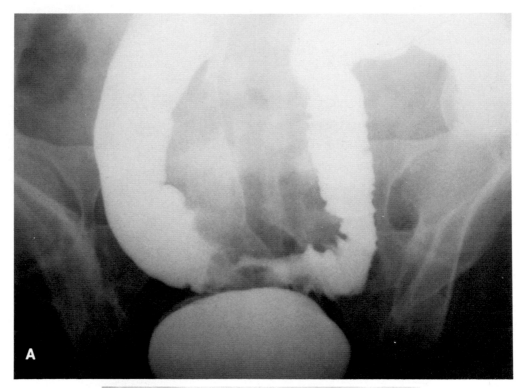

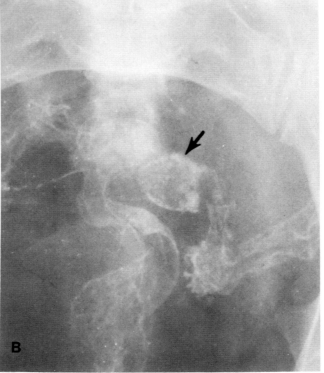

FIG. 17.19. EVOLUTION OF A POLYPOID TUMOR TO AN ANNULAR CARCINOMA
This 47-year-old woman with rectal bleeding was found to have an 8.0 cm annular carcinoma of the sigmoid colon, best seen on the Chassard-Lapiné view (**A**). Review of a barium enema done 3 years earlier, also for rectal bleeding, showed a 3.5 cm polypoid mass (arrow) that was overlooked (**B**).

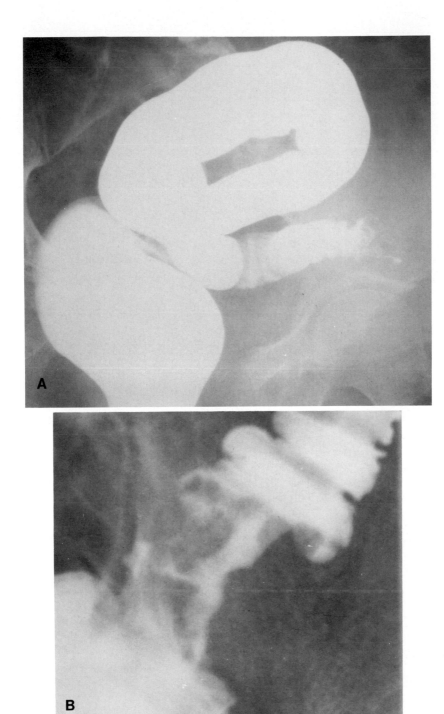

FIG. 17.20. USE OF AN ANTISPASMOTIC DRUG TO OVERCOME SPASM AND DEFINE A
LESION
   (A) Apparent retrograde obstruction to the flow of barium in the sigmoid colon.
(B) Immediately after the intravenous administration of 1 mg of glucagon, there is
relaxation of the bowel with definition of an annular carcinoma.

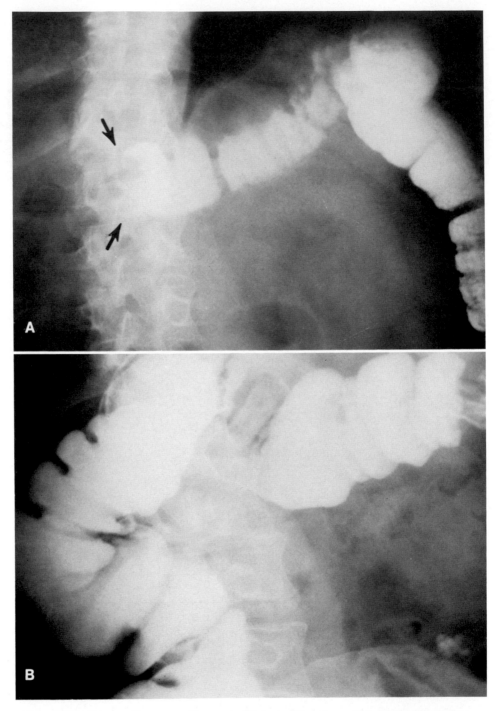

FIG. 17.21. FALSE-POSITIVE BARIUM ENEMA DUE TO A COLON SPHINCTER
(CANNON'S POINT)

(A) Apparent retrograde obstruction of barium consistent with an annular carcinoma (arrows). The patient underwent an exploratory laparotomy and no lesion
was found. (B) Normal barium enema 2 months after the negative surgical procedure.

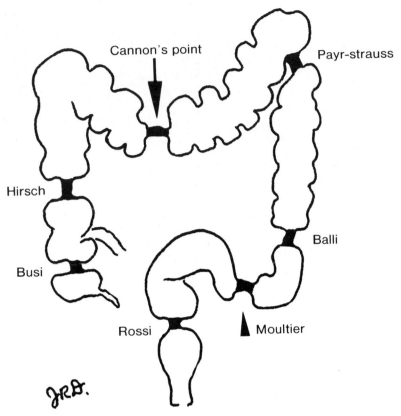

FIG. 17.22. SCHEMATIC REPRESENTATION OF THE "COLON SPHINCTERS"
Any of the so-called colon sphincters may simulate an annular carcinoma. The rather constant location of these sphincters is shown, together with their eponyms. Cannon's point is the most frequently encountered area of transient spasm during a barium enema.

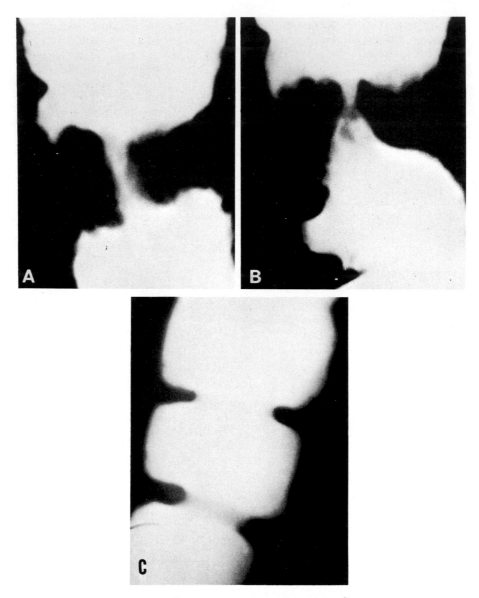

FIG. 17.23. PSEUDOSPHINCTER OF THE COLON

Three fluoroscopic spot-films of the mid-descending colon taken at 2-min intervals and showing the changeability of the proximal and distal margins of this apparent stenosing lesion. The final film (C) defines a normal bowel lumen.

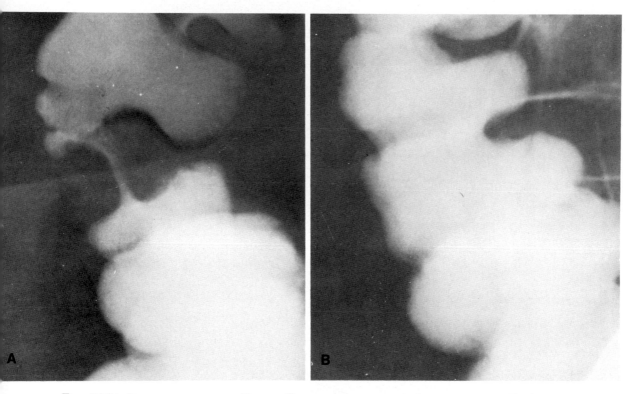

FIG. 17.24. RELAXATION OF A COLON SPHINCTER WITH AN ANTISPASMOTIC DRUG
(A) Sustained spasm of the mid-ascending colon, simulating an annular carcinoma.
(B) One minute after the intravenous injection of 1 mg of glucagon, there is complete
relaxation of this transient area of spasm.

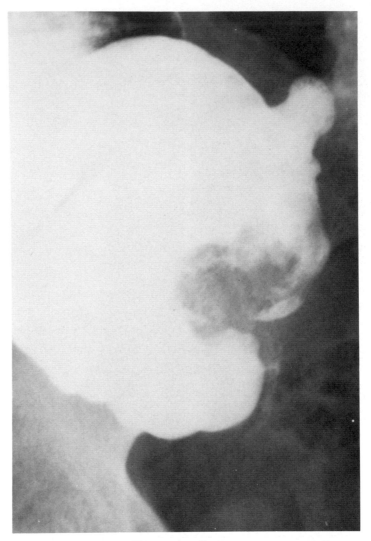

FIG. 17.25. A 3-CM POLYPOID CARCINOMA OF THE CECUM

Note the lobulated contour of this tumor and the irregularity of the colon wall at the point of origin.

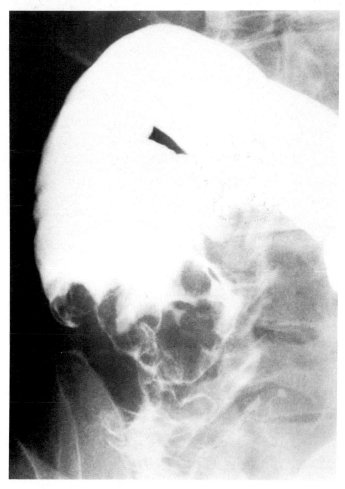

FIG. 17.26. A 12-CM POLYPOID (FUNGATING) CARCINOMA OF THE CECUM
Note how the bulk of this lobulated tumor widens the diameter of the cecum
beyond normal.

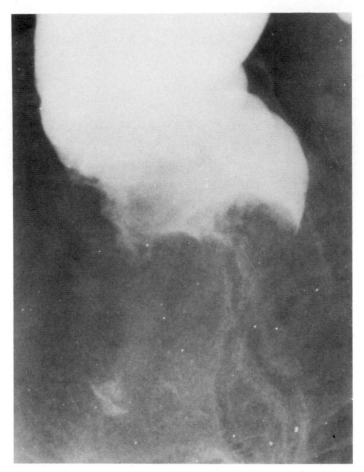

FIG. 17.27. A 15-CM OBSTRUCTING POLYPOID CARCINOMA OF THE CECUM
    The bulk of this huge, lobulated cancer has obstructed the retrograde passage of
barium.

carcinoma distends the bowel locally, while all other segments are collapsed and
show a normal, contracted mucosal pattern (Fig. 17.28). When there is doubt, or
when fecal material is present elsewhere in the colon, it is best to repeat the barium
enema at once or after a 3-day bowel preparation. For thorough coverage of the
colon, special x-ray views are recommended in Chapter 3, and these will aid
immeasurably in visualizing easily obscured areas of the rectosigmoid, sigmoid, and
the two flexures.

Scirrhous Carcinoma

A rare variant of annular or infiltrating carcinoma of the colon, scirrhous carcinoma, extends over a much longer segment and is characterized by the striking
amount of desmoplastic reaction which it stimulates. It is also known as linitis
plastica of the colon. The marked increase in fibrous tissue associated with this
tumor frequently results in a long, stiff lesion that may simulate an area of burned-
out ulcerative colitis or a segment of Crohn's colitis. Some additional characteristics
of scirrhous carcinoma are that the mucosa may not be effaced completely by the
underlying tumor, and there is rarely a marked sharp demarcation between normal
bowel and the area of malignancy. When a segment of the rectosigmoid or sigmoid
colon is involved by scirrhous carcinoma, it is likely to appear rigid, fixed in position
with unchanging mucosal detail and measuring 4–12 cm in length (Fig. 17.29).

Clinically, this tumor is notorious for its insidious presentation. Since there is rarely mucosal disruption, there is no bleeding to alert the patient. The lesion grows slowly causing gradual narrowing of the bowel lumen, intermittent constipation, diarrhea, lower abdominal cramps, progressive decrease in caliber of the stools and, later, weight loss. Scirrhous carcinoma of the colon tends to occur 5–10 years earlier than other types of colorectal cancer, the average age at diagnosis being 55 years. It is a particularly virulent tumor with a poor prognosis.

The rarity of primary scirrhous carcinoma of the colon has been stressed, the incidence being under 1% of all colonic cancers. Secondary or metastatic scirrhous carcinoma of the colon, although relatively rare, is more often seen than the primary type. It may be found as a secondary tumor in patients with scirrhous cancer, or linitis plastica, of the stomach or, less commonly, of the breast or gallbladder. The transverse colon is the most frequent site of secondary involvement. Patients with long-standing ulcerative colitis, who develop carcinoma as a late complication of their disease, often have the scirrhous form of tumor (Fig. 17.30).

Derivation of Term: Linitis Plastica

By way of historical interest, it should be noted that most physicians use the term *linitis plastica* without knowing what it actually means. Over the years, the assumption has developed that it is synonymous with "leather bottle," "rigid," or "wood-like." This is not correct. When Brinton first used the term linitis plastica in

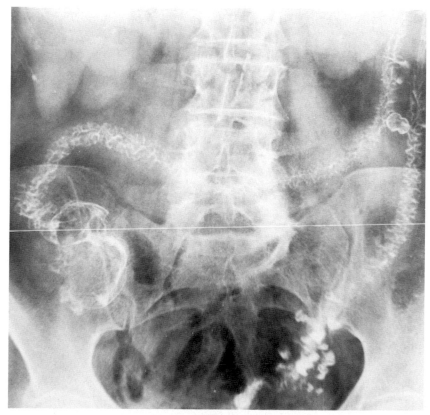

FIG. 17.28. POLYPOID CARCINOMA OF THE CECUM AS SEEN ON A POSTEVACUATION FILM

While the remainder of the colon has contracted, the cecum remains distended by a large fungating tumor.

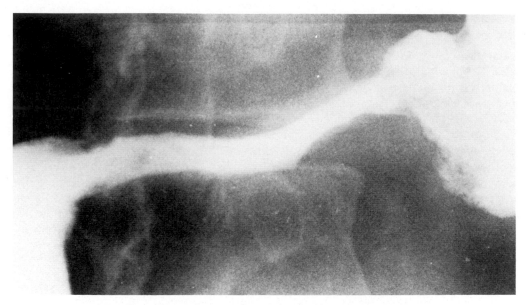

FIG. 17.29. SCIRRHOUS CARCINOMA OF COLON
There is a long area of narrowing with sharp proximal and distal shelves.

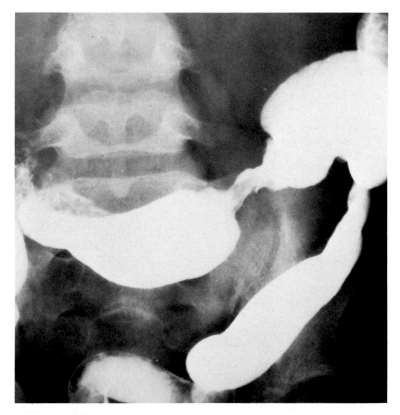

FIG. 17.30. SCIRRHOUS CARCINOMA IN THE COLON OF A CHILD WITH ULCERATIVE
COLITIS
This 12-year-old girl had ulcerative colitis from the age of 3. (Reproduced with
permission from Symposium on Radiology of the Alimentary Tract, Radiologic
Clinics of North America, April 1969, W. B. Saunders Co.)

1865, he did so because the extensive, interwoven connective tissue fibers so characteristic of the lesion he was describing in the stomach reminded him of the grid-like pattern of fibers in a net or cloth. And that is what the term linitis plastica connotes—derived from the Greek words *linon* (which means flax, the fibers of which were used to make fish nets and linen cloth) and *plastikos* (which means formed).

Brinton reported what he thought was a severe form of benign interstitial gastritis, and it was not until 1933 that Howard recognized the malignant nature of this lesion. The histology of primary linitis plastica of the colon is identical to that seen in the stomach.

LYMPHOMA

Involvement of the large bowel by lymphosarcoma, reticulum cell sarcoma, and Hodgkin's disease is extremely rare. Symptoms are anorexia, fatigue, weight loss, and fever. Generalized abdominal discomfort and alternating diarrhea and constipation may be among the patient's complaints. Lymphoma may be limited to the colon or may be a part of systemic involvement with generalized lymphadenopathy. Rectal bleeding from lymphoma of the colon is not as common as in patients with adenocarcinoma of the colon. Lymphoma may involve any part of the gastrointestinal tract, but the stomach and small bowel are affected more often than is the esophagus or colon. There are two radiologic types of lymphoma of the colon.

Polypoid Lymphoma

The polypoid form of lymphoma is a discrete lesion indistinguishable by x-ray examination from a fungating carcinoma (Fig. 17.31). When there are differential features, the tumor due to lymphoma may appear to be unusually bulky and may extend over a longer segment of the colon than does carcinoma. Lymphoma may be suspected when a large lesion of the colon characterized by extremely thickened and distorted mucosal fold pattern is present but does not cause significant obstruction. The bowel lumen at the site of the lesion may be markedly widened by the mass or the mass may have a considerable extrinsic (extracolonic) component which displaces adjacent abdominal structures. Polypoid lymphoma more often occurs in the right or proximal transverse colon segments.

Diffuse Lymphoma

The second type of lymphoma of the colon is even more rare, but has a more specific x-ray pattern. Large segments or even the entire colon is involved by a diffuse infiltration and thickening of the submucosa which results in a nodular mucosal relief pattern; the lumen of the bowel is widened and in addition to the thickened fold pattern, the mucosa appears to be studded with countless polypoid defects which are actually islands of lymphomatous infiltration, varying in size from several millimeters to several centimeters and best seen on the postevacuation film (Fig. 17.32). Because of the marked thickening of the mucosa and submucosa, the colon shows little contraction on the evacuation film and this is the most striking radiographic feature (Fig. 17.33). Ulceration and perforation are uncommon. The appearance of diffuse lymphosarcoma of the colon may mimic nodular lymphoid hyperplasia (described at the end of this chapter), familial adenomatous colonic polyposis, or the hyperplastic mucosal phase of ulcerative colitis and Crohn's colitis. Careful attention to the history is essential, but endoscopic biopsy may be necessary to make the correct diagnosis.

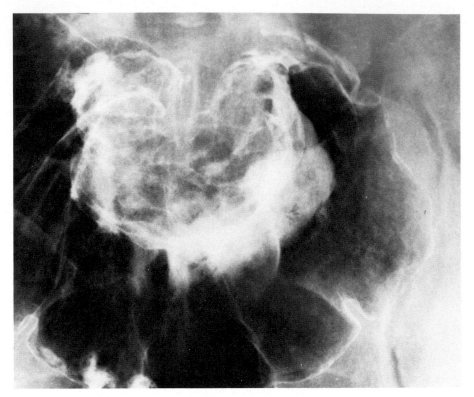

FIG. 17.31. RETICULUM CELL SARCOMA
This large, multilobulated tumor cannot be distinguished from a polypoid carcinoma.

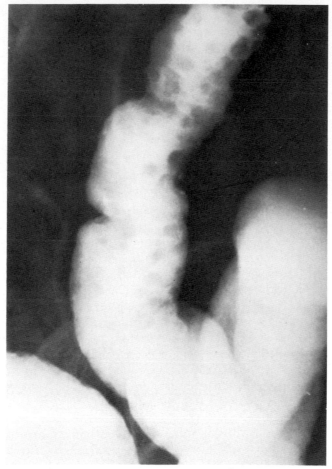

FIG. 17.32. DIFFUSE NODULAR LYMPHOMA

The mucosa is studded with nodules of lymphomatous infiltration which measure from 3 mm to 1 cm in size, indistinguishable radiographically from adenomatous polyps.

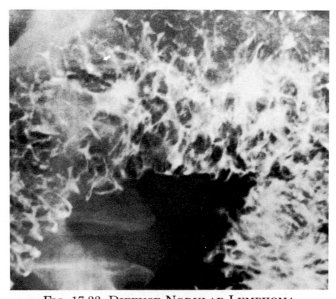

FIG. 17.33. DIFFUSE NODULAR LYMPHOMA

Note the failure of the colon to contract completely due to the bulk of the countless nodules of lymphoma.

OTHER TUMORS OF THE COLON

In addition to the adenomatous polyp, villous adenoma, carcinoma, and malignant lymphoma, there are a variety of other tumors that may involve the colon directly or indirectly in a small percentage of cases. These tumors are: lipoma; carcinoid; spindle cell tumors, such as leiomyoma and fibroma; endometrioma; and metastatic carcinoma.

Lipoma

A submucosal lipoma is the next most common benign tumor of the colon after adenomas. Since a lipoma does not usually cause symptoms, it is more likely to be a fortuitous finding on barium study of the large bowel. A lipoma has a characteristic sharply defined outline and an unusually lucent appearance as compared to other bowel tumors. This lucency is due in part to the fat content and also to the very smooth surface of the mucosa stretched over the mass which does not remain as well coated with barium as does the more crenated mucosa of an adenomatous polyp.

The most important diagnostic feature of a lipoma is changeability of size and shape during the course of a barium enema examination. This is a reflection of the very soft nature of the tumor and can be readily demonstrated by palpation or compression spot-films. A lipoma may appear round or oval on the full barium film, but sausage shaped on the postevacuation film as the contracting colon squeezes and elongates this malleable tumor (Fig. 17.34).

Lipomas most commonly occur in the right colon, are usually single and measure 1–4 cm in diameter. They are true mural tumors but almost invariably appear as sessile protrusions into the bowel lumen. If there seems to be a stalk, it is never a true pedicle, but rather the dragging of a broad and thick pseudopedicle of mucosa. Bleeding may occur and is due to superficial traumatic erosion of the mucosa stretched over the mass.

In order to dramatize its lucency within a water column, films made after a tap-water enema were once recommended, but this is an unnecessary procedure if the other x-ray criteria are looked for on barium enema examination.

When the ileo-cecal valve is involved by benign fatty infiltration, it may appear as a slightly irregular and larger-than-normal valve, but its smooth surface is maintained (Fig. 17.35) and it also is changeable in size and shape. A very lobulated, asymmetrical, rigid, or eccentric ileo-cecal valve must be considered suspect of carcinoma and surgical exploration is then warranted (Fig. 17.36).

Rarely, a large lipoma may cause colo-colic intussusception or obstruction. Continued oozing of blood from the surface of a lipoma may also require that it be resected. Because of its soft nature, a lipoma may not be palpated by the surgeon at laparotomy, and colotomy is mandatory if this tumor is suspected on barium enema examination.

Carcinoid

Accounting for less than 1% of all gastrointestinal neoplasms, the carcinoid tumor is an uncommon entity. Ninety percent of these tumors will be in the distal ileum or appendix and only 10% in the rectum, cecum, or other colon segments.

The vast majority of colonic carcinoids are asymptomatic, under 1 cm in size, and found only incidentally on barium enema or sigmoidoscopic examination. They arise from the submucosa but present as polypoid luminal protrusions, usually in the rectum or cecum. Although far more common in the appendix, they are rarely demonstrable by x-ray in this location. However, an appendiceal carcinoid is one of the several causes of an extrinsic pressure defect against the medial wall or tip of the cecum and this may be the only clue to its presence.

The malignant potential of a carcinoid in the appendix is very low, but the incidence increases slightly for rectal and cecal tumors and may approach 20% for small bowel carcinoids. Even when metastasis to the liver occurs, the clinical course may be indolent for many years. Mid-gut tumors which drain into the portal circulation may be responsible for the "carcinoid syndrome" (episodic cutaneous flushing, diarrhea, respiratory, and cardiac symptoms) due to the release of serotonin and other endocrine substances from hepatic metastases.

For some unknown reason, small colonic carcinoids do not often invade locally, metastasize to the liver, or precipitate the carcinoid syndrome as do the small ileal tumors. However, a large colonic carcinoid may be very aggressive locally, invade the muscularis, extend beyond the serosa and result in an extracolonic component that is more impressive than the protrusion into the lumen.

These larger, more aggressive carcinoids may occur in the cecum, transverse or sigmoid segments of the colon and be indistinguishable by x-ray from a bulky villous adenoma, adenocarcinoma, or lymphoma. Abdominal pain, bleeding, fatigue and weight loss are the usual complaints which prompt diagnostic attention. Because of their size (3–5 cm) necrosis, intussusception and obstruction may occur (Fig. 17.37).

Spindle Cell Tumors

A leiomyoma is a rare tumor of the colon, as are fibroma and neurofibroma. These tumors may appear as either small or relatively large intramural, extramucosal masses, or their size may cause such marked intraluminal protrusion that they appear as large, sessile, polypoid lesions and differentiation from carcinoma may be impossible. Intussusception may occur.

One of the x-ray features of a benign spindle cell tumor is the tendency for the overlying mucosa to be stretched but intact. Occasionally, the mucosa may ulcerate. A leiomyosarcoma is a very rare tumor of the colon, less than 0.1% of all colonic malignancies; it is prone to ulcerate. Both benign and malignant spindle cell tumors may have a large extracolonic component (Fig. 17.38), the "ice-berg" phenomenon.

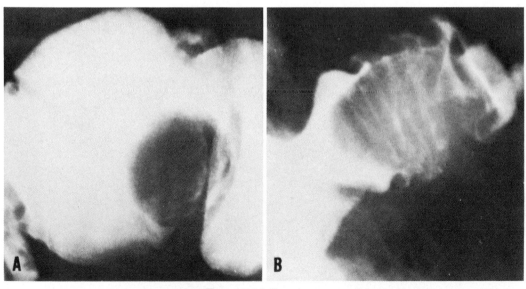

FIG. 17.34. LIPOMA
Note the change in size and shape of this soft tumor between the full colon film (**A**) and the postevacuation film (**B**).

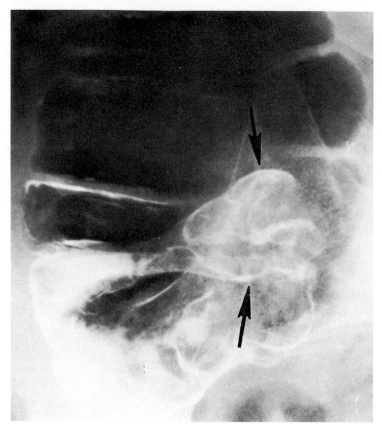

FIG. 17.35. FATTY INFILTRATION OF ILEO-CECAL VALVE

The lips of the valve are irregularly enlarged (arrows), but a smooth surface is maintained.

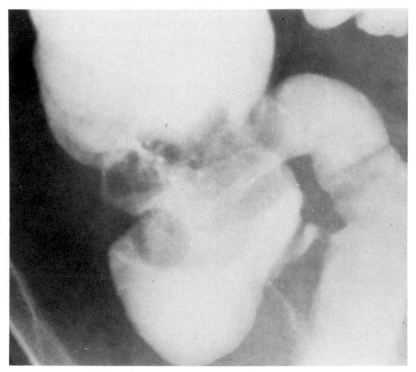

FIG. 17.36. CARCINOMA OF THE ILEO-CECAL VALVE

The valve is enlarged, lobulated, and asymmetrical.

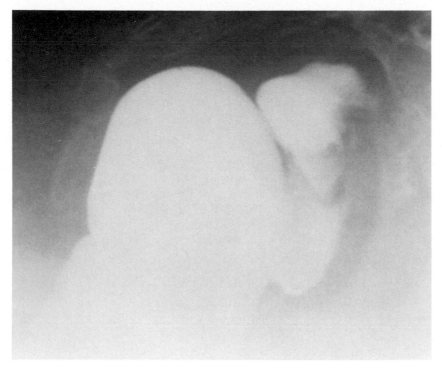

FIG. 17.37. CARCINOID CAUSING RETROGRADE OBSTRUCTION TO THE FLOW OF BARIUM IN THE SIGMOID
There are no specific radiographic signs to suggest that the obstructing lesion is a carcinoid tumor.

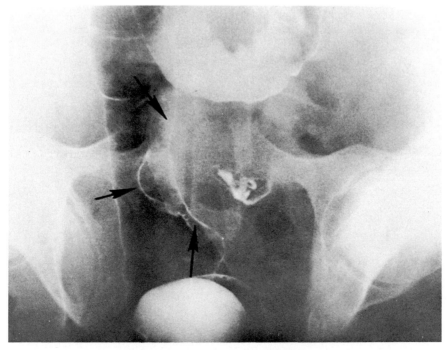

FIG. 17.38. LEIOMYOSARCOMA
Chassard-Lapiné view demonstrating a large extramucosal lesion of the rectum (arrows).

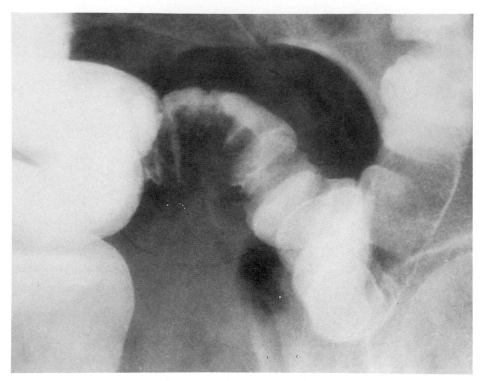

FIG. 17.39. ENDOMETRIOMA

On an angled view of the distal sigmoid, the tumor shows as a curved, sharply defined, extrinsic defect on the inferior margin of the bowel. The overlying but stretched mucosa appears intact in contrast to the ulcerated appearance of a flat, saddle cancer.

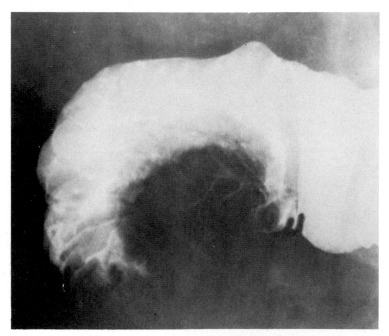

FIG. 17.40. METASTATIC CARCINOMA

An extrinsic pressure defect against the under surface of the hepatic flexure is caused by an ovarian metastasis implanted on the serosa of the colon. There was also invasion of the muscularis.

Endometrioma

Menstrual irregularity, constipation, tenesmus, and pelvic pain in the 25–45 year age group are the symptoms of endometriosis, although they may be present in under 5% of patients with the disorder. When an endometrioma is implanted on the serosal surface of the colon, usually the rectosigmoid or sigmoid, there may be abdominal cramps and diarrhea during the menstrual period. Intermittent constipation is common between periods. As the endometrioma grows, it may partially obstruct the bowel by gradually increasing fibrosis and infiltration of the muscularis. The area of relative narrowing is apt to be most marked during a menstrual period.

The x-ray appearance of an endometrioma may suggest a primary plaque-like carcinoma or a metastatic serosal implant or it may mimic localized inflammatory disease. The serosal implant of endometriosis is frequently best seen on the lateral and posteroanterior angled view as a curved, sharply defined, and fixed defect against the wall (Fig. 17.39). In contrast to primary malignancy or inflammatory disease, the mucosa in the area of the lesion usually is intact and for this reason rectal bleeding is rare. An endometrioma may extend to the submucosa and cause the lesion to have a polypoid or stenosing appearance.

An endometrioma may also occur in postmenopausal women. Because its roentgen appearance so closely simulates an adenocarcinoma, the preoperative diagnosis of endometriosis in this group of women is almost never considered or made.

Metastatic Carcinoma

Metastatic tumor of the colon may simulate a sharply demarcated primary flat or annular neoplasm or it may appear as a longer, concentric, scirrhous lesion with tapered edges. Metastatic lesions may also cause shallow, extrinsic pressure defects against the bowel wall (Fig. 17.40) or the overhanging edge of uninvolved bowel may mimic an intramural, extramucosal tumor. The mucosa is rarely effaced but may show marked transverse ridging. Nodular filling defects, mucosal ulceration, or obstruction may occur in the late stages.

In other cases, the presence of metastasis in the adjacent mesentery or on the serosal surface of the bowel may result only in spasm of the affected segment of the colon with no fixed narrowing or alteration in contour. The bowel wall may appear finely serrated at any point of fixation and otherwise normal mucosal folds will tend to radiate away from this area. Metastasis to the large bowel often occurs at multiple sites, a helpful sign in the differentiation from primary carcinoma (Fig. 17.41).

When a combination of the various forms of metastatic involvement of the colon occurs, the appearance may be confused with segmental inflammatory bowel disease. Eccentric strictures, mucosal nodularity, marginal spiculation, and rigidity may all be present. Metastatic encasement of a segment of colon may also occur, especially with contiguous spread of carcinoma from the stomach or ovary (Fig. 17.42).

COMPLICATIONS

The major complications of colonic tumors are bleeding, intussusception, obstruction, perforation, and proximal colitis.

Bleeding

The various types of bleeding associated with specific colonic neoplasms are covered in the chapters on polyps, polyposis disorders, and in this chapter.

Intussusception

The colon may be involved in an ileocolic, ileo-ileocolic or a colo-colic intussus-

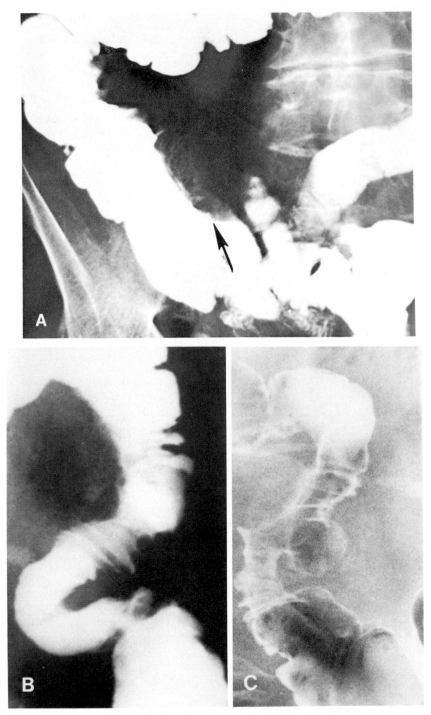

FIG. 17.41. METASTATIC CARCINOMA
(A) A shallow extrinsic pressure defect is present along the medial wall of the cecum (arrow) due to a plaque of metastatic tumor. (B and C) Detail films of the proximal descending colon filled with barium and air demonstrating transverse ridging of the mucosal folds adjacent to an extrinsic pressure defect along the medial wall.

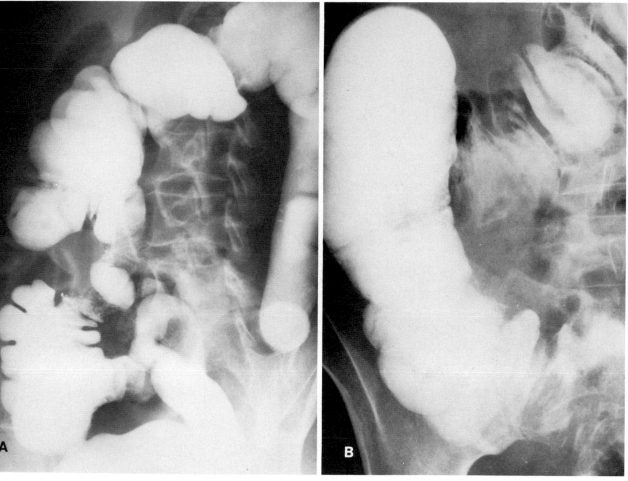

FIG. 17.42. METASTATIC CARCINOMA WITH ENCASEMENT OF THE COLON

Two cases with abdominal carcinomatosis secondary to ovarian tumor. (**A**) The mid-ascending colon is encased by metastatic cancer. (**B**) The entire cecum and ascending colon are encased by metastatic disease. The cecum is flattened and the medial side of the right colon is smooth and rigid.

ception. Only 5% of all intussusceptions occur in adults, and the leading cause is tumor, usually malignant, especially when there is a colo-colic intussusception in the transverse or sigmoid segments.

An intussusception is the telescoping of one segment of the bowel into another. The invaginating bowel is called the intussusceptum and the segment of bowel which receives it, the intussuscipiens. Symptoms of intermittent obstruction suggest recurrent intussusception which is more common in adults; sudden obstructive symptoms are more likely to occur in children under 2 years of age.

The diagnosis can often be made by the history alone, or by physical examination, a supine film of the abdomen, and a barium enema. In the typical case, the barium column abuts the rounded edge of the intussusception. As barium seeps around the intussusceptum, it outlines the telescoped mucosal folds of the segment of bowel into which the intussusception is taking place, giving the characteristic coiled-spring pattern (Fig. 17.43). It is rare to reduce an intussusception due to tumor with a barium enema. The subject is further covered in Chapters 5 and 19.

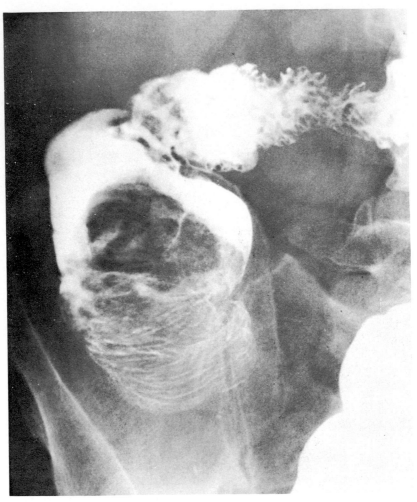

FIG. 17.43. INTUSSUSCEPTION

A nodular cecal tumor is outlined by the head of the barium column. The tumor has intussuscepted into the right colon as evidenced by the coiled spring pattern of barium.

Obstruction

Large bowel obstruction accounts for approximately 25% of all cases of intestinal obstruction. Carcinoma of the colon is the etiologic agent in about 65% of the cases while diverticulitis will be found in about 20%. A variety of other lesions, including volvulus, hernia, and secondary invasion from other sites of pelvic malignancy account for most of the remaining cases.

In the decade from 1966–1976, 8% of patients with a colonic cancer at the Massachusetts General Hospital presented with obstruction requiring emergency surgery. This group of patients tended to be elderly; the average age was 71. Abdominal pain, vomiting, and obstipation were the most frequent presenting symptoms, with a median duration of only 2 weeks.

The plain film of the abdomen will usually show only small bowel distention in patients with an obstructing cecal lesion. Obstructing tumors more distally in the colon will usually cause dilated large bowel up to the site of the lesion. In the Massachusetts General Hospital series, two-thirds of obstructing colonic tumors were distal to the splenic flexure and one-third were in the sigmoid segment. An emergency barium enema, without bowel preparation, may be necessary to define the exact site of obstruction.

Colonic obstruction due to carcinoma and other causes is described in detail in Chapter 19.

Perforation

Perforation of a malignant colonic tumor with localized abscess formation is relatively rare, occurring in under 5% of cases, and is secondary to necrosis, infection or both. Most such perforations are rapidly walled off and do not result in generalized peritonitis. However, free perforation and peritonitis may occasionally occur in markedly dilated segments of colon proximal to an obstructing carcinoma. A cecal "blow-out" is an example of such a situation; any distention of the cecum over 10 cm must be regarded as potentially dangerous.

The signs of localized perforation are pain, tenderness, fever and leukocytosis; they may precede or dominate symptoms due to the tumor itself. The x-ray appearance of a perforated carcinoma, particularly in the sigmoid segment, may mimic acute diverticulitis or segmental Crohn's disease. Because diverticulitis is often the leading clinical diagnosis on admission, a barium enema is usually done and is without danger if there is a walled-off perforated carcinoma. However, if free perforation into the peritoneal cavity is suspected, a water-soluble contrast enema is the examination of choice. When severe spasm is also present, an accurate x-ray diagnosis may be impossible unless some relaxation can be achieved by the intravenous injection of an antispasmotic drug.

Colitis Proximal to Obstructing Carcinoma

Experimental production of partially obstructing lesions in the colons of dogs suggests that the etiology of colitis proximal to stenosing cancers is most likely on the basis of an ischemic process with the decreased or absent mucosal blood flow resulting from stretching, spasm, and increased luminal pressure (Fig. 17.44). The possible role of bacterial proliferation due to stagnation of fecal material is uncertain. Similar changes of ulcerating colitis have been shown proximal to other partially obstructing lesions of the colon such as: volvulus, diverticulitis, impaction of a fecalith, and strictures due to ischemia, surgery, or radiation.

In the segment of bowel involved by proximal colitis, the wall is thickened; the mucosa is edematous, congested and covered by a hemorrhagic and purulent exudate. There are large, irregular ulcerations. Histologically there are areas of necrotic mucosa with marked acute and subacute inflammation and microabscesses. The inflammatory reaction may vary from edema and linear ulcerations to necrosis and perforation. Interestingly, there does not seem to be a correlation between the intensity of the inflammation and the degree of obstruction or distention of the colon.

It is important to recognize this entity at the time of radiographic evaluation so that the surgeon may plan the correct anastomosis. It has been recommended that after the obstructing tumor is resected, the proximal segment of colon should be examined through a sigmoidoscope and resection be extended to normal bowel. Anastomosis to inflamed bowel may lead to leakage at the suture line, delayed healing or stricture formation.

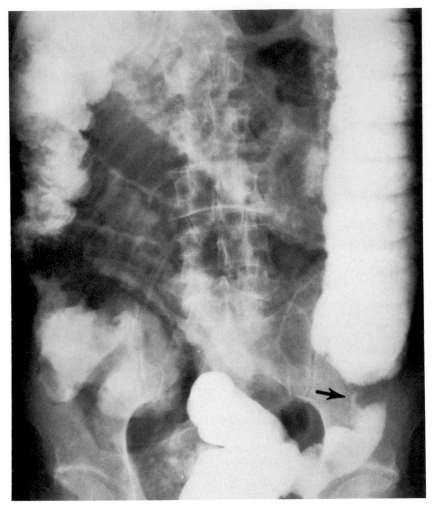

FIG. 17.44. COLITIS PROXIMAL TO AN OBSTRUCTING CARCINOMA

Proximal to the carcinoma (arrow) the entire colon is dilated with multiple ulcerations and mucosal edema extending around to the cecum. The small bowel is also dilated.

RECURRENT CARCINOMA

With the performance of more extensive surgical resections, residual or recurrent tumor at the anastomotic site has become relatively rare. When it does occur, it is likely the result of implantation of tumor cells at the time of anastomosis.

Recurrent carcinoma at the site of anastomosis will appear as an irregular nondistensible defect, frequently asymmetric (Fig. 17.45) and may show a tumor shelf or ulceration. A small unilateral indentation may also be seen if a foreign body granuloma has formed in reaction to the suture material. If there is any question about the diagnosis, a repeat examination should be done at once. If there is still doubt, exploratory laparotomy should be considered.

The site of anastomosis is usually apparent in the sigmoid and descending colon, but may be difficult to identify more proximally; in a few cases the exact site of the anastomosis is not identifiable. An end-to-side anastomosis will appear as a localized area of minimal constriction involving both sides of the bowel wall. The margin should be smooth and the area should be changeable; the mucosal pattern, although

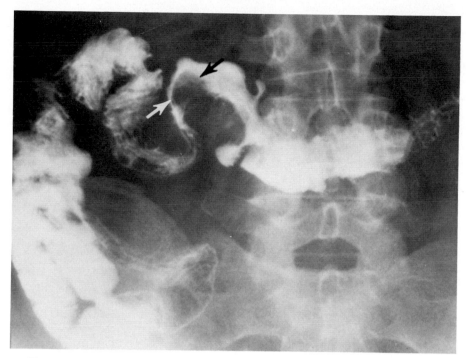

FIG. 17.45. RECURRENT CARCINOMA AT AN ILEOCOLIC ANASTOMOSIS
An asymmetrical defect (arrows) distorts the under surface of the ileocolic anastomosis, 14 months after a right colon resection for cancer.

not entirely normal, should not appear destroyed. If the ileum has been anastomosed to the colon, the transition from normal colon to normal ileum is easily detected. Any departure from the above findings should be considered potentially abnormal, especially any fixed decrease in size of the bowel lumen at the anastomotic line on subsequent examinations.

It is a good general rule to perform a barium enema approximately 2–3 months after surgery for carcinoma of the colon in order to have a baseline for future studies. By this time the edema and spasm will have subsided. Since local recurrence may occur in about 10% (Fig. 17.46) and a second primary (metachronous tumor) will be found in about 3%, there is ample reason for subsequent follow-up examinations, which should be done at yearly intervals for 5 years.

MISCELLANEOUS CONSIDERATIONS

Calcification in Carcinoma

Although rarely seen, calcification may be detectable by x-ray in a colonic cancer. The observation is always made on the plain film of the abdomen, but usually only after the tumor has been identified on barium enema. When present, the calcification is stippled or mottled and since mucous producing glands are prone to form stones, the tumor is invariably a mucoid adenocarcinoma.

Metastatic carcinoma of the colon involving the liver may also show a stippled form of calcification and, again, the tumor of origin is almost invariably a colloid cancer (Fig. 17.47).

Carcinoma vs Diverticulitis

At times, a partially obstructing, stenotic cancer, particularly in the sigmoid colon,

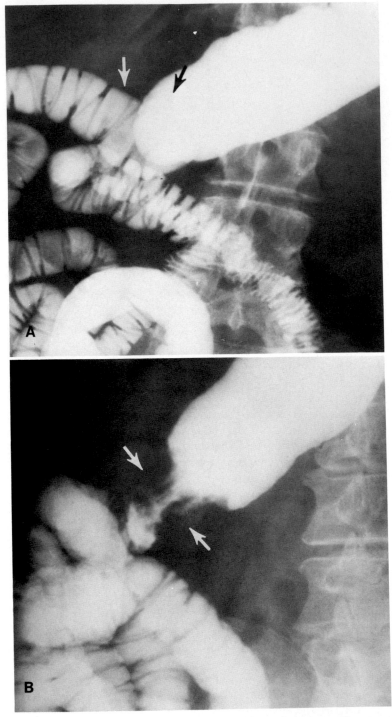

FIG. 17.46. RECURRENT CARCINOMA 12 MONTHS AFTER SURGERY
(A) The distal ileum (white arrow) and the mid-transverse colon (black arrow) appear normal on a baseline barium enema performed 2 months after a right colectomy. (B) Ten months later, a follow-up barium enema shows recurrent tumor at the ileocolic anastomosis (arrows) marked by irregular narrowing, nodularity, and mucosal destruction.

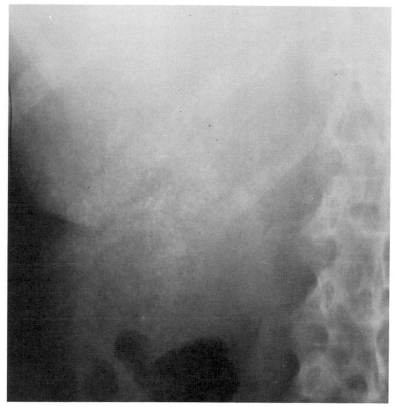

FIG. 17.47. METASTATIC CARCINOMA TO THE LIVER
The areas of stippled calcification are in a huge hepatic metastasis from a colloid carcinoma of the colon.

may resemble an area of acute diverticulitis. Careful attention to the predominant features of each lesion will most often allow a differential diagnosis to be made.

An annular, stenotic cancer usually involves only a short segment of the colon, the proximal and distal edges (shelves) of the tumor mass are sharply demarcated from adjacent normal bowel, and the central core is without mucosal detail due to ulceration.

The differential points in favor of acute diverticulitis with spasm are the longer area of involvement, tapered proximal and distal margins, and the fact that some mucosa is preserved through the narrowed segment. With complete obstruction, a differential diagnosis may be impossible by barium enema.

Colon Carcinoma Following Ureterosigmoidostomy

Patients who have had a ureterosigmoidostomy are at 100 times the normal risk of developing colon cancer. This appears to hold true whether the indication for urinary diversion was a benign or malignant condition. The colonic cancer develops at the site of the ureteral implant in the colon and is usually polypoid or exophytic in type. There is also an increased incidence of benign polyps developing at the ureterosigmoidostomy. In younger patients, whose diversion was done for a benign condition, the median time interval between original surgery and the diagnosis of colonic cancer is reported at 21 years, and the median age at diagnosis 33 years. In older patients, whose original surgery was for bladder cancer, the mean time before development of cancer is reported at 5.6 years and the median age at diagnosis 63 years.

To date, the explanation for this heightened risk of colon cancer in patients who have undergone ureterosigmoidostomy is unknown. The risk seems to continue even after a subsequent ileal conduit procedure is done, leaving the old ureterosigmoid anastomosis in place, although no longer in contact with urine or any carcinogen that urine may contain.

Fortunately, the ileal conduit operation is now a more popular primary procedure than ureterosigmoidostomy. However, there are a large number of individuals at risk of developing a colonic malignancy because they underwent the older procedure. These patients require careful surveillance; any sign of rectal bleeding, abdominal pain, or change in bowel habits must be investigated promptly. Periodic x-ray studies of the colon and testing for occult blood in the stool should also be carried out.

Carcinoma of the Colon and Inguinal Hernia

There is no statistically valid relationship between carcinoma of the colon and inguinal hernia, although it has been the tradition for decades "to order a barium enema" as part of the preoperative work-up of patients about to undergo inguinal hernia repair.

It should be stressed that there is waste in cost, time and radiation exposure when such a preoperative barium enema is done on asymptomatic inguinal hernia patients as a screening procedure for cancer; the examination is simply not productive enough to warrant its routine use in this group of patients any more than it is in the asymptomatic general population.

Colitis Cystica Profunda and Pneumatosis Coli

There are two benign conditions of the colon which have been confused radiologically with malignant disease or polyps. They are described in more detail in Chapter 20.

Colitis cystica profunda is a rare lesion that can cause the rectum and sigmoid to have a markedly irregular contour with an exaggerated mucosal pattern. Pathologically, the mucosa is intact, but markedly elevated and irregular secondary to the deposition of large amounts of mucus in a myriad of small cystic spaces in the submucosa. Few cases of this entity have been reported and its development and significance are not understood.

When pneumatosis intestinalis involves the colon (Fig. 17.48) the collections of intramural gas are usually cystic in appearance and more often distributed along the distal transverse colon and the descending colon or in the sigmoid. Pneumatosis coli is the preferred term when only the colon is involved; an underlying disease of the gastrointestinal tract is rarely found.

Pseudotumor of the Colon Due to Adhesions

Intra-abdominal adhesions and fibrous bands are difficult to diagnose radiologically. They may occasionally be suspected as the cause of partial or complete intestinal obstruction in a patient with a history of previous abdominal surgery. In such cases, a band-like extrinsic defect crossing the bowel, an area of fixation and narrowing or a point of complete obstruction are the more common x-ray manifestations.

However, adhesions may also simulate the contour defect of a primary colonic cancer, a metastatic serosal implant or an endometrioma (Fig. 17.49). This type of pseudotumor defect due to adhesion is more often seen in the transverse or sigmoid segments and cannot be differentiated from a true tumor by any barium enema technique.

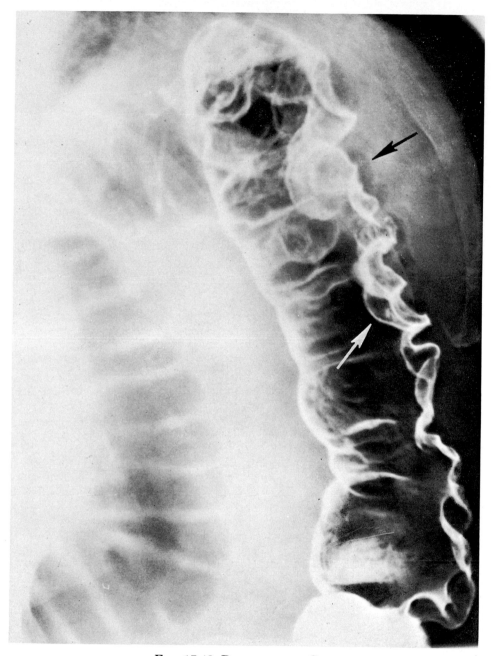

FIG. 17.48. PNEUMATOSIS COLI
The lobulated contour of the colon is due to multiple air cysts, which appear both
to indent the lumen (white arrow), and project beyond the bowel wall (black arrow).

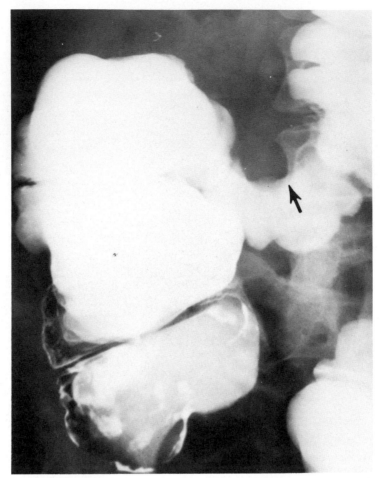

FIG. 17.49. PSEUDOTUMOR, PROXIMAL TRANSVERSE COLON

Simulating a primary cancer of the colon or a large serosal metastatic implant (arrow), this deformity was found at surgery to be caused by a fibrous band adherent to the stomach and transverse colon. The patient had surgery for a perforated duodenal ulcer 14 years previously.

Nodular Lymphoid Hyperplasia

Lymphoid hyperplasia is a frequent normal finding in the terminal ileum of children or may be an abnormal pattern in the small bowel of patients with giardiasis or dysgammaglobulinemia. Rarely, the colon may show lymphoid hyperplasia in the latter condition.

Diffuse, nodular lymphoid hyperplasia of the colon, however, is usually a nonspecific entity that may simulate diffuse, nodular lymphoma, the pseudopolyps of ulcerative colitis, or familial adenomatous colonic polyposis, particularly in adolescents. Representing aggregates of lymphoid tissue, the number and size of the nodules may reflect adjacent inflammatory disease in some cases, but the pattern is inconstant and nearly always reverts to normal in early adult life.

A differential diagnosis between benign lymphoid hyperplasia and nodular lymphoma, ulcerative colitis or multiple polyps can usually be made by excluding other systemic or gastrointestinal manifestations of these diseases. Since in the younger patient the presence of lymphoid hyperplasia rarely can be correlated with any specific symptomatology or disease state, there should be no radical therapy without biopsy confirmation of some more ominous diagnosis.

BIBLIOGRAPHY

American Cancer Society, New York: Cancer statistics. CA *28:* 17, 1978.

Bockus, H. L.: *Gastroenterology*, 3rd Ed., Vol. 2, pp. 1021–1033. W. B. Saunders, Philadelphia, 1976.

Brendel, T. H., and Kirsh, I. E.: Lack of association between inguinal hernia and carcinoma of the colon. N. Engl. J. Med., *284:* 369, 1971.

Dreyfuss, J. R., and Benacerraf, B.: Saddle cancers of the colon and their progression to annular carcinomas. Radiology, *129:* 289, 1978.

DeSmet, A. E., Tubergen, D. G., and Martel, W.: Nodular lymphoid hyperplasia of the colon associated with dysgammaglobulinemia. Am. J. Roentgenol., *127:* 515, 1976.

Ekelund, G., Lindström, C., and Rosengren, J.-E.: Appearance and growth of early carcinomas of the colon-rectum. Acta Radiol. (Diagn), *15:* 670, 1974.

Elliott, G. B., and Elliott, K. A.: The roentgenologic pathology of so-called pneumatosis cystoides intestinalis. Am. J. Roentgenol., *89:* 720, 1963.

Falterman, K. W., Hill, C. B., Markey, J. C., Fox, J. W., and Cohn, I.: Cancer of the colon, rectum, and anus: A review of 2313 cases. Cancer, *34:* 951, 1974.

Fenlon, J. W., and Margulis, A. R.: Current concepts in cancer. Cancer of the GI tract: Colon, rectum, anus. The radiologic diagnosis. J.A.M.A., *231:* 752, 1975.

Fleischner, F. G., and Berenberg, A. L.: Recurrent carcinoma of colon at site of anastomosis. Roentgen observations. Radiology, *66:* 540, 1956.

Franken, E. A.: Lymphoid hyperplasia of the colon. Radiology, *94:* 329, 1970.

Hurwitz, A., and Khafif, R. A.: Acute necrotizing colitis proximal to obstructing neoplasms of the colon. Surg. Gynecol. Obstet., *111:* 749, 1960.

Janower, M. L.: Vanishing lesion of the colon. X-ray Seminar Number 39. J.A.M.A., *189:* 942, 1964.

Janower, M. L., Dreyfuss, J. R., and Weber, A. L.: Cancer of the gastrointestinal tract in young people. Radiol. Clin. North Am., 7: 121, 1969.

Khilnani, M. T., Marshak, R. H., Eliasoph, J., and Wolf, B. S.: Roentgen features of metastases to the colon. Am. J. Roentgenol., *96:* 302, 1966.

Kyaw, M. M., and Koehler, P. R.: Pseudotumors of colon due to adhesions. Radiology, *103:* 597, 1972.

Laufer, I., and Joffe, N.: Roentgenologic aspects of chronic perforating carcinoma of the colon. Dis. Colon Rectum, *16:* 127, 1973.

Marshak, R. H., Lindner, A. E., and Maklansky, D.: Adenomatous polyps of the colon. A rational approach. J.A.M.A., *235:* 2856, 1976.

Meyers, M. A., Oliphant, M., Teixidor, H., and Weiser, P.: Metastatic carcinoma simulating inflammatory colitis. Am. J. Roentgenol., *123:* 74, 1975.

McCartney, W. H., and Hoffer, P. B.: The value of carcinoembryonic antigen (CEA) as an adjunct to the radiological colon examination in the diagnosis of malignancy. Radiology, *110:* 325, 1974.

Miller, R. E.: The cleansing enema. Radiology, *117:* 483, 1975.

Miller, S. F.: Colorectal cancer: Are the goals of early detection achieved? CA *27:* 338, 1977.

Moertel, C. G., Schutt, A. J., and Go, V. L. W.: Carcinoembryonic antigen test for recurrent colorectal carcinoma. Inadequacy for early detection. J.A.M.A., *239:* 1065, 1978.

Pochaczevsky, R., and Sherman, R. S.: Diffuse lymphomatous disease of the colon: Its roentgen appearance. Am. J. Roentgenol., *87:* 670, 1962.

Raskin, M. M., Viamonte, M., and Viamonte, M., Jr.: Primary linitis plastica carcinoma of the colon. Radiology, *113:* 17, 1974.

Robbins, S. L.: *Pathologic Basis of Disease*, 4th Ed., p. 968. W. B. Saunders, Philadelphia, 1974.

Schatzki, R.: The roentgenologic appearance of intussuscepted tumors of the colon, with and without barium examinations. Am. J. Roentgenol., *41:* 549, 1939.

Spratt, J. S., Jr., and Ackerman, L. V.: Small primary adenocarcinomas of the colon and rectum. J.A.M.A., *179:* 337, 1962.

Shulman, H., and Giustra, P.: Invasive carcinoids of the colon. Radiology, *98:* 139, 1971.

Schwartz, S. S., and Boley, S. J.: Ischemic origin of ulcerative colitis associated with potentially obstructing lesions of the colon. Radiology, *102:* 249, 1972.

Sooriyaarachchi, G. S., Johnson, R. O., and Carbone, P. P.: Neoplasms of the large bowel following ureterosigmoidostomy. Arch. Surg., *112:* 1174, 1977.

Wanebo, H. J., Rao, B., Pinsky, C. M., *et al.:* Preoperative carcinoembryonic antigen level as a prognostic indicator in colorectal cancer. N. Engl. J. Med., *299:* 448, 1978.

Welch, C. E., and Burke, J. F.: Carcinoma of the colon and rectum. N. Engl. J. Med., *266:* 211, 1962.

Welch, J. P., and Donaldson, G. A.: Recent experience in the management of cancer of the colon and rectum. Am. J. Surg., *127:* 258, 1974.

Welch, J. P., Donaldson, G. A., and Welch, C. E.: Carcinoma of the colon and rectum. Curr. Probl. Cancer *1:* 5, 1976.

Welin, S., Youker, J., Spratt, J. S., Jr., Linnell, F., Spjut, H. J., Johnson, R. E., and Ackerman, L. V.: The rates and patterns of growth of 375 tumors of the large intestine and rectum observed serially by double contrast enema study (Malmo technique). Am. J. Roentgenol., *90:* 673, 1963.

Wolf, B. S.: Lipoma of the colon. J.A.M.A., *235:* 2225, 1976.

Youker, J. E., and Welin, S.: Differentiation of true polypoid tumors of the colon from extraneous material: A new roentgen sign. Radiology, *84:* 610, 1965.

Zimmer, G., Kurzban, J. D., Maklansky, D., and Marshak, R. H.: The radiology corner. Colonic endometriosis: Roentgen studies with a five-year follow-up. Am. J. Gastroenterol., *64:* 410, 1975.

18

The Appendix

JOHN A. LONG, M.D.

The human vermiform appendix arises from the posteromedial aspect of the cecum at the junction of the three tenia coli. It is a narrow and hollow organ that lacks sacculations and a true mesentery and which is supplied by the appendicular artery, a branch of the ileocolic artery. It is wormlike in appearance and is contained in a peritoneal fold which is called the mesentery of the vermiform appendix.

The appendix first appears in the 6th to 8th weeks of life and is usually fully developed by the 12th week. Agenesis or absence of the appendix is very rare. It usually ranges in size from 1.5–24 cm in length but the average length is 5–10 cm. On cross-section it has a starlike passageway and a diameter in the range of 6 mm. Its distal end has been described as being bulbous, a fact used to determine complete filling during radiographic examinations with the barium enema or barium meal.

The abdominal position of the appendix may vary, but it is found in the right lower quadrant 96% of the time. When it is in the right lower quadrant, it is found anterior to the cecum in 74% of cases. Of these 74%, it is found caudad toward the pelvis in 30%, medial to the cecum in 38%, and lateral to cecum in 6%.

The other position in which it may be found in the right lower quadrant is retrocecal (Figs. 18.1 and 18.2). When it is here, diagnostic difficulties may arise. Of the 26% of appendicies which are retrocecal, 10% are free in position and 16% are fixed in position.

Other positions in which the appendix may be located include the right upper quadrant (3.9%), the left lower quadrant (0.04%), the left upper quadrant (0.056%), and positions that are due to excessive length, malrotations of the colon, cecal mobility, and hernias.

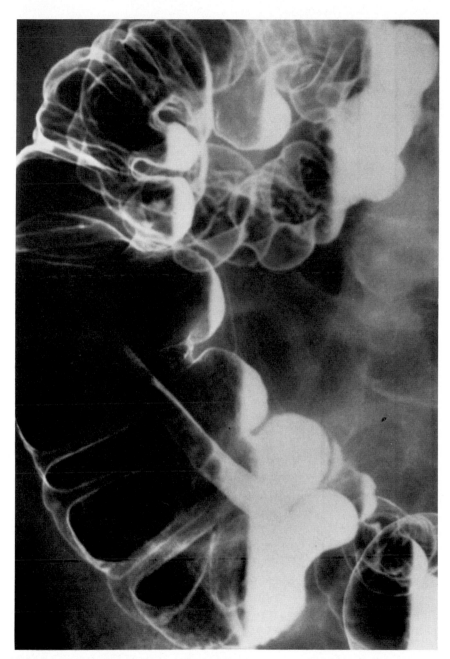

FIG. 18.1. ANTEROPOSTERIOR VIEW OF A RETROCECAL APPENDIX SEEN DURING AN
AIR-CONTRAST EXAMINATION

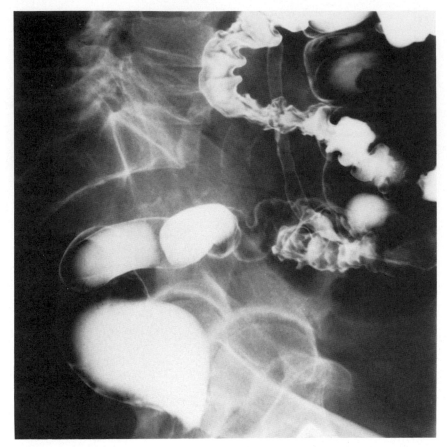

FIG. 18.2. LATERAL VIEW OF A RETROCECAL APPENDIX, AIR CONTRAST
EXAMINATION

APPENDICITIS

Introduction

Appendicitis is found in the United States in 200,000 patients a year with a
resultant 2,000 deaths. The maximal incidence is between the ages of 10 and 12 and
it is rare below the age of 2 years but reported. It is of great interest that 20% of
cases occur after the age of 50.

Incisions of large encysted collections of pus from the abdomen, most probably
appendiceal in origin, have been documented historically from early Christian times.
The first successful appendectomy was performed by the English surgeon, Claudius
Amyand in 1735. He removed a pin from an appendix of an 11-year-old boy which
was present in a scrotal hernia sac. The present day recognition of appendicitis as
a clinical entity is due to the efforts of Reginald H. Fitz of Harvard who described
it in 1886. After this, prompt diagnosis and early surgery helped to decrease the
mortality and morbidity associated with the disease.

Pathology

Obstruction and inflammation are major factors in the pathogenesis of appendicitis. With obstruction, the appendix becomes a closed space which serves as a
breeding ground for bacteria as there can be no adequate drainage of the exudate
formed. The most common cause of obstruction is fecalith formation, or stenosis

due to previous inflammation. Theoretically, lymphoid hyperplasia can cause obstruction also. Quite commonly fecaliths are found in the lumen of the appendix and
represent fecal concretions without calcification. With impaction there will be
enhancement of the inflammatory process in the obstructed segment (Figs. 18.3 and
18.4). The histologic criterion for acute appendicitis is polymorphonuclear leukocytic
infiltration of the muscularis. Neutrophils and ulcerations may also be present in
the mucosa.

Clinical Features

Usually, the patient is below the age of 40 and a male. There is often a history of
indigestion, gastric complaints, or flatulence prior to the attack. Pain is most often
the first symptom followed by nausea, vomiting, and anorexia. The symptoms are
usually classic enough to allow the diagnosis to be made on physical exam if there
is tenderness in the right lower abdomen. There may be a low grade fever with a
slight leukocytosis. The radiologic exam is not needed for the classic case but in up
to 18% of cases the preoperative diagnosis of acute appendicitis may be uncertain
and the symptomatology may not be straightforward. The radiologic examination
may then be very helpful in establishing the diagnosis.

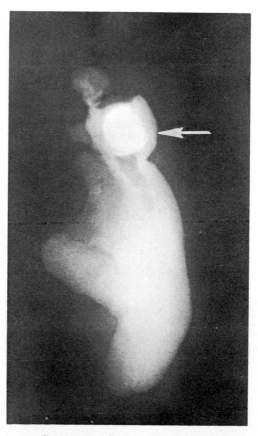

FIG. 18.3. X-RAY FILM OF SURGICAL SPECIMEN DEMONSTRATING APPENDICOLITH
IMPACTED IN ORIFICE OF DILATED APPENDIX (ARROW)

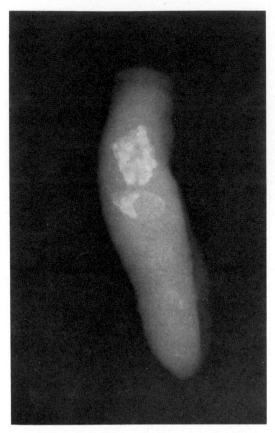

FIG. 18.4. EXAMPLE OF TWO CALCIFIED APPENDICOLITHS IN A SURGICAL SPECIMEN

Roentgen Findings

Plain Film

The findings on the plain film will correspond to the degree of inflammatory reaction present; *i.e.*, early acute, localized perforation or generalized peritonitis. A number of x-ray findings will be considered below which may be helpful in establishing the diagnosis.

Appendicolith

A calcified fecalith, or appendicolith, may be present in the right lower quadrant (Figs. 18.5 and 18.6) or elsewhere on the abdominal film (Fig. 18.7). The appendicolith may be single or (in 5% of cases) multiple (Figs. 18.8 and 18.9). It consists of a nidus of inspissated fecal material which is covered by a layer or layers of calcium phosphate or calcium carbonate. This is derived from the mucous glands of the appendix and causes a laminated appearance.

The appendicolith is composed of 50% fats and fatty derivatives, 25% inorganic residue such as calcium phosphate, and 20% organic residues. In size the appendicolith will range from 2–40 mm with a usual size of from 5–20 mm. Occasional giant appendicoliths have been reported which measure up to 2 × 4 cm. The appendicolith is usually of a much softer consistency than a gallstone.

When appendicitis is present, radiographic examinations of the excised appendix will show a calcified appendicolith 33% of the time. However, only 10% of cases of acute appendicitis in which preoperative abdominal series are obtained will show a calcified appendicolith.

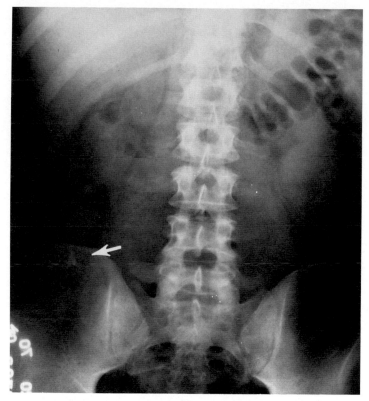

FIG. 18.5. A RIGHT LOWER QUADRANT APPENDICOLITH (ARROW)

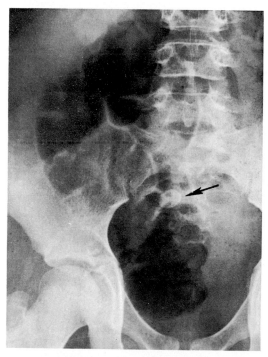

FIG. 18.6. SINGLE APPENDICOLITH IS SUPERIMPOSED ON RIGHT UPPER SACRUM
(ARROW)

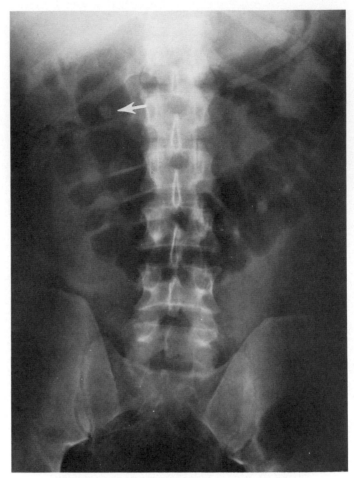

FIG. 18.7. RIGHT UPPER QUADRANT APPENDICOLITH SEEN IN APPENDICITIS IN A
PATIENT WITH NONROTATION OF THE COLON (ARROW)

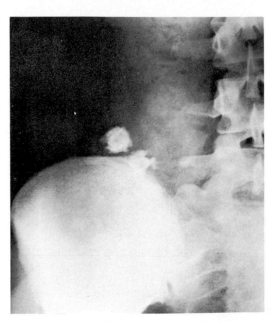

FIG. 18.8. TWO APPENDICOLITHS

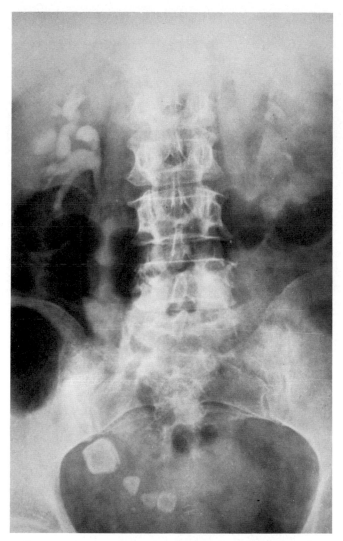

FIG. 18.9. FOUR LARGE APPENDICOLITHS SEEN IN THE RIGHT LOWER QUADRANT
DURING AN INTRAVENOUS UROGRAM

The presence of an appendicolith in a patient with the appropriate symptoms is virtually diagnostic of acute appendicitis (90% accuracy). Also, in such cases there is a higher than usual incidence of complications, particularly perforation or abscess formation. These complications are present in one-half of the cases in which an appendicolith is present in acute appendicitis. In less than 1% of asymptomatic people will an appendicolith be found and in this instance there is strong argument in the literature for an elective appendectomy. Foreign bodies will also occasionally be seen in the appendix and cause appendicitis (Fig. 18.10).

The differential diagnosis of an appendicolith includes a bone island, gallstone, calcified lymph node, phlebolith, ureteral calculus, gynecologic and vascular calcification. However, lamination of the calcification in an appendicolith helps to establish its true nature except in the patient with gallstone ileus in which case other evidence such as air in the bilary tree may be present.

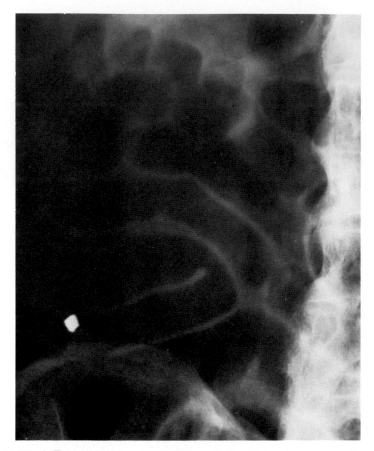

FIG. 18.10. A DENTAL AMALGAM IMPACTED IN THE APPENDIX CAUSING
APPENDICITIS

Cecum and Terminal Ileum

Abnormalities of the cecum and terminal ileum will also help in establishing the diagnosis. Air-fluid levels in the terminal ileum may be present in about 50% of cases of acute appendicitis. A sentinal loop of terminal ileum may also be present. Cecal air-fluid levels are also present in 40% of cases and may be shown more clearly with a lateral decubitus film (Fig. 18.11). Sometimes a persistent cecal deformity may be visualized on the plain film of the abdomen indicating the presence of an appendiceal abscess and its location. The walls of the cecum and the terminal ileum may be thickened because of the adjacent inflammatory process and if a perforation or peritonitis is present there may be a generalized paralytic ileus present which causes confusion in radiographic interpretation (Fig. 18.12).

Obliteration of Soft Tissue Landmarks

The periappendiceal inflammatory response may cause obliteration of certain landmarks normally visualized on a plain film of the abdomen. There may be broadening of the properitoneal fat line due to abnormal contraction of the abdominal muscles or this landmark may be lost. The lower margin of the right psoas muscle may become indistinct as may the outlines of the obturator or levator muscles. An ill defined density may be present in the right lower quadrant sometimes best noted when comparing the sharpness of the sacroiliac joints. If perforation with abscess formation has occurred, a more clearly defined mass, sometimes containing gas, may be seen (Figs. 18.13 and 18.14).

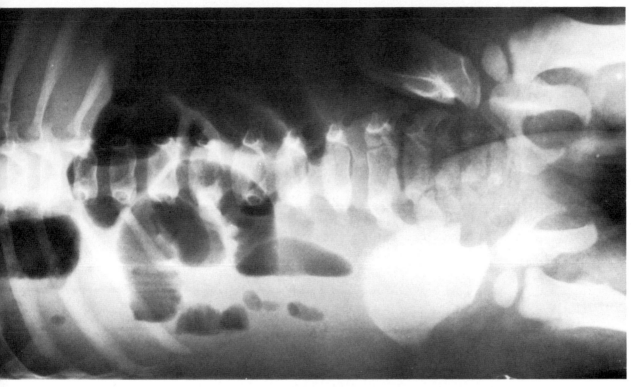

FIG. 18.11. FLUID LEVELS IN SMALL BOWEL AND CECUM IN CASE OF APPENDICITIS
IN A CHILD (LATERAL DECUBITUS FILM)

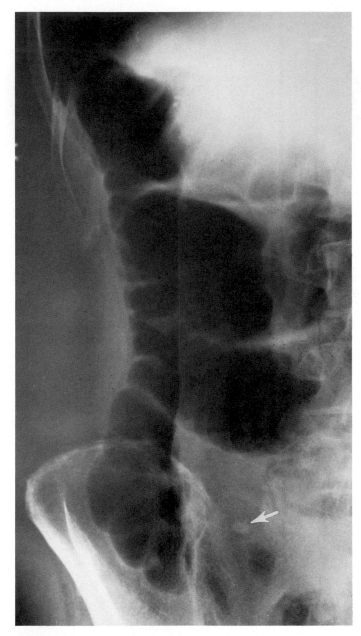

FIG. 18.12. DILATED RIGHT COLON AND SMALL BOWEL AND AN APPENDICOLITH
(ARROW) IN A CASE OF APPENDICITIS IN AN ADULT

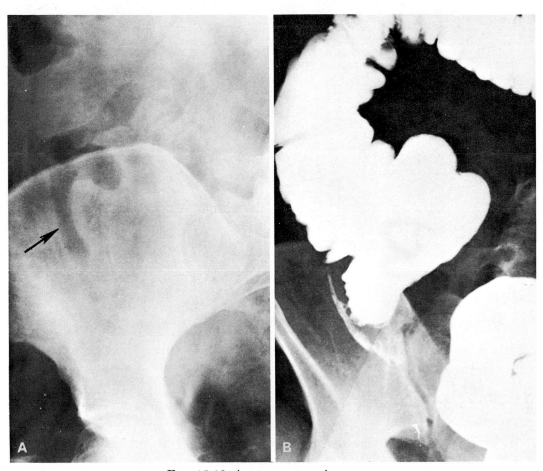

FIG. 18.13. APPENDICEAL ABSCESS

(A) Plain film demonstrating a right lower quadrant soft tissue mass overlying the pelvic brim and a collection of extracolonic gas (arrow). (B) The barium-filled cecum is indented by the mass and barium has extravasated into the right gutter.

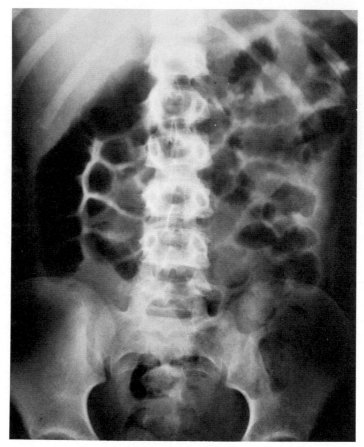

FIG. 18.14. AN APPENDICEAL ABSCESS PRESENTING AS A RIGHT LOWER QUADRANT
MASS IN A CHILD

Lumbar Scoliosis

In one-third of cases of acute appendicitis a lumbar scoliosis may be present, but, unfortunately, this may be a very nonspecific finding.

Gas-Filled Appendix or Pneumoperitoneum

The normal appendix may occasionally be filled with air especially if the cecum is in an abnormal position so that the tip of the appendix is located superiorly. The diseased appendix may rarely be filled with air and if an air-fluid level is present and recognized, the diagnosis of gangrenous appendicitis is assured. However, in the presence of symptoms of appendicitis this sign takes on more meaning particularly if it is persistent. Even more rarely pneumoperitoneum may occur. This does not happen more often because of the rapidity with which the appendiceal lumen becomes occluded and no longer communicates with the intestinal lumen, and because the perforated appendix is usually walled off immediately.

The Use of the Barium Enema in Appendicitis

In addition to plain films of the abdomen a barium enema may be required for further clarification. It should be stressed that the presence of an acute (nonperforated) appendix is not a contraindication to the performance of the examination.

The barium enema may be the best means of establishing the diagnosis. In one-fifth of cases of suspected appendicitis the preoperative diagnosis has been found to be incorrect and the appendix shown to be normal. Diagnostic difficulty is present particularly in patients over 50 years of age in whom 20% of appendicitis occurs. When the clinical diagnosis is obscure, great help may be obtained by performing this examination.

Useful signs

The correct diagnosis of appendiceal inflammatory disease can be made from a barium enema when changes are demonstrated in the cecum. The cecal wall in the immediate region of the appendiceal stoma may become irregular or indented because of edema (Figs. 18.15 and 18.16); a thin track of barium may point into the incompletely filled lumen of the appendix (Fig. 18.17). If perforation and abscess formation have occurred, the cecum or terminal ileum may show either a smooth or an irregular extrinsic pressure deformity (Fig. 18.18). These findings will have to be considered with the history in attempting a differential diagnosis between other entities such as an ameboma, cecal polyp, or carcinoma, postoperative appendiceal stump (Fig. 18.19), mucocele, carcinoid, or some other adjacent mass.

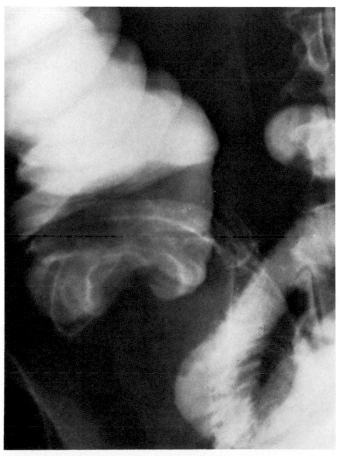

FIG. 18.15. MASS IMPRESSION AGAINST THE CECUM DUE TO APPENDICITIS

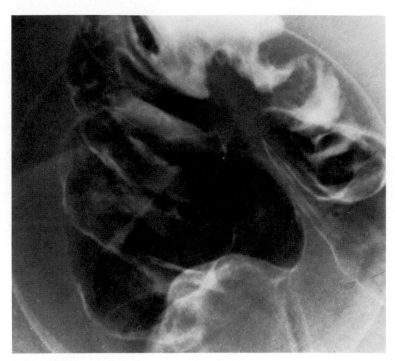

FIG. 18.16. MASS IMPRESSION AGAINST THE CECUM DUE TO APPENDICITIS (AIR-CONTRAST EXAMINATION)

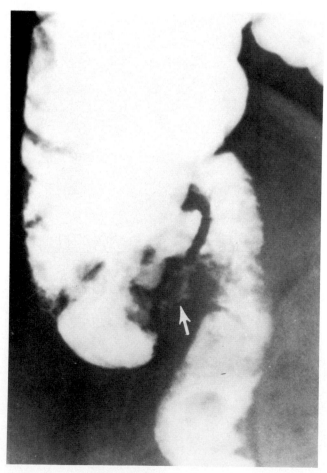

FIG. 18.17. APPENDICITIS

Irregularly filled appendix (arrow) surrounded by an inflammatory mass which indents the cecum and terminal ileum.

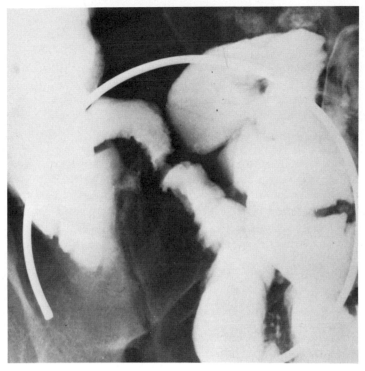

FIG. 18.18. MASS IMPRESSION AGAINST THE MEDIAL WALL OF THE CECUM AND THE LATERAL WALL OF THE TERMINAL ILEUM DUE TO APPENDICITIS

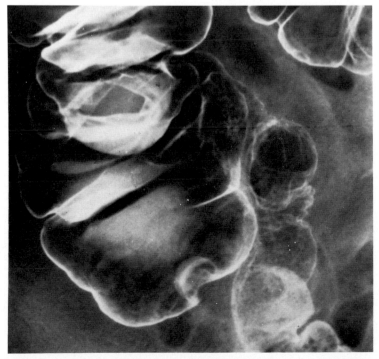

FIG. 18.19. INVERTED APPENDICEAL STUMP (AIR-CONTRAST EXAMINATION)

Useless signs

A variety of signs have also been noted pertaining to the unfilled or barium-filled appendix. Many of these have proven worthless and are mentioned here only that they may finally be put to rest. Such findings as failure of filling of the appendix with barium, kinking, a shortened lumen, filling defects within the lumen, lack of mobility (fixation), tenderness on palpation, and retention of barium within the appendix for prolonged periods of time are of limited usefulness. The normal appendix is frequently not seen during a barium enema examination. If the lumen is filled, its length will vary depending on the quantity of fecal material within it; feces may appear as small filling defects. The appendix may be mobile or nonmobile; acute angulation may occasionally occur. On palpation of the right lower quadrant, the normal patient may complain of tenderness during a barium enema examination. Barium is frequently retained in the appendix after the cecum is emptied for varying periods of time ranging from weeks to months; this does not indicate a diseased appendix. While it is theoretically possible that the barium may become impacted in the appendiceal lumen and cause a secondary appendicitis, this must be extraordinarily rare, if it occurs at all.

DIVERTICULOSIS

Diverticulosis of the appendix is seen in 1% of surgical specimens, and it is frequently associated with appendicitis and perforation. In slightly over one-half of the cases there is a single diverticulum. Asymptomatic people with diverticulosis of the appendix should be closely watched and possibly should be considered for an elective appendectomy (Fig. 18.20).

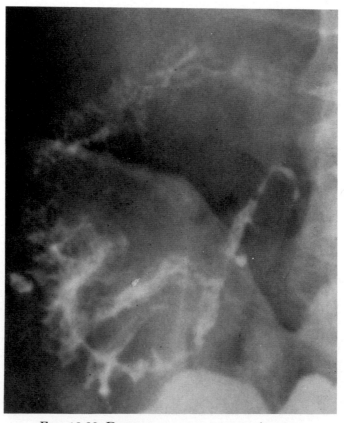

FIG. 18.20. DIVERTICULOSIS OF THE APPENDIX

MUCOCELE

Introduction

A mucocele is a benign cystic dilatation of the appendix seen infrequently in surgical and autopsy specimens. It is an unusual lesion and may vary in size from 1–10 cm. The term mucocele was first used by Fere who dissected a fusiformly enlarged appendix containing a gelatinous mass.

Pathology

With a mucocele there is either complete or partial obstruction of the appendiceal lumen. The mucosa demonstrates globular dilatation of the glands of Lieberkühn, papillary formation, and epithelial atrophy. All of these findings are the result of increased intraluminal pressure. Mucin is produced distal to the obstructed lumen.

Clinical Features

The symptoms vary and are chronic in nature unless complications occur. The patient complains of vague lower abdominal discomfort which is recurrent in nature. Physical examination may reveal a right lower quadrant mass.

Roentgen Findings

The radiologist is often called upon to clarify the nature of the discomfort or the mass. A plain film may be normal or may reveal a well defined right lower quadrant mass of varying size; if surgery is not performed the mass may increase in size. Calcification, either mottled or rimlike, occurs infrequently but is helpful in establishing the diagnosis.

A barium enema will fail to demonstrate the appendix and the barium-filled cecum will be indented usually on its medial side by a smooth-walled mass (Fig. 18.21). The cecum will be distensible but inseparable from the mass and the terminal ileum may also be displaced. A few cases have been reported in which barium has entered the mucocele through what is presumed to be a recanalized lumen. The defect must be differentiated from an appendiceal abscess or other pericecal inflammatory disease as well as other right lower quadrant masses.

Complications include pseudomyxoma peritonei which is due to multiple collections of mucinous material scattered throughout the peritoneal cavity. A similar condition results from the rupture of certain types of ovarian cysts in the female. The origin of the intraperitoneal mucus is not completely settled, but is probably discharged into the peritoneum from a small perforation of the mucocele. A mucocele may also cause ureteral or ileal obstruction, become inflamed, twist on itself, or intussuscept.

Myxoglobulosis

Myxoglobulosis of the appendix is an uncommon form of mucocele of the appendix in that it is made up of many round or oval globules mixed with mucus. The overall effect has been described as resembling tapioca or fish eggs. Why they develop is unknown but a high concentration of calcium is also present which may precipitate on the globules. Radiologically there is a mass adjacent to the cecum and many calculi may also be seen. The differential diagnosis includes gynecologic calcifications, phleboliths, and metastatic calcified lesions applied to the cecum.

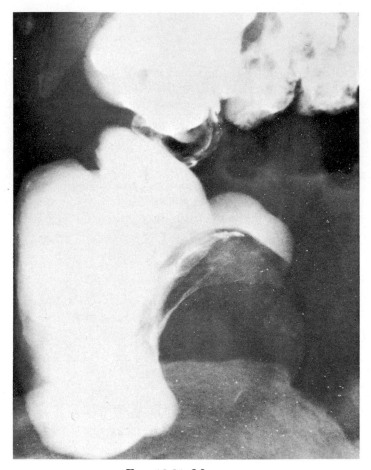

FIG. 18.21. MUCOCELE

A well defined, calcified mass smoothly indents the medial aspect of the cecum in the expected position of the appendix.

TUMORS

Tumors of the appendix occur in 6% of surgical and autopsy specimens. Roentgen studies may show a right lower quadrant mass but usually the tumor is not diagnosed because of its small size or the complication of appendicitis. Benign tumors are encountered in 5% of specimens while malignant tumors occur in 1%.

The most common tumor is the carcinoid tumor which arises from the Kulchitsky (argentaffin) cells of the crypts of Lieberkühn. Ninety percent of carcinoids arise in the appendix, and 90% of all tumors of the appendix are carcinoids. They are essentially benign tumors and only about 0.01% metastasize. The carcinoid syndrome does not occur unless there has been metastasis to the liver. Usually the carcinoid tumor is found in an appendix removed incidentally at surgery for another procedure or because appendicitis supervened. The occurrence of appendicitis explains the earlier age at which the carcinoid tumor is found in the appendix, 25 years vs 55 years in the ileum; the onset of appendicitis also interrupts the natural life history of the tumor and this explains why metastasis is unusual.

Other appendiceal tumors include benign lymphoma, neuroma, and fibroma. Malignant tumors include adenocarcinoma or lymphoma which are usually recognized only after surgery (Figs. 18.22 and 18.23).

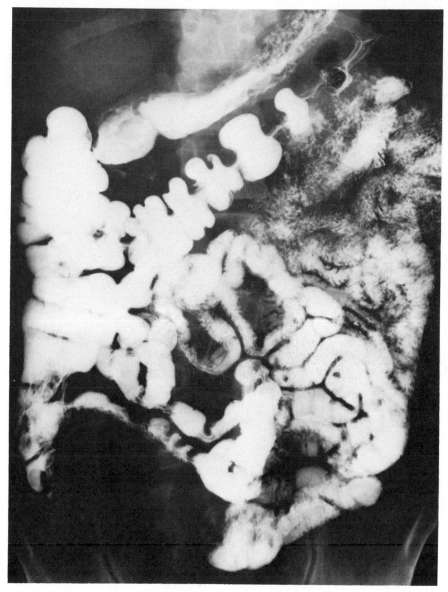

FIG. 18.22. APPENDICEAL CARCINOMA PRESENTING AS A MASS IN THE RIGHT
LOWER QUADRANT

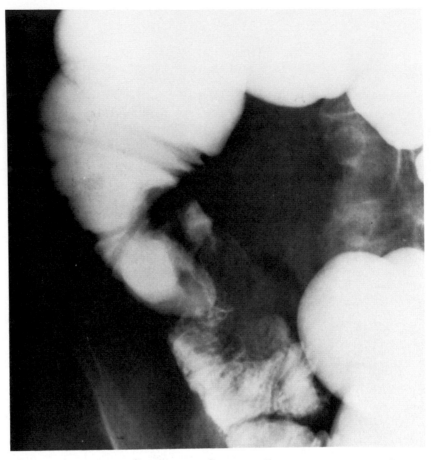

FIG. 18.23. APPENDICEAL CARCINOMA CAUSING DEFORMITY OF THE CECUM AND
TERMINAL ILEUM

BIBLIOGRAPHY

Balthazar, E. J., and Grade, M.: The normal and abnormal development of the appendix. Radiology, *121:* 599, 1976.

Barnes, B. A., Behringer, G. E., Wheelock, F. C., and Wilkins, E. W.: Treatment of appendicitis at the Massachusetts General Hospital (1937–1959). J.A.M.A., *180:* 122, 1962.

Berk, R. N.: Barium enema examination in acute appendicitis. J.A.M.A., *236:* 394, 1976.

Benventano, T. C., Schein, C. J., and Jacobson, H. G.: The roentgen aspects of some appendiceal abnormalities. Am. J. Roentgen. Radium Therapy Nucl. Med., *96:* 344, 1966.

Carleton, C. C.: Mucocele of the appendix and peritoneal pseudomyxoma. Arch. Pathol., *60:* 39, 1955.

Collins, D. C.: 71,000 human appendix specimens: A final report, summarizing forty years' study. Am. J. Protol., *14:* 365, 1963.

Faegenburg, D.: Fecaliths of the appendix: Incidence and significance. Am. J. Roentgen. Radium Therapy Nucl. Med., *89:* 752, 1963.

Felson, B., and Bernhard, C. M.: The roentgenologic diagnosis of appendiceal calculi. Radiology, *49:* 178, 1947.

Felson, B., and Wiot, J. F.: Some interesting right lower quadrant entities: Myxoglobulosis of the appendix, ileal prolapse, diverticulitis, lymphoma, endometriosis. Radiol. Clin. North Am., *7:* 83, 1969.

Figiel, L. S., and Figiel, J. J.: Barium examination of cecum in appendicitis. Acta. Radiol., *57:* 569, 1962.

Graham, A. D., and Johnson, H. F.: The incidence of radiographic findings in acute appendicitis compared to 200 normal abdomens. Mil. Med., *131:* 272, 1966.

Joffe, N.: Radiology of acute appendicitis and its complications. CRC Crit. Rev. Clin. Radiol. Nucl. Med., *7:* 97, 1975.

Norman, A., Leider, S., and Del Carman, J.: Mucocele of the appendix. Am. J. Roentgenol. Radium Therapy Nucl. Med., *77:* 647, 1957.

Shaw, R. E.: Appendix calculi and acute appendicitis. Br. J. Surg., *52:* 451, 1965.

Soter, C. S.: The contribution of the radiologist to the diagnosis of acute appendicitis. Semin. Roentgenol., *8:* 375, 1973.

19

Obstruction, Trauma, and Surgery

JAMES J. McCORT, M.D.

OBSTRUCTION

Large bowel obstruction accounts for approximately 25% of all cases of intestinal obstruction. Colon obstruction may quickly lead to cecal perforation, peritonitis, and septic shock. For the patient with suspected colon obstruction, immediate consultation between the radiologist, surgeon, and emergency room physician facilitates the therapeutic decision.

Patient Examination—Plain Film, Chest Film, and Barium Enema

The plain film series and chest radiographs form the first line of investigation. When the history and plain film suggest colon obstruction, an immediate barium enema should be done. Delay can impair the patient's chance of recovery.

Plain Film

Positioning and film sequence

Three films in different projections show the presence of intraperitoneal air, the degree of distention, the location of intraluminal air-fluid levels, and bowel loop mobility. The left lateral decubitus, the upright, and the supine are obtained in that order. The patient remains on his left side for 5 min before the technician exposes the left lateral decubitus film. This allows small amounts of intraperitoneal (free) air to rise over the liver. The technician then elevates the table for the upright abdominal film. This causes free intraperitoneal air to enter the subdiaphragmatic space. The patient is returned to the horizontal position for the final supine abdominal film.

Exposure factors

Radiographic visualization of the abdominal viscera depends on the differential photon absorption by air, fat, viscera, and bone. Photoelectric scattering varies with the cube of the absorbing medium density and increases at lower kilovoltages. A film taken at 60–65 kV gives good contrast with a sufficiently short exposure time and adequate penetration. Using 500 mA, three-phase equipment, the shortest possible time and a 12:1 movable grid shows anatomical detail with visualization of the properitoneal fat lines.

Gas pattern

The information available on the plain abdominal study depends upon the distribution of gas and fluid. Most intestinal gas is swallowed and carried through the intestinal tract by peristalsis. Only a small increment arises from intraluminal fermentation or nitrogen diffusion from the blood.

Some bowel fluid is ingested. In a 24-hr period secretions of intestinal mucus glands, liver and pancreas augment this fluid by 4–11 liters. In strangulating obstruction, fluid and electrolytes exude into the bowel. Peristalsis and fluid absorption empties the colon distal to an obstruction.

Small bowel contents (succus entericus) entering the colon are semiliquid. Hence air-fluid levels appear normally in the cecum and ascending colon. The unobstructed colon efficiently absorbs water and sodium. In the absence of diarrhea, air-fluid levels beyond the hepatic flexure strongly suggest mechanical colon obstruction. A cleansing enema nullifies these findings and should be withheld before filming.

Chest Film

Abdominal pain and distention may reflect intrathoracic disease such as pneumonia or heart failure. A chest film excludes this possibility.

Barium Enema

In suspected large bowel and/or distal ileum obstruction, the emergency barium enema can confirm the diagnosis, localize the point of obstruction, and define its cause. (A water-soluble media is used if perforation is suspected or believed to be impending.) Toxic megacolon or free intraperitoneal air contraindicate enema examination.

If stool fills the rectosigmoid, preliminary digital disimpaction or tap-water enema will dislodge it. Cathartics are never used. Often the unprepared bowel study supplies diagnostically valuable information.

Digital and sigmoidoscopic examinations should precede the barium enema as 40% of carcinomas lie within range of the sigmoidscope. Biopsy of suspicious lesions should be deferred until the barium study has been completed to minimize the risk of perforation.

Under fluoroscopic control, the examiner introduces barium into the rectum with low pressure and discontinues the examination when he identifies the obstruction site and the nature of the lesion. To avoid the risk of barium impaction, he should allow only a small amount to pass proximal to a constricting lesion.

Mechanical Obstruction

Patients with mechanical large bowel obstruction complain of distention, colicky pain, nausea, and constipation. Vomiting may be absent or occur late. Mechanical causes of colon obstruction include: carcinoma 65%, diverticulitis 20%, volvulus 5%, and miscellaneous including intussusception, hernia, and obturation 10%.

Carcinoma

Colon carcinoma rarely causes acute large bowel obstruction. Usually these patients have neglected the prodromal signs and symptoms of rectal bleeding, pain, weight loss, anemia, and gradual change in bowel habits. More commonly the patient with colon carcinoma develops chronic obstruction. Plain film findings vary with tumor location, the amount of swallowed air and ileo-cecal valve function.

Carcinoma at the ileo-cecal valve

Cecal carcinoma produces a mechanical small bowel obstruction and the large bowel is usually empty (Fig. 19.1). In the patient with distal small bowel obstruction a barium enema should be done to exclude an ileo-cecal lesion. Barium should not be given by mouth until the physician is sure the colon contains no obstructing lesion.

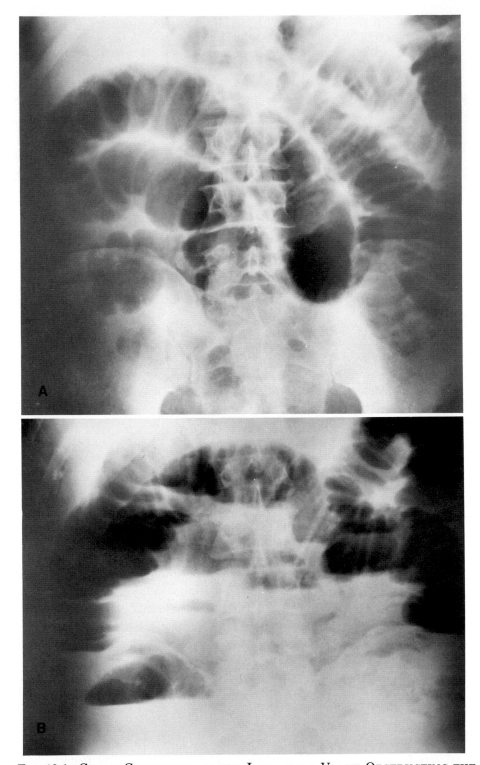

FIG. 19.1. COLON CARCINOMA AT THE ILEO-CECAL VALVE OBSTRUCTING THE
SMALL BOWEL
This 62-year-old man had continuous cramping abdominal pain with intermittent
diarrhea and constipation. (**A**) The abdominal film shows dilated small bowel loops.
(**B**) On the erect film these loops contain multiple fluid levels.

Carcinoma distal to the ileo-cecal valve

On plain film examination, food residues, fluid, and gas distend the colon. Because fluid rather than gas accumulates behind the constricting lesion, the visible end of the gas column rarely corresponds to the obstruction site.

The combination of carcinomatous bowel occlusion and a contracted ileo-cecal valve produces a closed loop type obstruction and an enormously dilated cecum. Cecal distention obliterates the characteristic haustral sacculations (Fig. 19.2). Concomitant small bowel distention occurs when the patient continues to swallow air.

Most large bowel ruptures occur in the cecum. No measurement can predict potential rupture with accuracy but a distended, thin walled cecum exceeding 10 cm in diameter foretells a possible rupture and calls for decompression regardless of the cause (Fig. 19.3).

On enema, the barium column arrests at the obstructing carcinoma which characteristically constricts the lumen over several centimeters. Colon carcinoma has shelf-like margins, a nodular, irregular lumen and may be ulcerated.

Pelvic tumors

Within the closed pelvic space, malignant tumors arising in the vagina, uterus, ovaries, bladder, or prostate may compress and on rare occasions invade the rectum and sigmoid to produce a chronic low grade obstruction (Fig. 19.4). Pelvic tumors are more likely to obstruct the ureters than the rectosigmoid.

Metastatic tumors and endometriosis

Hematogenous metastases from tumors arising outside the pelvis occasionally cause mechanical bowel obstruction (Fig. 19.5). Gastric or pancreatic carcinoma may directly invade the transverse colon or gravitate into the vaginal or rectovesical pouch. The examiner may palpate a shelf on rectal examination.

On barium enema, endometriosis may produce a filling defect in the rectosigmoid wall that usually does not completely obstruct. The patient relates cyclic pain, constipation, and occasionally rectal bleeding.

Inflammation

Intrinsic inflammatory lesions, *i.e.,* ulcerative and Crohn's colitis or lymphogranuloma venereum may rarely obstruct the colon and have been discussed in Chapters 9, 10 and 11.

Diverticulitis

The pathologic changes of this disease are described in Chapter 6.

Diverticula occur most commonly in the sigmoid and lower descending colon. Herniation of the colonic mucosa through the muscle wall shortens and narrows the sigmoid but rarely produces mechanical obstruction. Obstructing intramural or intraperitoneal abscesses arise from diverticular erosion and perforation. In sigmoid diverticulitis symptoms have a gradual onset and the obstruction is usually incomplete. Chills, fever, leukocytosis, and left lower abdominal pain accompanies obstructive signs and symptoms. Often the patient gives a history of previous symptomatic diverticulitis.

On plain film examination the colon contains varying amounts of gas and stool down to the sigmoid. Multiple gas-filled diverticula can occasionally be seen in the descending colon (Fig. 19.6). With perforation, an inflammatory mass may surround the sigmoid and displace adjacent small bowel loops. Entrapment of a small intestinal loop in the inflammatory mass can cause small bowel obstruction. Air

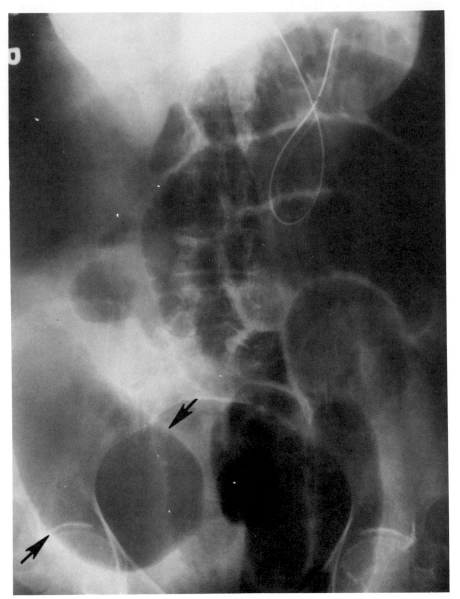

FIG. 19.2. CARCINOMA OF TRANSVERSE COLON CAUSING CECAL AND SMALL
BOWEL DISTENTION

This 88-year-old woman was vomiting and constipated. The cecal gas collection
measures 10 cm in transverse diameter (between arrows). Since the cecum and
ascending colon also contain fluid, the true diameter is larger. On barium enema a
carcinoma obstructed the transverse colon.

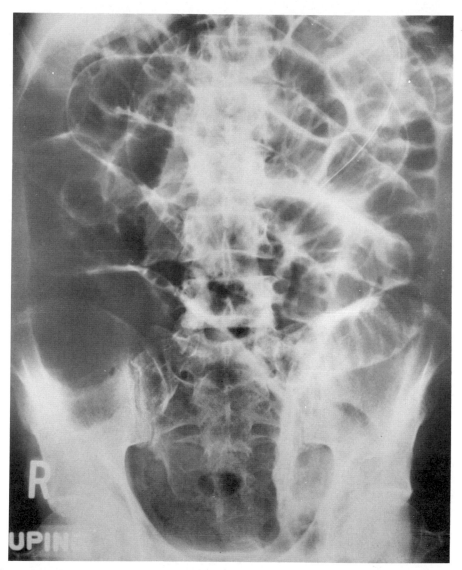

FIG. 19.3. OBSTRUCTING CARCINOMA OF THE DESCENDING COLON LEADING TO
CECAL PERFORATION AND PNEUMOPERITONEUM
This 68-year-old man had had no bowel movements for 5 days. The plain film shows a markedly distended cecum. Free intraperitoneal air outlines the outer wall of the bowel and indicates perforation.

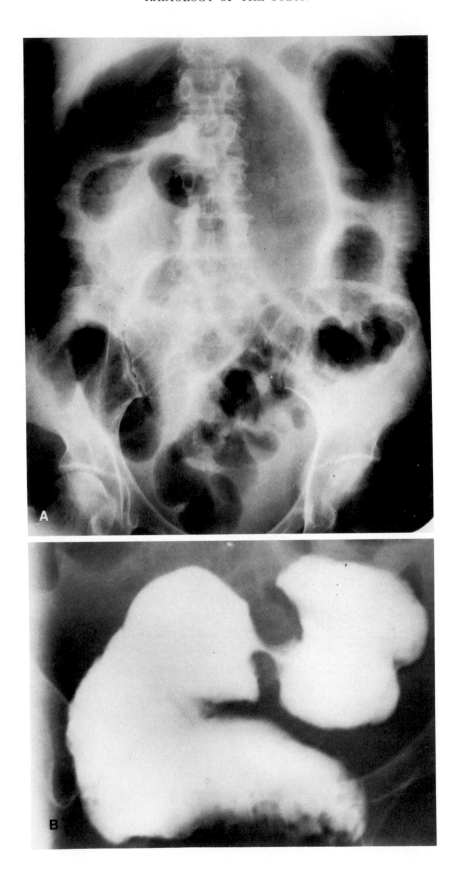

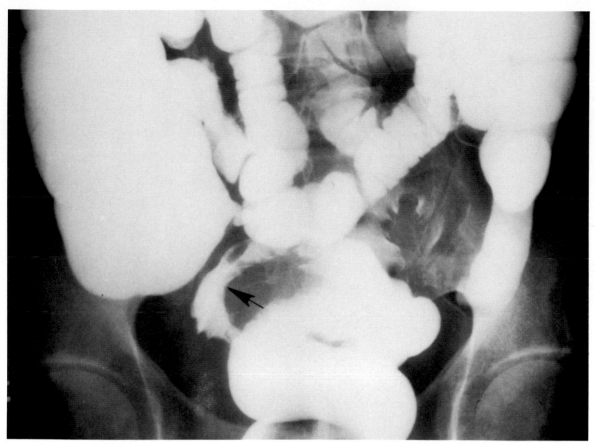

FIG. 19.5. HEMATOGENOUS METASTASIS FROM LUNG CARCINOMA TO SIGMOID.
PARTIAL COLON OBSTRUCTION

One year following pneumonectomy for carcinoma, this 65-year-old man developed abdominal distention, constipation, and rectal bleeding. Barium enema shows a mass (arrow) compressing the sigmoid.

FIG. 19.4. OVARIAN CYSTADENOCARCINOMA—PERITONEAL SEEDING CAUSING
CHRONIC LOW GRADE OBSTRUCTION

This 63-year-old woman had an anaplastic ovarian cystadenocarcinoma with peritoneal seeding. (A) Plain film shows the colon distended down to the rectum. (B) The barium enema shows two lesions: a napkin ring constriction in the distal sigmoid and a complete obstruction proximal to this ring. Despite radiation and chemotherapy, the patient expired and autopsy showed tumor implants invading the sigmoid.

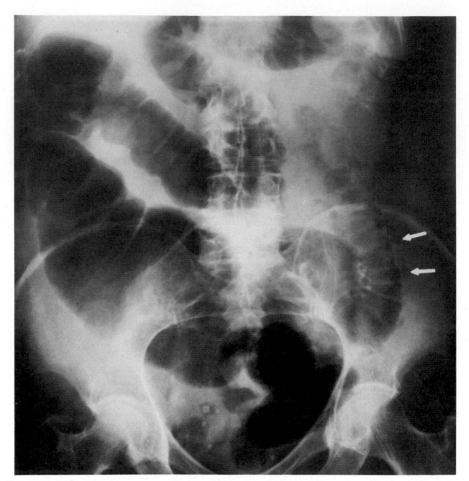

FIG. 19.6. OBSTRUCTION OF LARGE BOWEL DUE TO SIGMOID DIVERTICULITIS
This elderly woman complained of abdominal distention and constipation with
left lower quadrant pain and tenderness. The entire colon is distended and measures
11 cm in diameter. Air-filled diverticula (arrows) line the descending colon. Barium
enema showed diverticulitis, which subsided on medical management.

within the inflammatory mass indicates abscess. Fistula formation between bladder
and sigmoid causes intravesical gas and the attendant symptom of pneumaturia.

A barium enema shows an irregular constriction with tapered margins. Glucagon
(0.5–1 mg intravenously) will minimize bowel spasm and irritability. Barium-filled
diverticula may appear on both sides of the constricted area. The two certain signs
of sigmoid diverticulitis are: (1) intramural or subserosal abscesses constricting the
bowel lumen (Fig. 19.7) and (2) diverticular perforation with extravasation of barium
into an abscess, fistula, or sinus. The radiology of diverticulitis is also discussed in
Chapter 7.

Carcinoma and diverticulitis occur in the same age group and cannot always be
differentiated by barium study. Two percent of patients with colon carcinoma have
concomitant acute diverticulitis. The final diagnosis may rest on surgical extirpation.

Pelvic abscess

Inflammation of the uterus, tubes, and ovaries usually follows gonococcus infection
or less frequently streptococcus, staphylococcus, and tuberculosis. Abscesses develop
within the tubes and the pelvic recess. Less commonly a pelvic abscess follows
perforation of the appendix.

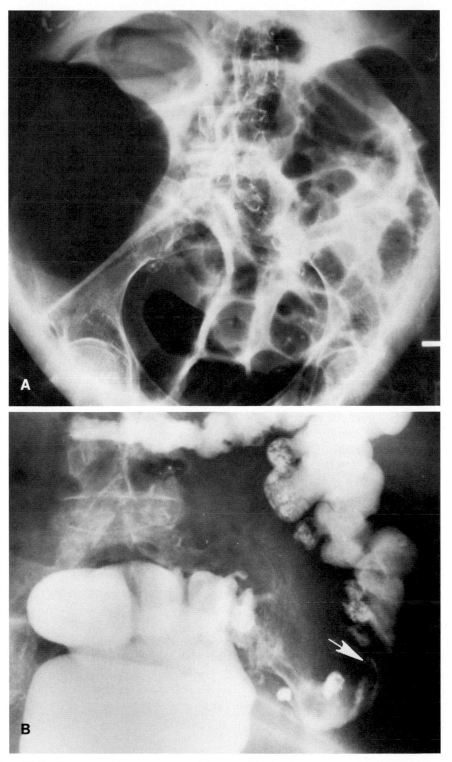

FIG. 19.7. COLONIC OBSTRUCTION DUE TO DIVERTICULITIS AND INTRAMURAL ABSCESS

This 76-year-old woman had a 2-day history of abdominal distention. (**A**) The plain film shows large and small bowel distention with a massively dilated cecum. (**B**) On barium enema, an intramural abscess (arrow) constricts the bowel lumen.

Adnexal tenderness, cervical discharge, and a tender pelvic mass characterize abscess. Dilatation of the small bowel and the colon down to the rectosigmoid with increased intraperitoneal fluid is found on the plain film. Barium study shows an inflammatory mass compressing the bowel, giving the bowel wall a spiculated or serrated margin. The abscess may contain gas (Fig. 19.8) and show a fistulous rectal communication. Ultrasound study can delineate echo-free adnexal abscesses. Obstruction of the colon disappears on antibiotic treatment and/or surgical drainage.

Pancreatitis

In pancreatitis, a rare cause of colon obstruction, blood, pus, and secretions escape from the inflamed pancreas and extend between the transverse mesocolon leaves to involve the transverse and proximal descending colon. In the bowel wall, pancreatic enzymes incite an inflammatory reaction causing constriction, necrosis, and intraluminal hemorrhage (Fig. 19.9).

Volvulus

In order of frequency, volvulus in an adult involves those areas possessing a mobile mesentery: sigmoid, cecum, and transverse colon. Symptoms are usually acute but may be chronic and recurrent. Colon volvulus produces marked distention. The usual elderly patient complains of nausea, vomiting, and abdominal pain. Twisting of the bowel invariably compromises the blood supply and uncorrected, leads to bowel necrosis, colonic pneumatosis and perforation.

Sigmoid volvulus

Postoperative ileus, fecal impaction, or carcinoma may predispose the patient to sigmoid volvulus. From the anterior aspect, the sigmoid colon twists either clockwise or counterclockwise about its mesentery. The twisted sigmoid undergoes massive dilatation, projects into the upper abdomen, and folds upon itself forming a proximal and distal segment. On the upright and decubitus films the two segments show separate fluid levels. As classically demonstrated by Frimann-Dahl, the walls of the dilated, obstructed segments converge on the twisted mesentery (Fig. 19.10) as three separate lines. The adjacent medial walls of the proximal and distal segments form the denser central line and the lateral walls the lateral lines. The colon proximal to the twist dilates while the lower sigmoid and rectum contain little gas and stool.

Barium study will show the exact point of obstruction, the length of the involved segment, and the completeness of the obstruction. At the point of twist the barium column terminates in a characteristic "beak" (Fig. 19.11). Passage of barium beyond the twist indicates incomplete obstruction.

By turning the patient into the prone position during the barium enema, the radiologist can sometimes hydrostatically untwist an incomplete obstruction. If this maneuver is ineffective, passing a well lubricated, rubber rectal tube into the distal segment under fluoroscopic control may reduce the volvulus. Preoperative reduction facilitates the subsequent surgical repair. Signs or symptoms of colon ischemia and/ or perforation contraindicate an attempt at hydrostatic or tube reduction.

Cecal volvulus

Incomplete fixation to the posterior abdominal wall allows the right colon to twist. Some writers consider "right colon volvulus" a more appropriate name.

From the anterior aspect the colon twists in a clockwise manner, obstructing the ascending colon. The dilated cecum lies in the left mid-abdomen or upper quadrant. The walls of the bowel converge on the point of twist in the right mid-abdomen

(Fig. 19.12). Liquid stool and gas distend the cecum and ascending colon. A long single fluid level will be seen on horizontal beam films of the left lateral decubitus patient. Marked small bowel distention accompanies cecal volulus. The ileum follows the cecum through its 180° twist so that the dilated ileum encircles the cecum and the ileo-cecal valve usually lies cephalad.

In the questionable case a barium enema shows the typical beak-like obstruction. Hydrostatic reduction of cecal volvulus has not been reported.

Transverse colon volvulus

The rare transverse colon volvulus occurs in association with an abnormality of mesenteric fixation or a nonrotation, carcinoma, inflammatory stricture, submucosal hematoma, or congenital megacolon.

Gas and stool distend the ascending colon proximal to the volvulus. The dilated transverse colon has a double fluid level.

Barium enema shows the beak-like point of twist and rules out other forms of obstruction.

Intestinal knot (compound volvulus)

Intestinal knot occurs when two separate loops of bowel twist about each other. Usually a loop of jejunum will encircle a previously twisted loop of sigmoid.

The patient experiences a rapid onset of pain and vomiting as compared with the gradual onset of symptoms in single volvulus. On plain film, air and fluid distend the upper small bowel (Fig. 19.13). Barium enema shows sigmoid obstruction.

Intussusception

Eighty-five percent of intussusceptions occur in children between 6 months and 2 years of age. Usually the ileum invaginates into the colon to produce an ileocolic intussusception. Rarer types are ileo-ileal or colo-colic.

Fewer than 10% of intussusceptions result from a mass lesion. More commonly, contraction of the longitudinal muscle buckles and invaginates a preexisting inflamed bowel segment. Peristalsis carries this segment, the intussusceptum, forward into the distal small bowel or the ascending colon, the intussuscipiens. Subsequent peristaltic waves, increasing in tone as the gut attempts to overcome the obstruction, further telescopes the bowel and can propel the intussusceptum into the descending colon.

Plain film

The dilated small bowel has a nipple or beak-like termination at the intussusception site. No gas appears in the right side of the abdomen since only invaginated bowel fills the ascending colon. The intussuscepted mass produces a concave defect in the air column of the transverse colon.

Barium enema and hydrostatic reduction

A smooth defect encountered by the head of the barium column marks the leading edge of the intussuscepted bowel. Barium seeps around the intussusceptum and outlines the telescoped mucosal folds of the intussuscipiens, giving the mucosa a "coiled spring" pattern (Fig. 19.14).

The hydrostatic method reduces the intussusception in 80–90% of patients. Clinical or radiographic signs of perforation absolutely contraindicate hydrostatic reduction.

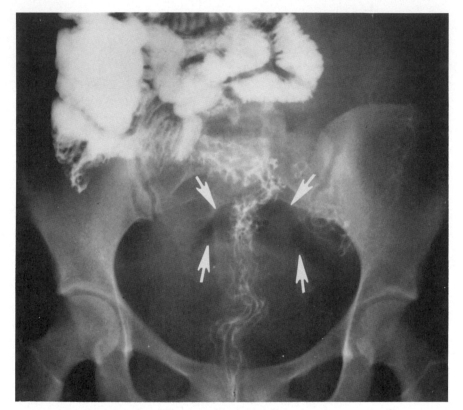

FIG. 19.8. GAS-CONTAINING PELVIC ABSCESS COMPRESSING AND CONSTRICTING
THE RECTOSIGMOID

This 24-year-old woman had a purulent vaginal discharge, fever, and pelvic pain.
A palpable pelvic mass shows a semilunar collection of gas (arrows) on the postevacuation film. On barium enema the mass compressed the rectosigmoid colon and
displaced it cephalad and posteriorly.

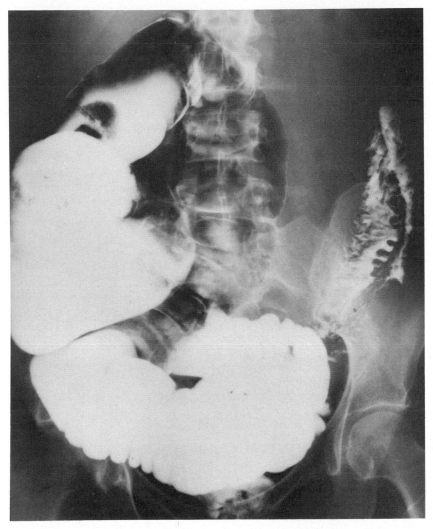

FIG. 19.9. PANCREATITIS EXTENDING INTO AND OBSTRUCTING THE TRANSVERSE
AND DESCENDING COLON

This 41-year old known alcoholic had cramping abdominal pain, nausea, and
vomiting. The barium enema shows constriction of the transverse and descending
colon and dilatation of the cecum and proximal colon. Mucosal swelling in the
constricted area gives the colon wall a spiculated appearance.

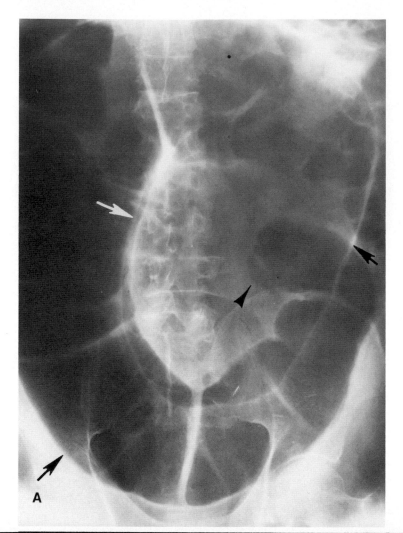

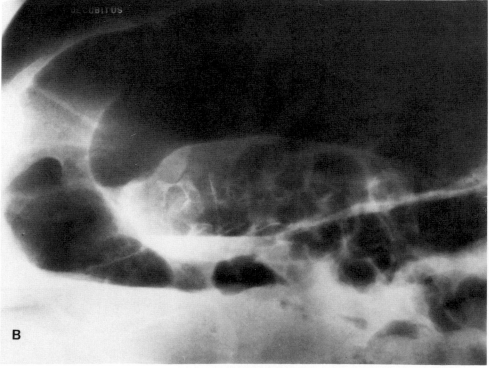

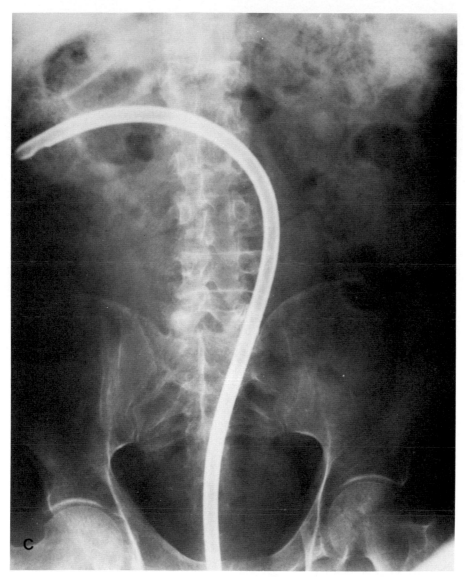

Fig. 19.10 (C)

Fig. 19.10. Sigmoid Volvulus—Convergence of Bowel Walls on Sigmoid Mesentery—Double Fluid Level on Decubitus Film. Long Tube Reduction

This 72-year-old man with severe hypothyroidism (a known cause of large bowel atony and dilatation) had abdominal pain and distention. (**A**) The supine film shows marked sigmoid dilatation. The walls of the dilated sigmoid converge on the twist in the sigmoid mesentery. Overlapping central walls (white arrow). Single lateral walls (black arrows). Tapered end of twisted colon (black arrow head). (**B**) Left lateral decubitus projection with horizontal beam. Separate fluid levels occur in the two segments of the sigmoid volvulus. (**C**) Supine radiograph of the abdomen after proctoscopic insertion of a long rubber rectal tube shows the deflated sigmoid.

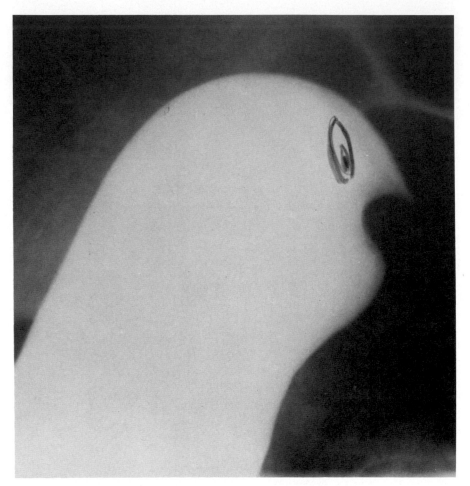

FIG. 19.11. BEAK SIGN IN SIGMOID VOLVULUS

This 77-year-old man had not had a bowel movement for 3 days. Plain film suggested sigmoid volvulus. On barium enema the point of obstruction resembles a bird's beak.

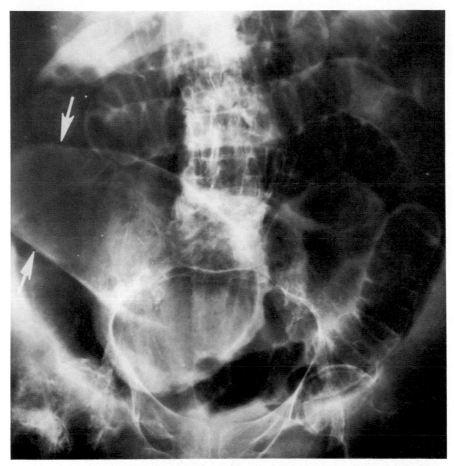

FIG. 19.12. RIGHT COLON (CECAL) VOLVULUS POSTPERFORATION

This 96-year-old woman had a 3-day history of vomiting, abdominal distention, and fever. On the plain film a distended cecum tapers to the right mid-abdomen (arrows). Dilated small bowel and terminal ileum are twisted around the distended cecum. Intraperitoneal air outlining the exterior bowel wall indicates antecedent perforation. The colon distal to the volvulus is empty.

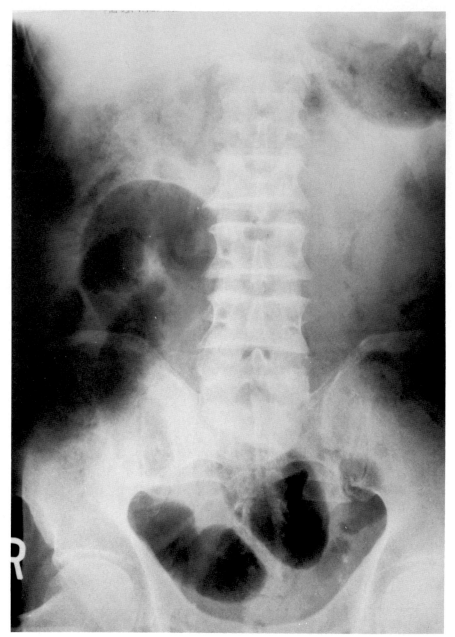

FIG. 19.13. COMPOUND VOLVULUS OR INTESTINAL KNOT

Following an episode of vomiting, this 76-year-old man developed cramping abdominal pain. The supine film shows a dilated small bowel loop in the right mid-abdomen and a mass on the left. The dilated small bowel has a figure-eight configuration, separate fluid levels, and did not change in position on upright and decubitus films. The surgeon found a primary sigmoid volvulus about which the small bowel had twisted.

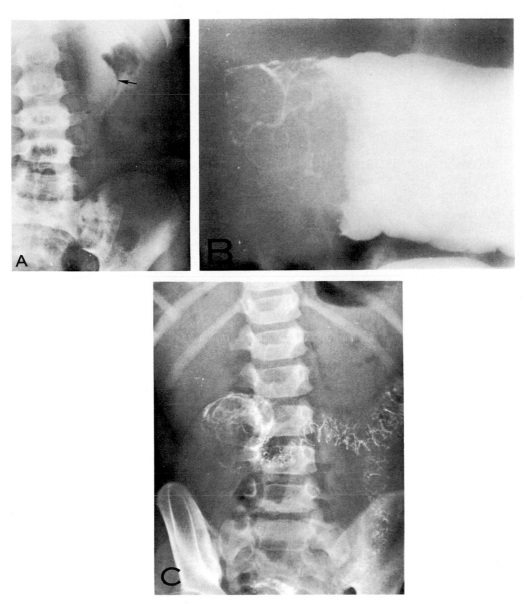

FIG. 19.14. INTUSSUSCEPTION
(A) Plain film of the abdomen demonstrating the head of the intussusception
(arrow), outlined by gas in the splenic flexure. (B) Obstruction of the barium column
in the transverse colon with beginning definition of the opposing mucosal surfaces
of the intussusceptum and the intussuscipiens. (C) Postevacuation film with further
definition of the intussusceptum.

Hematochezia or dehydration are not contraindications. Symptoms of over 24 hr duration make reduction less likely.

Certain precautions reduce the incidence of complications and enhance the chances of success.

(a) The surgeon should agree with the plan to attempt hydrostatic reduction.

(b) As a rule the barium container need not be raised more than 1 m above the table top. Successful reduction requires patience rather than a large head of pressure.

The intramuscular or intravenous administration of 0.5 mg of glucagon relaxes smooth muscles and aids hydrostatic reduction.

(c) An inflated balloon can damage the child's rectum and is best avoided. Insertion of a large rubber catheter and taping the buttocks together produces a tight seal.

(d) A normal saline barium suspension minimizes the possibility of water intoxication in the dehydrated child.

(e) Only with barium reflux well into the ileum can the radiologist be certain he has reduced the intussusception.

(f) Evidence of recurrence on the postevacuation film calls for a repeat hydrostatic reduction. Recurrent intussusception after 2 hydrostatic reductions usually requires surgical repair.

(g) The child should remain under medical observation for 24 hr following reduction as 4–6% experience recurrence. By comparison 3–4% recur following surgical reduction.

In less than 10% of intussusceptions a local lesion such as Meckel's diverticulum, lymphoid hyperplasia, lymphoma, polyp, or cecal duplication causes bowel invagination. Rarely intussusception complicates Henoch-Schoenlein purpura or spontaneous hemophilic intestinal hemorrhage. Beyond 2 years of age the incidence of local lesions increases. For the child over 6 years, primary surgical reduction should be considered because lymphosarcoma or other tumors usually initiate intussusception.

Following other abdominal surgery, children may develop ileo-ileal intussusception. A small bowel obstruction in the postoperative child suggests this possibility.

In the adult, benign and malignant tumors, especially polypoid lesions, occasionally cause colo-colic intussusception.

Hernia

Normally only the sigmoid and transverse colon possess sufficient mobility to herniate.

External hernia

External hernias commonly develop in the inguinal, femoral, umbilical, and obturator canals or in old surgical incisions (Fig. 19.15). They comprise 95% of intestinal obstructions due to hernias. Most patients report an existing hernia, a sudden increase in hernia size, or an inability to reduce a known hernia. A painful, tender, and tense swelling in one of the susceptible areas suggests incarceration.

In suspected inguinal hernia, the film is positioned to include the scrotal areas. Air-containing bowel within the scrotum indicates herniation and a barium enema shows the extent of entrapment (Fig. 19.16).

On the supine abdominal film, incisional hernias appear as oval densities containing a cluster of gas-filled bowel loops. On the lateral film, the bowel projects outside the anterior abdominal wall (Fig. 19.17). Rarely the descending colon will herniate through the lumbar muscles at Petit's triangle.

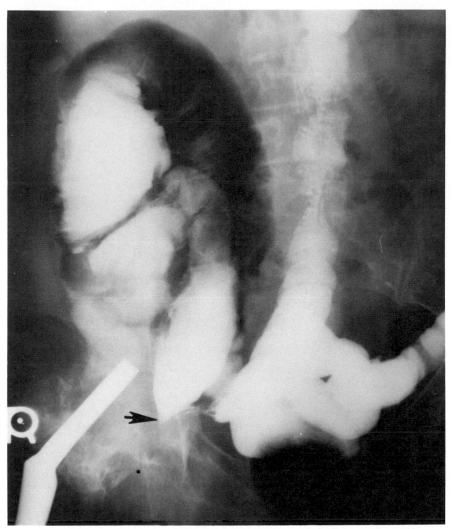

FIG. 19.15. RIGHT FEMORAL HERNIA—RICHTER TYPE

This 72-year-old man had right lower quadrant distention and diffuse abdominal pain. Supine plain film showed marked right colon and mild small bowel distention. Barium enema shows right colon obstruction by entrapment of a knuckle of the transverse colon in a right femoral hernia (arrow).

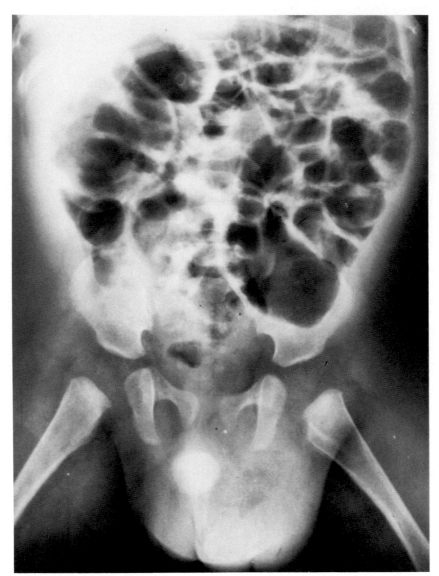

FIG. 19.16. INGUINAL HERNIA

This 6-month-old child had a left inguinal hernia which previously had been reducible. He had a 5-day history of no bowel movements and an increase in hernia size. The hernia was hard and not reducible. On plain film the enlarged left scrotum contains a loop of air and stool-filled bowel.

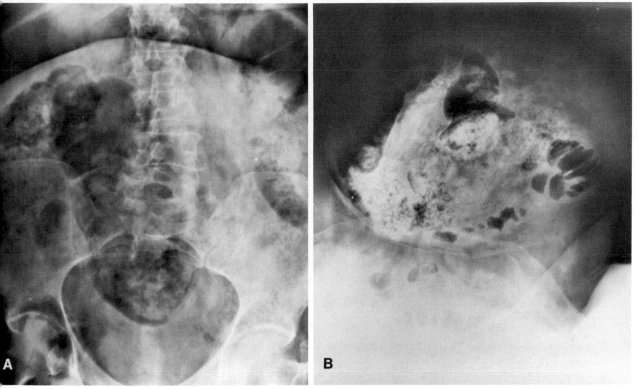

FIG. 19.17. VENTRAL HERNIA CONTAINING LARGE AND SMALL BOWEL
For many years this 73-year-old woman was known to have a large ventral hernia.
She was admitted with abdominal pain, tenderness over the hernia, and vomiting.
The anteroposterior (**A**) and cross-table lateral (**B**) films show both large and small
bowel entrapped within the ventral hernia.

Internal hernia

Internal hernias constitute only about 5% of intestinal obstructions due to hernia.
The herniated colon appears to be enclosed in a bag with a narrow neck. Occasionally
internal hernias reduce spontaneously during barium examination.

In order of descending frequency internal hernias include the following: (1)
diaphragmatic; (2) foramen of Winslow; (3) paraduodenal fossa; (4) persistent
mesenteric defect; (5) intersigmoid fossa; and (6) pericecal. Bowel twisting or
entrapment compromises the blood supply and leads to necrosis and perforation.

Diaphragmatic hernia

Diaphragmetic hernias comprise the most common type of internal hernia. The
transverse colon may herniate through the esophageal, the pleuroperitonealis (Bochdalek), and the anterior vascular (Morgagni) foramina, or through a traumatic rent
in the diaphragm. Bochdalek hernias result from protrusion of an incompletely
rotated gut through a posterolateral diaphragmatic defect. Therefore, they appear
more frequently in the newborn period and contain both large and small bowel.

On the chest film the herniated transverse colon often with the omentum projects
above the diaphragm. Barium enema shows an entrapped loop of large bowel (Figs.
19.18 and 19.19).

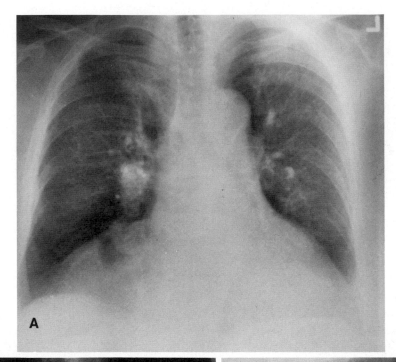

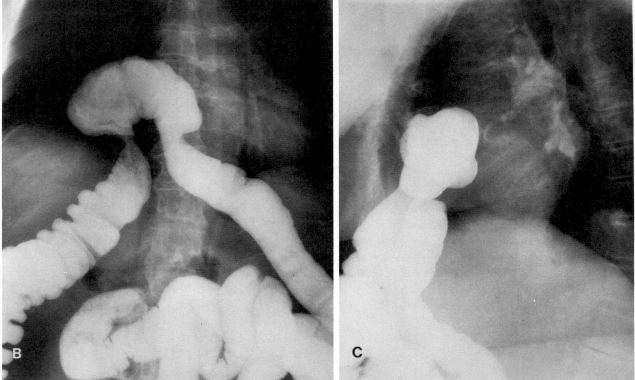

FIG. 19.18. FORAMEN OF MORGAGNI HERNIA

This 82-year-old woman had chronic constipation. (A) The chest film shows a soft tissue, gas-containing mass in the right cardiophrenic angle. (B) On the barium enema anteroposterior film a loop of transverse colon extends into the mediastinum. The hernia orifice constricts the colon. (C) Lateral film of the barium enema shows that the colon has protruded through the anterior vascular foramen. Because of the presence of the heart on the left, Morgagni hernias usually project into the right thorax.

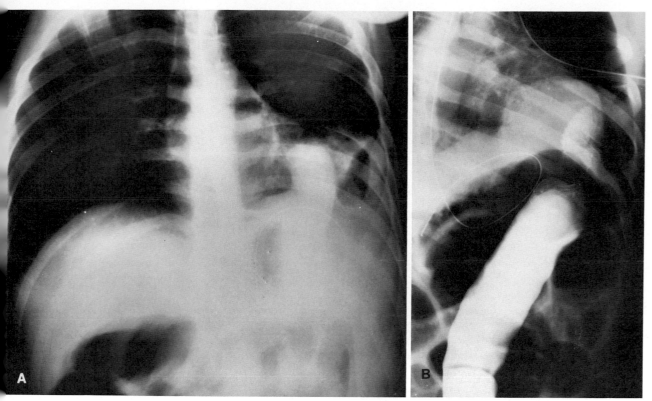

FIG. 19.19. FORAMEN OF BOCHDALEK HERNIA (PLEUROPERITONEALIS)
This 22-year-old man had left lower chest pain, vomiting, and abdominal distention. (**A**) On chest film an air-containing density is present in the posterolateral
aspect of the left lower thorax. (**B**) Barium enema—a segment of left transverse
colon constitutes the left supradiaphragmatic mass. The colon is acutely narrowed
at the hernia orifice.

Epiploic foramen hernia (Winslow)

In order of descending frequency the organs which will herniate through the
foramen of Winslow are (a) the small bowel (approximately 68%); (b) the cecum and
terminal ileum; (c) the transverse colon; (d) the omentum and (e) the gallbaldder.

Plain film signs of cecal herniation are: (a) a collection of gas and/or fluid in the
lesser sac; (b) anterior and medial displacement of the stomach; (c) absence of the
cecum from its original position; and (d) leftward displacement of the 2nd and 3rd
portion of the duodenum (Fig. 19.20).

Other types of internal hernias rarely, if ever, incarcerate the large bowel.

Obturation

Foreign body

In children, the mentally retarded, and individuals with unusual sexual proclivi-
ties, bizarre foreign objects occasionally appear in the rectum (Fig. 19.21).

Fecal impaction

Elderly, cachetic, bed-ridden patients, and the mentally retarded are susceptible
to fecal impaction. Paradoxically the patient may complain or the nursing home

attendant may report small episodes of diarrhea, as the colon attempts to pass stool around the obstruction.

On plain film examination the large mottled mass of stool fills the rectosigmoid or other colon segments and causes distention of the proximal large bowel and the small intestine (Fig. 19.22).

Gallstone

A gallstone extruded from a chronically inflamed and eroded gallbladder may enter the intestinal tract and lodge in the small bowel, but on rare occasions may obstruct the colon, usually the sigmoid.

Functional Large Bowel Obstruction

Functional colonic obstruction due to impaired contractility has many causes including: anticholinergic medication, aganglionosis, toxic megacolon, bowel ischemia, central nervous system defects, sprue, myotonic dystrophy, peritonitis, hypokalemia, psychogenic, diabetes, Chagas' disease, cathartic habituation, uremia, urticaria, hypothyroidism, porphyria, lead poisoning, amyloidosis, congestive heart failure, and idiopathic.

Diffuse dilatation of the large bowel with stasis of stool and gas characterizes functional obstruction. Usually the small bowel is also dilated. Impairment of neuromuscular integrity causes most functional large bowel obstructions. In comparison to mechanical obstruction, the patient with "adynamic ileus" does not have cramping, colicky abdominal pain. Barium enema excludes mechanical obstruction. In rare instances functional obstruction can cause cecal perforation. Aganglionosis (Hirschsprung), end-stage bowel ischemia, Chagas' disease, toxic megacolon, and cathartic colon have been discussed in other sections.

Psychotrophic and Anticonvulsant Medication and Autonomic Nervous System Blocking Agents

Drugs such as chlorpromazine, amytriptyline, nortriptyline, diazepam, benztropine, thioridazine, imipramine, and hexamethonium bromide exert a parasympatholytic effect and produce a clinical and radiologic picture of large bowel obstruction. A history of taking this medication and a negative barium enema rule out mechanical obstruction.

Peritonitis

Peritoneal irritation reflexly inhibits both large and small bowel motor activity producing "adynamic ileus." Empyema of the gallbladder can produce localized dilatation of adjacent colon (Fig. 19.23).

FIG. 19.20. CECAL HERNIATION INTO THE LESSER OMENTAL BURSA THROUGH THE FORAMEN OF WINSLOW

This 84-year-old woman had abdominal pain and vomiting. The preliminary abdominal film showed a large oval air collection in the upper abdomen. (**A**) On upper gastrointestinal series, the air collection appears below and behind the stomach. It displaces the stomach medially, anteriorly and cephalad and the duodenum to the right. The gallbladder contains a large laminated calculus. (**B**) Barium enema shows a normal colon up to the hepatic flexure. A funnel-shaped narrowing indicates where the colon passes through the foramen of Winslow.

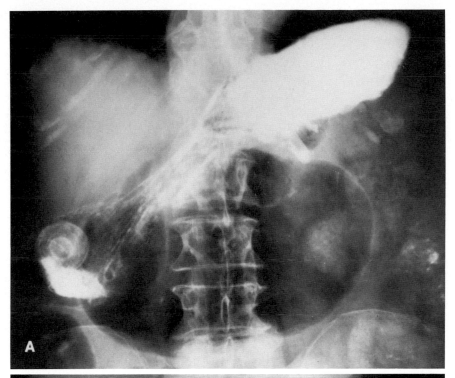

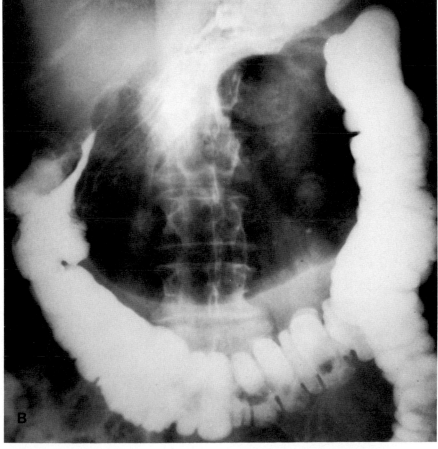

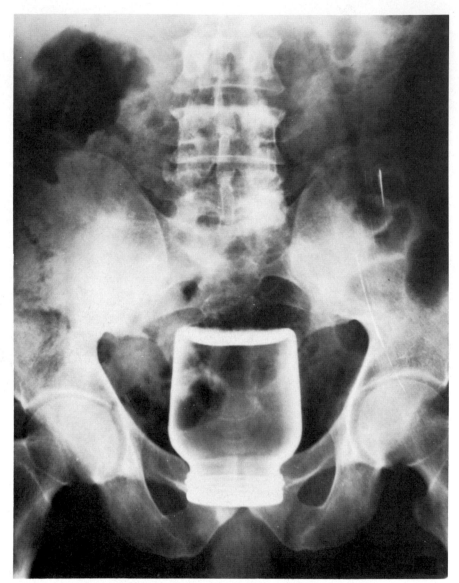

FIG. 19.21. RECTAL FOREIGN BODY OBTURATION

The patient complained of inability to have a bowel movement, rectal pain, and bleeding. The physician removed this intrarectal mustard jar intact by Piper forceps. The patient declined to say how the jar entered the rectum.

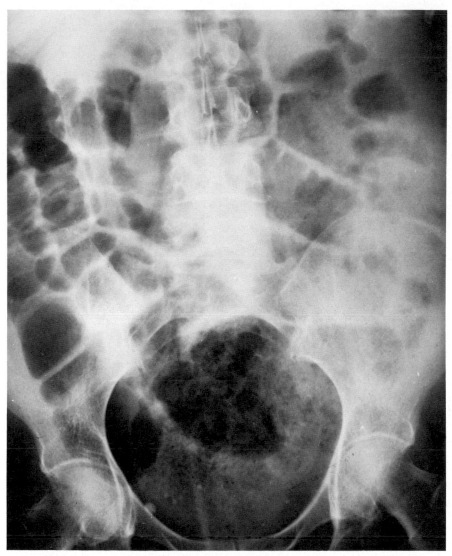

FIG. 19.22. LARGE BOWEL OBTURATION BY FECAL IMPACTION

Due to chronic schizophrenia, this 65-year-old woman had been a longtime resident of a state mental hospital. When seen she was having repeated episodes of nausea and vomiting. A massive amount of stool fills the rectosigmoid. The entire colon and multiple small bowel loops are dilated.

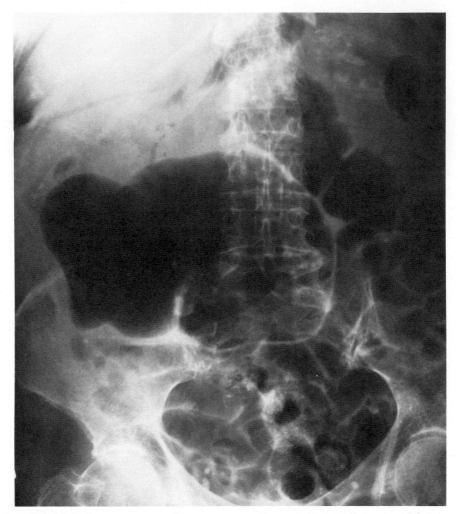

FIG. 19.23. A GANGRENOUS, PERFORATED GALLBLADDER CAUSING MARKED
DILATATION OF THE ASCENDING COLON

This 94-year-old woman had right upper quadrant pain and tenderness. The plain
film shows diffuse small bowel distention and a massively dilated ascending colon.

Central Nervous System

Abnormalities of the central nervous system such as tumors of the spinal cord
and cauda equina, paraplegia, quadriplegia, and spina bifida interrupt autonomic
nervous system control of the colon and produce a dilated and atonic bowel.

Psychogenic Constipation of Childhood

Distention of the colon by large quantities of feces develops in the child who
neglects or ignores the call to stool (Fig. 19.24). Digital exam shows a relaxed rectal
ampulla. On laxative stimulation the child will have a massive evacuation. The
child's ability to completely evacuate the barium enema usually excludes aganglionosis (Fig. 19.25).

Hypokalemia

Potassium depletion increases blood glucose, lowers neural conduction time, and
produces generalized muscle weakness. Colon dilatation will improve with correction
of the abnormal electrolytes.

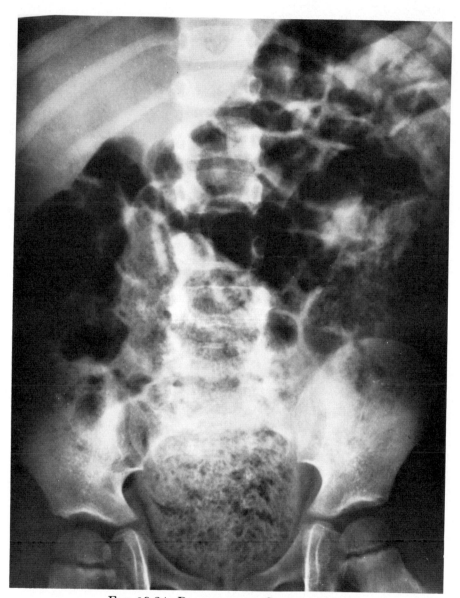

FIG. 19.24. PSYCHOGENIC CONSTIPATION

The mother of this 3½-year-old boy reported that he had bowel movements at 3–4 day intervals. Laxatives produced a massive bowel evacuation. The plain film of the abdomen shows stool distending the rectum, sigmoid, and descending colon. The problem responded to counseling by the pediatrician.

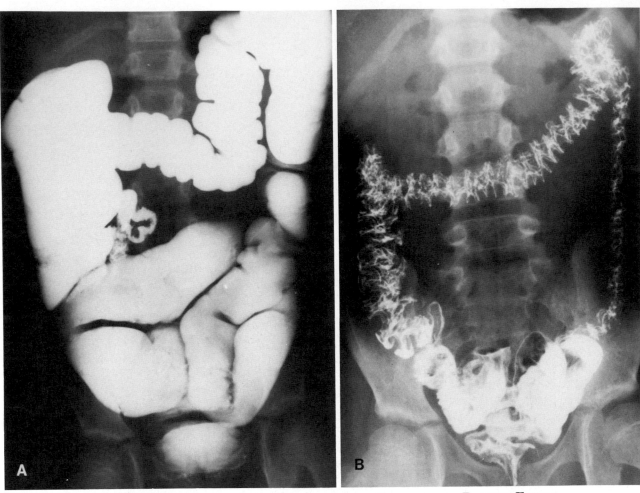

FIG. 19.25. PSYCHOGENIC CONSTIPATION—RESPONSE TO BARIUM ENEMA
This 11-year-old boy had been constipated for many years. When bowel movements occurred, they were very large. He had a history of emotional problems. (**A**) Filled film of barium enema shows a distended and redundant colon. (**B**) On evacuation the colon completely empties indicating an intact neuromuscular mechanism.

Urticaria

An allergic reaction of the colon mucosa to medication can cause large raised mucosal plaques in a grossly dilated bowel (Fig. 19.26). The changes in the colon regress on removal of the inciting medication.

Hypothyroidism

In patients with severely depleted thyroid hormones the intestine becomes atonic. This leads to abdominal distention and constipation. The atonic bowel dilates and appears obstructed, and this dilated atonic bowel may undergo volvulus. Bowel tone returns to normal following thyroxine replacement.

Myotonic Dystrophy Megacolon

Most authors postulate that smooth muscle atrophy causes functional obstruction.

The possibility of persistent local spasm causing obstruction has been suggested. The patients have known skeletal muscular disease, often familial. Abdominal distention compromises respiratory function.

Diabetic Megacolon

Extensive small vessel disease appears responsible for the neurovascular insufficiency in diabetes. Bowel distention improves with good medical control.

Idiopathic Intestinal Pseudo-Obstruction

In a small group of patients the physiologic response to intestinal distention is impaired and the colon does not evacuate its contents (Fig. 19.27). The disease has no detectable organic cause.

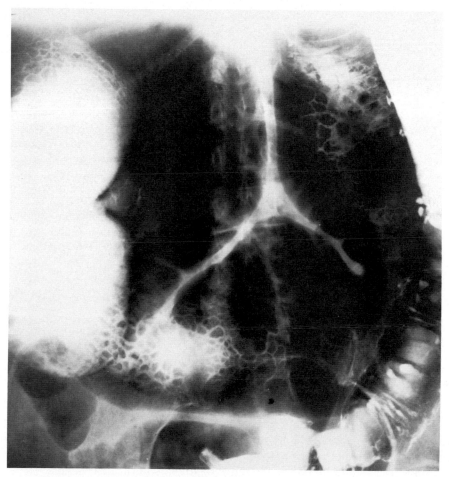

FIG. 19.26. FUNCTIONAL MEGACOLON WITH URTICARIA

This 67-year-old woman experienced diffuse abdominal pain with cramping and diarrhea. On the preliminary film the entire colon was distended. Barium enema demonstrates dilated bowel, no mechanical obstruction, and multiple mucosal bullae. Direct colon visualization showed marked mucosal reddening and edema, moderate serous exudations, and bullous lesions. The cause of the patient's urticaria was never determined and she recovered spontaneously.

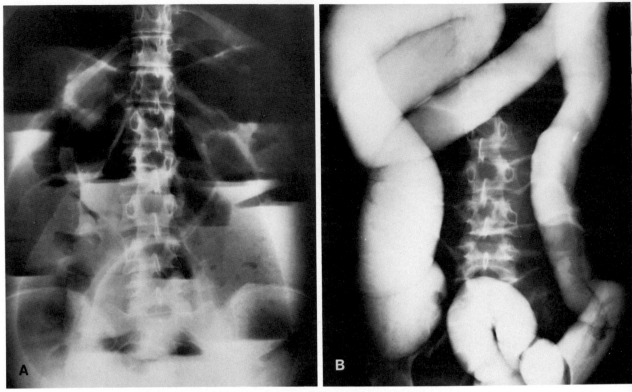

FIG. 19.27. CHRONIC IDIOPATHIC INTESTINAL PSEUDO-OBSTRUCTION
This malnourished 22-year-old woman with abdominal pain and weight loss had
had 5 negative surgical abdominal explorations for mechanical bowel obstruction.
Studies on the pharmacologic response of the bowel were within normal limits. No
drugs were detected in the patient's blood. Colon biopsy showed a normal complement of ganglion cells. (**A**) Upright abdominal film showing marked small and large
bowel distention with multiple fluid levels. (**B**) Subsequent barium enema shows no
obstructing lesion. (Reprinted with permission from Moss, A., Goldberg, H., and
Bratmen, M.: Idiopathic intestinal pseudo-obstruction. Am. J. Roentgenol. *65:* 312,
© 1972, American Roentgen Ray Society.)

TRAUMA

Examining the Traumatized Patient

In the emergency room, the physician (1) establishes an adequate airway; (2)
supports the circulation; (3) controls open bleeding, and (4) administers blood and
electrolytes as needed. Radiographic study is deferred until these measures have
succeeded and shock has been corrected.

Although three views of the abdomen are desirable, the nature and extent of the
associated injuries may restrict the study to a portable supine anteroposterior film.
All radiographs should be obtained before diagnostic peritoneal lavage.

In acute abdominal injuries a preliminary chest film serves: (1) to rule out
concomitant chest and diaphragmatic injury; (2) to document existing cardiac or
pulmonary disease; and (3) to provide a baseline if the patient subsequently develops
respiratory difficulty.

In all patients with hematuria or penetrating injuries, an infusion urogram with
tomography assures the integrity of retroperitoneal structures.

Blunt Abdominal Trauma

Blood found on digital rectal examination, hematochezia or blood on the under-clothing points to a possible colon injury. Blunt abdominal trauma produces a spectrum of colon injuries.

Intramural Hematoma

Bleeding in the submucosa or muscles induces a localized hematoma which appears as a smooth intramural filling defect on barium enema. Intramural hematomas rarely obstruct and most regress spontaneously.

Vascular Injury

Laceration of the mesenteric vessels produces hemoperitoneum shown by blood in the flank and pelvis (Fig. 19.28). Occlusion of the vessels may devitalize a segment of bowel. In the absence of collateral blood supply, the bowel wall undergoes necrosis. Intestinal gas may dissect into the bowel wall causing pneumatosis or actual perforation with resulting peritonitis. When there is an adequate collateral blood supply, the avascular segment of bowel undergoes healing. The resultant scar tissue may progressively stenose and obstruct the bowel.

Intraperitoneal Laceration

Peritoneum partially covers the vertical segments of the colon and completely covers the transverse and sigmoid colon. Blunt trauma may cause a shearing effect which lacerates the bowel wall allowing colon contents to spill into the peritoneal cavity. The patient has immediate signs and symptoms of peritonitis with the radiographic findings of free air, free fluid, and ileus.

Retroperitoneal Laceration

Colon contents can spill into the anterior pararenal space with laceration of a vertical colon segment (Fig. 19.29). The patient becomes febrile and experiences pain in the involved flank.

The supine abdominal film may show a collection of gas bubbles lateral and medial to the bowel and on a lateral abdominal film these appear behind the colon. Extravasation of intestinal gas and/or the action by gas-forming bacilli accounts for retroperitoneal gas (Fig. 19.30). The retroperitoneal gas bubbles do not change position on upright and lateral decubitus films.

Penetrating Abdominal Trauma

In civilian life assault by knives and hand guns can cause colon laceration. These weapons produce different types of injuries and require different handling. Impalement injuries can damage the perineum and rectum.

Stab Wounds

The patient with clinical signs of peritoneal irritation, progressive blood loss or hypovolemic shock, and with radiographic evidence of free air or fluid (Fig. 19.31) needs immediate surgery.

For the patient without the above findings, surgical care has gradually evolved. In the years following World War II, surgeons immediately explored most stab wounds. Lacerations requiring surgical repair were found in only one-half of these patients. In the patients without visceral injury, celiotomy prolonged hospitalization and carried a morbidity of 10–20%.

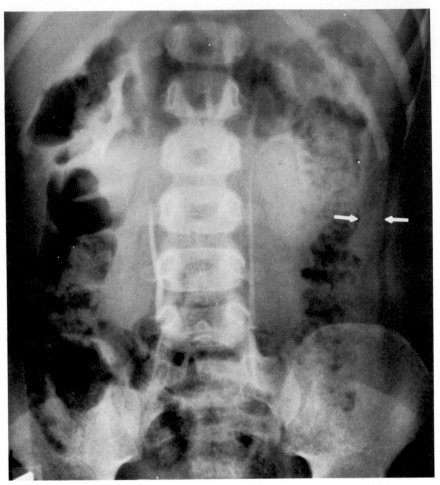

FIG. 19.28. AVULSION OF THE DESCENDING COLON FROM THE POSTERIOR
PERITONEUM. ACCUMULATION OF BLOOD IN THE LEFT LATERAL GUTTER
This 3-year-old child sustained multiple abrasions in an automobile accident and
complained of abdominal pain. The urogram shows normal kidneys. A soft tissue
density is noted between the descending colon and the lateral properitoneal fat line
(arrows).

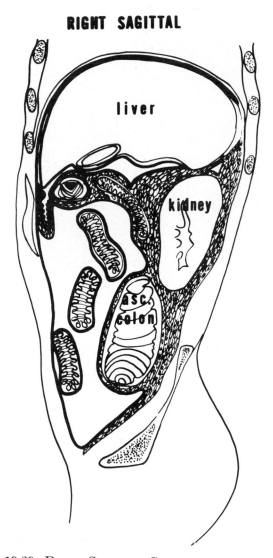

RIGHT SAGITTAL

FIG. 19.29. RIGHT SAGITTAL SECTION OF ABDOMEN

Peritoneum (heavy black line) partially covers the ascending colon. Laceration of the anterior colon wall allows colon contents to enter the peritoneal cavity—within the heavy black line. Laceration of the posterior colon wall contaminates the anterior pararenal space—lying between the posterior peritoneum and anterior layer of renal (Gerota's) fascia.

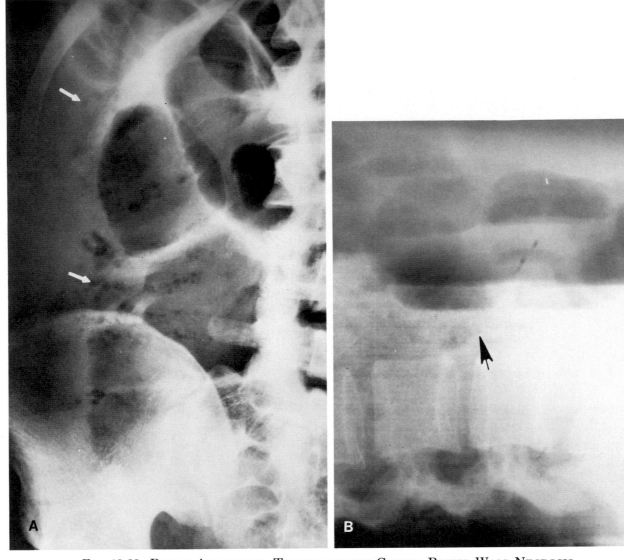

FIG. 19.30. BLUNT ABDOMINAL TRAUMA TO THE CECUM, BOWEL WALL NECROSIS
WITH INTRA- AND RETROPERITONEAL PERFORATION, ABSCESS WITHIN THE
ANTERIOR PARARENAL SPACE

In a motorcycle accident this 24-year-old man sustained multiple skeletal injuries
including traumatic amputation of the left leg. On the fourth hospital day the
patient became febrile and complained of right flank pain. (**A**) On the plain
abdominal film multiple small bubbles of gas in the anterior pararenal space (arrows)
extend cephalad between the posterior liver margin and right kidney. (**B**) The lateral
abdominal film with horizontal beam shows the bubbles of gas to lie behind the
ascending colon (arrow).

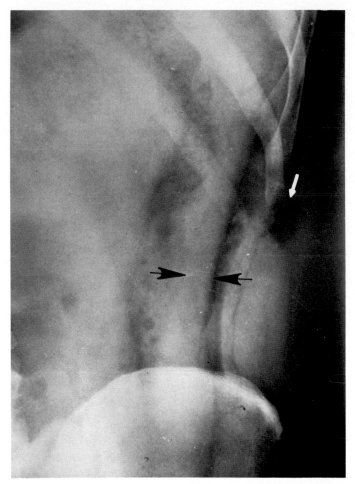

FIG. 19.31. LEFT ABDOMINAL STAB WOUND LACERATING THE DESCENDING
COLON MESENTERY, WITH BLOOD IN THE LEFT LATERAL GUTTER

This young man had a 2 cm long stab wound in the left upper abdomen. Air in the
intramuscular tissues outlines the knife track (white arrow). Blood was present in
the left lateral gutter (between black arrows) and was also found in the pelvic
recesses.

More recently the stab wound patient with absent clinical and radiographic signs
of visceral injury has been kept under close medical observation for 48 hr. If
peritoneal irritation develops, the patient has an immediate celiotomy, and the
visceral injuries are repaired. Conservative observation has not increased the mortality or morbidity and spares many patients needless exploration.

Bullet Wounds

Bullet wound damage varies with muzzle velocity. At higher velocity, bullets
induce shock waves that injure contiguous tissues. In civilian life low velocity hand
guns cause the majority of wounds.

Patients with abdominal gunshot wounds require exploratory celiotomy. Two
films of the abdomen at right angles, anteroposterior and lateral, with radiopaque
markers placed at the sites of entrance and exit will suggest the path of the bullet
and the structures likely to have been injured. With a retained bullet, the entrance
site alone is marked.

Perforating gunshot wounds of the colon contaminate both the intra- and retro-peritoneal tissues. Air and/or blood in the retro- or intraperitoneal space is a certain sign of gut perforation (Fig. 19.32 and 19.33) as is fecal drainage from the wound.

Impalement

Impalement injuries of the perineum and rectum contaminate the perirectal retroperitoneal tissues. The plain film may show streaks of air in the pelvic soft tissues. An enema should not be done. The extent of damage can be evaluated by proctoscopy.

Radiation Injury

High voltage radiation therapy units have enabled the radiation therapist to deliver cancerocidal doses to intra-abdominal tumors without skin damage. Increased tumor doses have prolonged survival and raised the cure rate.

Radiation injury appears when the dose exceeds 4,500 rads and occurs in 1–2% of patients. The rate increases markedly if the dose exceeds 6,000 rads or if a second course of radiation is given for recurrent tumor. The pelvic structures are radiated for malignant lesions of the cervix, endometrium, ovaries, bladder, and prostate. The majority of radiation injuries occur in women following cervical carcinoma radiation, and involve the sigmoid and rectum. Patients with diabetes, arteriosclerosis, and hypertension whose vessels are already compromised are more susceptable to radiation bowel injury.

Early Radiation Effects

Procto-colitis

Procto-colitis occurs in most patients receiving treatment and the symptoms vary in severity. The lining mucosa of the bowel becomes swollen, edematous, and superficially ulcerated. This acute mucosal injury appears toward the end of the treatment series. The patient complains of painful bowel movement with oozing of blood and mucus. The patients are not usually examined by barium enema. No relationship exists between the presence of proctitis and the development of late sequellae.

Late Radiation Effects

Ulceration and stricture formation

Within 6–24 months following radiation, obliterative arteritis develops in the bowel wall and causes chronic ischemia with mucosal atrophy, indolent ulceration, and fibrous tissue replacement. Gradual scarring shortens and contracts the bowel lumen. A long smooth stricture is usual (Fig. 19.34). A short irregular stricture may mimic primary or metastatic malignant disease, and surgical resection may be necessary to make a definitive diagnosis. Cancer can develop *de novo* after many years in the previously radiated bowel. The stenosed bowel impairs mobility causing recurrent abdominal pain and cramps with bloody diarrhea. On plain film the proximal colon is dilated and on barium enema the involved segment is contracted, ulcerated, and pipe-like. Because the stenosis and chronic ischemic changes are irreversible, cure usually requires a diverting colostomy followed by resection.

Recto-vaginal fistula

Recto-vaginal fistula develops when radiation destroys tumor invading the recto-vaginal septum.

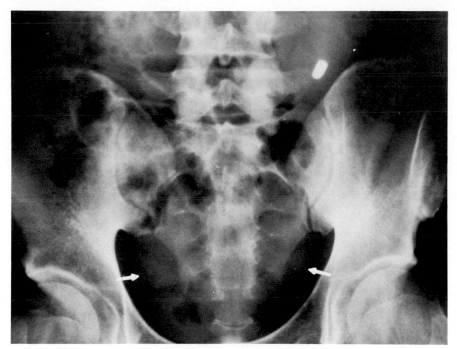

FIG. 19.32. BULLET WOUND PERFORATING SIGMOID AND TRANSVERSE COLON MANIFEST BY INTRAPERITONEAL HEMORRHAGE

This 25-year-old man allegedly shot himself in the abdomen. Blood filled the pelvic recesses (white arrows) and the lateral pericolic gutters.

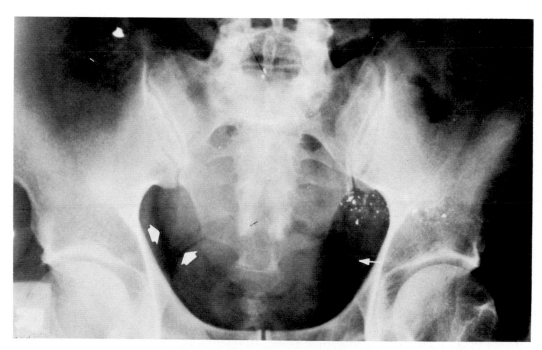

FIG. 19.33. GUNSHOT WOUND PERFORATING THE COLON AND SMALL BOWEL WITH INTRA- AND RETROPERITONEAL HEMORRHAGE

An assailant shot this 44-year-old man in the left side of the pelvis. Multiple small metallic fragments outline the bullet track in the soft tissues. A retroperitoneal hemorrhage in the left side of the pelvis obscures the outline of the obturator internus muscle, displaces the properitoneal fat medially, and compresses the left side of the bladder (white arrow). Blood filled the right pelvic recess (white arrow heads) and the flank.

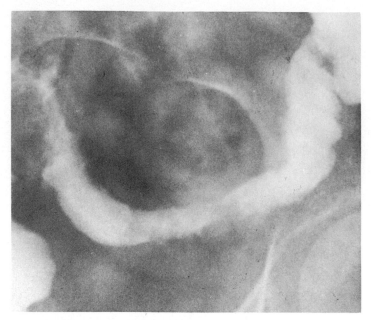

FIG. 19.34. LATE RADIATION CHANGES IN THE RECTOSIGMOID
This 50-year-old woman was treated with intravaginal radium and external radiation for cervical carcinoma. Nine months later she developed a rectal discharge and hematochezia. The proctoscopist found an area of ulcerated and inflamed mucosa. Barium enema reveals an extensive area of fixed narrowing involving the entire sigmoid colon.

SURGERY

Postoperative Ileus

After many major abdominal surgical procedures the patient develops abnormal bowel distention called "adynamic ileus." Characteristically, both large and small bowel show symmetrical dilatation and contain multiple air and fluid levels. There are no isolated or asymmetrically dilated loops. The patient complains of distention but not colicky pain. Inadequate nasogastric decompression aggravates this condition. Postoperative distension usually resolves by the 4th postoperative day and the patient begins to pass gas and stool. Distention lasting beyond the 7th postoperative day and characterized by isolated, dilated bowel loops, suggests the possibility of early adhesions, hernia, intussusception, volvulus or anastomotic leak. A cautiously administered barium enema can be helpful in this evaluation.

Postoperative Colon

Most patients presenting for a barium enema examination following colon resection have had their surgery either for carcinoma or diverticulitis. The remaining colon may be anastomosed to colon or ileum in an end-to-end (Fig. 19.35), side-to-side, or side-to-end (Fig. 19.36) fashion. In the more common end-to-end anastomosis, the apposition of the serosal surfaces by mattress sutures results in the invagination of a thin, well formed collar of colon wall into the bowel lumen (Fig. 19.37). A double-contrast enema will frequently define a thin rim of barium between the inverted ends of the bowel wall. Edema and spasm may also contribute to narrowing of the bowel lumen at the anastomotic site, if studied within several weeks of surgery.

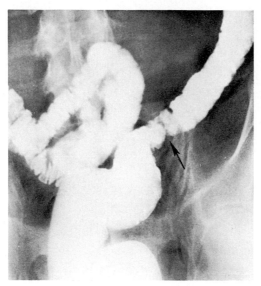

FIG. 19.35. END-TO-END ANASTOMOSIS
The area of relative narrowing marks the site of sigmoid anastomosis (arrow).

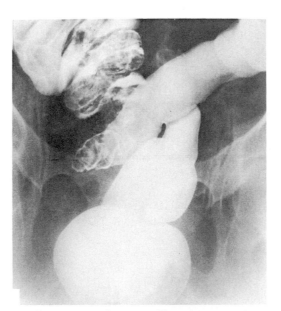

FIG. 19.36. SIDE-TO-END ANASTOMOSIS
Anastomosis of the sigmoid colon to the rectosigmoid.

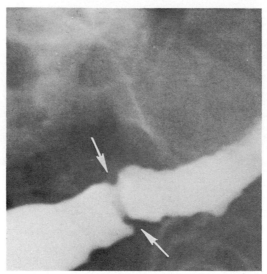

FIG. 19.37. INFOLDING OF COLON WALL AT SITE OF END-TO-END SIGMOID
ANASTOMOSIS (ARROWS)

Examination Technique

Colostomy

A soft rubber catheter carries less potential for harm than a metal tip. The patient
holds the inflated balloon of the catheter tightly against the outside of stoma. A
balloon is never inflated inside the stoma! An alternate method is to use a soft
catheter which has been passed through the cut tip of a nursing nipple, the latter
acting as a tampon while being held in the colostomy stoma by the patient.

Postoperative colon anastomosis

Barium examination of the colon between the 8th and 12th postoperative weeks
provides a baseline study of the anastomotic site. By then the postoperative edema
and spasm have subsided and the patient has regained bowel function.

Complications

Postoperative Stricture

Narrowing of the colon at the anastomotic site occurs in practically all patients.
Fortunately this narrowing rarely causes functional impairment. Postoperative
narrowing is smooth and concentric.

Recurrent Cancer

Local recurrences appear in 10% and metachronous colon carcinomas in 3% of
patients who have had a colon resection for carcinoma.

In the early stage, anastomotic recurrence causes an asymmetric narrowing. In
the later stage the anastomosis becomes nodular and ulcerated. Comparison with
the postoperative baseline study helps in evaluation of early subtle changes.

How often and how long should the postoperative patient have follow-up colon
studies? Opinions vary. As a minimum most authorities recommend the asymptomatic postsurgical cancer patient have a barium study yearly for 5 years.

Postoperative Leaks

The anastomosis

Devitalized or infected tissues account for most anastomotic leaks which develop in the intra- or retroperitoneal spaces (Fig. 19.38).

Colostomy site

Instrumentation may tear the colon or a recurrent tumor at the colostomy may perforate. Either can allow gas and stool to enter the retroperitoneal tissues. (Fig. 19.39).

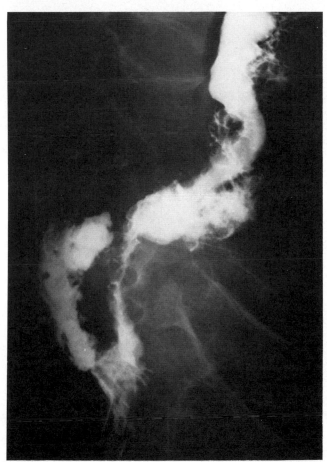

FIG. 19.38. PRESACRAL ABSCESS FOLLOWING ANASTOMATIC BREAKDOWN
This 62-year-old woman with severe rheumatoid arthritis had an anterior resection for rectal carcinoma. Lateral rectal film of the barium enema shows an abscess cavity filled with barium through a communication at the anastomatic site.

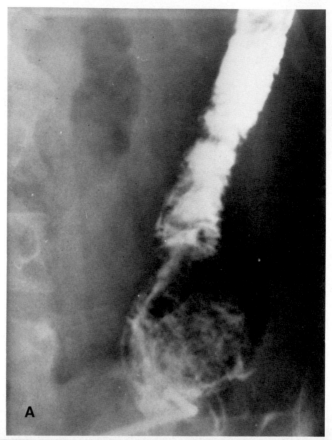

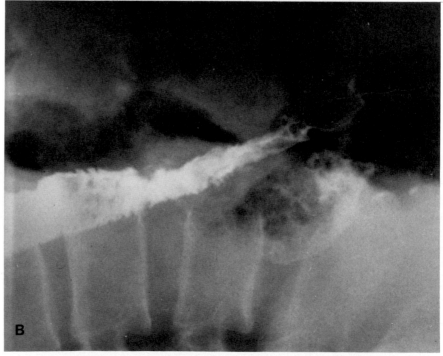

BIBLIOGRAPHY

Obstruction

Berk, R. N., and Millman, S. J.: Urticaria of the colon, Radiology, *99:* 539, 1971.

Botsford, T. W., and Wilson, R. E.: *The Acute Abdomen—An Approach to Diagnosis and Management,* 2nd Ed. W. B. Saunders, Philadelphia, 1977.

Bryk, D., and Soong, K. Y.: Colonic ileus and its differential diagnosis. Am. J. Roentgenol., *101:* 329, 1967.

Dunphy, J. E., and Way, L. W.: *Current Surgical Diagnosis and Treatment,* 3rd Ed. Lange Medical Publications, Los Altos, Calif., 1977.

Diner, W. C., and Barnhard, H. J.: Acute diverticulitis. Semin. Roentgenol., *8:* 415, 1973.

Ein, S. H., and Stephens, C. A.: Intussusception: 354 cases in 10 years. J. Pediatr. Surg., *6:* 16, 1971.

Frimann-Dahl, J.: *Roentgen Examination in Acute Abdominal Diseases,* 3rd Ed. Charles C Thomas, Springfield, Ill., 1974.

Laufer, I.: The left lateral view in the plain film assessment of abdominal distension. Radiology, *119:* 265, 1976.

Lowman, R. M.: The potassium depletion states and post operative ileus. Radiology, *98:* 691, 1974.

Miller, R. E.: The radiological evaluation of intraperitoneal gas. CRC Crit. Rev. Radiol. Sci., *4:* 61, 1973.

Miller, R. E.: The technical approach to the acute abdomen. Semin. Roentgenol., *8:* 267, 1973.

Moss, A. A., Goldberg, H. I., and Brotman, M.: Idiopathic intestinal pseudo-obstruction. Am. J. Roentgenol., *115:* 312, 1972.

Novy, S., Rogers, L. F., and Kirkpatrick, W.: Diastatic rupture of the cecum in obstructing carcinoma of the left colon. Am. J. Roentgenol., *123:* 281, 1975.

Phillips, J. C.: A spectrum of radiologic abnormalities due to tubo-ovarian abscess. Radiology, *110:* 307, 1974.

Raymond, R. D.: A mechanism of the kink formation which preceeds intussusception, Invest. Radiol., *6:* 61, 1971.

Warnes, H., Lehmann, H. E., and Bon, T. A.: Adynamic ileus during psychoactive medication: A report of 3 fatal and 5 severe cases. J. Can. Med. Assoc. *96:* 1112, 1967.

Weiner, M. J.: Myotonic megacolon in myotonic dystrophy. Am. J. Roentgenol., *138:* 177, 1978.

Whelan, J. P.: *Radiology of the Abdomen—Anatomic Basis.* Lea & Febrger, Philadelphia 1976.

Trauma

De Cosse, J. J., *et al.:* The natural history and management of radiation injury of the gastrointestinal tract. Ann. Surg., *170:* 369, 1969.

Freeark, R. J.: Current concepts—Penetrating wounds of the abdomen. N. Engl. J. Med., *291:* 185, 1974.

Howell, H. S., Bartizal, J. F., and Freeark, R. J.: Blunt trauma involving the colon and rectum. J. Trauma *61:* 624, 1976.

McCort, J. J.: Intraperitoneal and retroperitoneal hemorrhage. Radiol. Clin. North Am., *14:* 391, 1976.

Nance, F. C., Wennar, M. H., Johnson, L. W., *et al.:* Surgical judgement in the management of penetrating wounds of the abdomen. Experience with 2,212 patients. Ann. Surg. *179:* 639, 1974.

Rogers, L. F., and Goldstein, H. M.: Roentgen manifestations of radiation injury to the gastrointestinal tract. Gastrointest. Radiol., *2:* 281, 1977.

Wescott, J. L., and Smith, J.: Mesentery and colon injuries secondary to blunt trauma. Radiology, *114:* 597, 1975.

Wilder, J. R., Lotfi, M. W., and Paterno, J.: Comparative study of mandatory and selective surgical intervention in stab wounds of the abdomen. Surgery, *69:* 546, 1971.

Worth, M. H.: Abdominal trauma. J.A.M.A., *235:* 853, 1976.

Surgery

Bartram, C., and Hale, J. E.: Radiological diagnoses of recurrent colonic carcinoma at the anastomosis. Gut, *11:* 778, 1970.

Polk, H. C., and Pratt, J. S.: Recurrent colo-rectal carcinoma: Detection, treatment and other considerations. Surgery, *69:* 9, 1971.

FIG. 19.39. RECURRENT CARCINOMA AT COLOSTOMY SITE. RETROPERITONEAL PERFORATION AND ABSCESS FORMATION

This 64-year-old man with adenocarcinoma of the rectosigmoid was treated by anteroposterior resection and permanent colostomy. Two years later he developed pain, tenderness, and guarding in the left lower quadrant adjacent to the colostomy site. (**A**) Anteroposterior film shows irregular constriction of the lumen by recurrent tumor. (**B**) On the lateral film there was extravasation into an abscess in the posterior retroperitoneal tissues.

20

Other Colonic Disorders

CHARLES S. LANGSTON, M.D.

PNEUMATOSIS COLI

Introduction

Pneumatosis intestinalis is a term used to describe intramural collections of gas in the small and large bowel. It is useful to distinguish between linear and cystic pneumatosis. When the small bowel is involved, the collections of gas are nearly always linear in distribution and often secondary to some basic bowel disorder, such as infarction and necrosis, ulceration, or obstruction and perforation. These same grave diagnostic possibilities must also be considered when linear pneumatosis involves the large bowel (Fig. 20.1A).

Cystic pneumatosis more often occurs in the colon alone (Fig. 20.1B) in which case pneumatosis coli is the preferred term. This is a benign condition; underlying disease of the gastrointestinal tract is rarely found.

Pathology

The gross appearance of colonic pneumatosis is of air-filled bubbles under the serosa of the involved segment of the bowel wall. If the bubbles are large enough, or are located within the submucosa, the opened lumen of the bowel wall will appear to be covered with small cysts or polyps, and a cut section through the wall will show it to be honeycombed with thin-walled fragile cysts ranging in size from about 1 mm to several centimeters.

Microscopically, the cysts have an endothelial lining and often a low-grade inflammatory response in or around them. They do not obviously communicate with one another or with the bowel lumen. Occasionally, they are clearly formed from dilated lymphatic channels but usually this is not the case.

The pathophysiology of this disorder is still unclear, although gas-containing cysts of the colon have been known to anatomists and pathologists since the 18th century. Because many, but not all, of the early reports of pneumatosis coli were in patients with serious underlying abdominal disease, it was not clear whether the pneumatosis was merely an incidental finding or the cause of the patient's symptoms.

Mechanical, bacterial, and neoplastic theories have been advanced to explain the origin of the intramural gas, but the mechanical explanation seems to fit most cases best. Several researchers have been able to create pneumatosis coli experimentally by injecting air into the perivascular stroma of the mesenteric vessels, and occasionally by injecting air into the stroma surrounding the thoracic aorta. It is now thought that the majority of cases are caused by air forced into the bowel wall either through a breach in the mucosa, as in the case of intestinal obstruction or of traumatic sigmoidoscopy, or that the air dissects along the vascular sheaths of the aorta and mesenteric vessels from the chest after an episode of forceful vomiting or coughing. The resulting pneumomediastinum is decompressed by the downward passage of gas through the supporting structures of the mediastinal and retroperitoneal vessels and ultimately into the intestinal wall.

Clinical Features

Clinically, this is a disorder of middle age, and of men more than women (3.5 to 1). The patient may present with symptoms of intestinal obstruction, or gastric obstruction, or may have a history of forceful vomiting or coughing, perhaps with respiratory insufficiency. However, it is more common that the patient will not have any evidence of underlying disease, and the symptoms, if any, are not striking, usually consisting of vague abdominal discomfort with diarrhea or constipation. The stool may contain occult blood and is sometimes slimy or frothy.

Roentgen Findings

The diagnosis of pneumatosis coli is usually made by the radiologist. A cluster of radiolucent bubbles or curvilinear densities will be seen on a plain film of the abdomen, or beneath the diaphragm on a chest film. The cysts tend to be more obvious when the colon is involved, appearing larger and rounder than in the small bowel. On barium enema examination, the lumen of the bowel does not fill out completely since the cysts, which are under some tension, protrude into the lumen. Because of their subserosal location, they often seem to be half in and half out of the bowel (Fig. 20.2). If they are large, the cysts may simulate a so-called thumbprint pattern of the colon which might be confused with intestinal infarction (Fig. 20.3). However, when viewed tangentially, the cysts will be outlined on the mucosal side by barium and on the serosal side by the soft tissue density of the cyst wall against the air within it. Usually the colon remains relatively pliable and empties normally, although it may be slightly stiffened. The postevacuation film often shows the cysts to better advantage than do the filled films. Occasionally, pneumomediastinum or pneumoperitoneum are noted as ancillary signs.

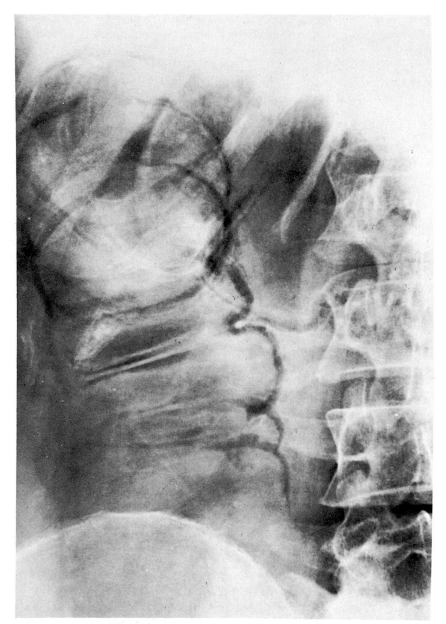

FIG. 20.1. PNEUMATOSIS INTESTINALIS
(A) Linear pneumatosis. Detail of the dilated ascending colon from a plain film of the abdomen in which dead bowel wall is outlined by intramural gas in a patient with inferior mesenteric artery thrombosis. (B) Cystic pneumatosis. The plain film shows multiple gas "bubbles" in the distribution of the ascending colon.

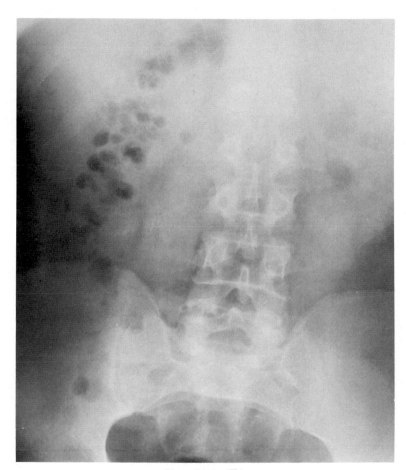

FIG. 20.1. (**B**)

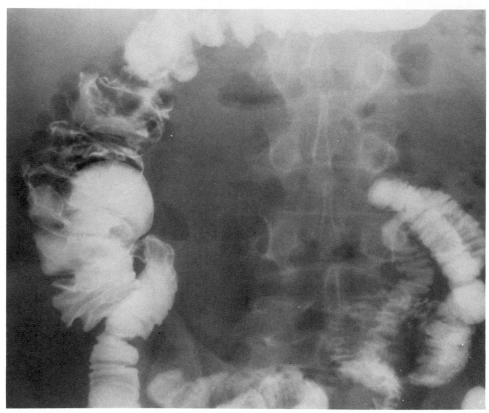

FIG. 20.2. PNEUMATOSIS COLI

Barium enema shows the gas cysts to be subserosal projecting half in and half out of the intestinal lumen. See also Fig. 17.48.

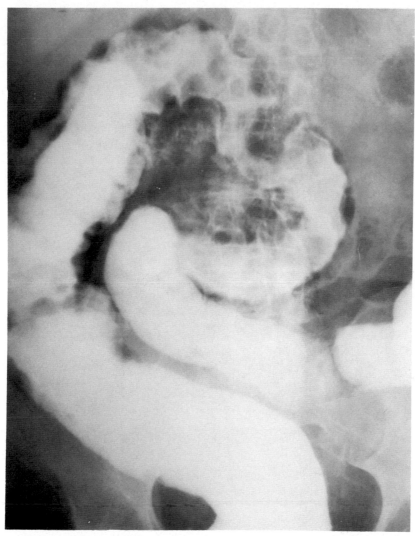

FIG. 20.3. PNEUMATOSIS COLI

Large cysts result in extensive "thumbprinting" in the sigmoid. However, the correct diagnosis can be deduced from the clearly visible subserosal gas collections.

Differential Diagnosis

The clustered bubbles seen on the plain film may simulate an intra-abdominal abscess (Figs. 20.4 and 20.5). The barium enema is usually unequivocal, but pneumatosis coli may be confused with multiple polyps, Crohn's colitis, colonic infarction, colitis cystica profunda, lymphoma, or multiple lipomas. Since intramural gas is seen in necrotizing colitis and toxic megacolon, both of these diagnoses may be considered. However, in these cases, intramural gas, probably produced at least in part by bacteria, is more typically linear and uniform in width rather than cystic. In the small bowel and stomach, this distinction does not hold since here pneumatosis is more likely to have a linear than cystic appearance.

Treatment and Prognosis

When pneumatosis is associated with serious disease, the prognosis depends upon the underlying condition. In the more usual asymptomatic case the prognosis is excellent and the process resolves slowly over a period of weeks or months. There is some evidence that symptomatic cases may be helped by treatment with nasal oxygen.

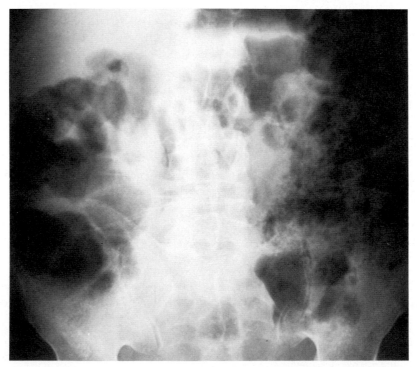

FIG. 20.4. INTRA-ABDOMINAL ABCESS SIMULATING PNEUMATOSIS COLI
Note multiple gas bubbles in the left flank.

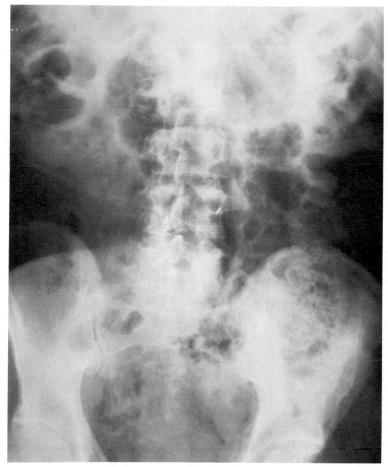

FIG. 20.5. PNEUMATOSIS COLI SIMULATING AN INTRA-ABDOMINAL ABSCESS
Note the multiple gas cysts to the left of the spine which were in the (redundant) transverse colon.

COLITIS CYSTICA PROFUNDA

Introduction

Colitis cystica profunda is a poorly understood disorder in which large mucous cysts form beneath the submucosa of the colon. Although this condition was described by Virchow, it was not until the 1950's that it received attention, culminating with an Armed Forces Institute of Pathology review in 1967. The main import of the disease is that it not be mistaken for colloid carcinoma of the colon.

Pathology

Grossly, the cysts are submucosal and measure from about 0.1–2.0 cm in diameter. If large enough, they elevate the overlying mucosa and have an appearance much like a polypoid tumor. The surrounding tissues are often inflamed and although the mucosa is usually intact, it may be ulcerated.

The majority of published reports describe single lesions in the rectum, but there is a second form of the disorder in which multiple mucous cysts are found throughout the colon, sometimes in association with chronic diarrhea or ulcerative colitis.

Microscopic sections of the mucosa typically show irregular, distorted glands interspersed among more normal areas. Some of the abnormal glands extend through the muscularis mucosa where they become dilated and then form submucosal cysts surrounded by chronic inflammatory cells and fibrosis. The cyst wall in many cases resembles the mucosa of the colon, but may show only columnar or cuboidal epithelium. It is important to note that cellular atypia and anaplasia are not seen.

The pathogenesis of the disorder is not understood, but a strong association with proctitis or colitis has led to the hypothesis that the cysts are formed when surface mucosa is implanted into the submucosa during the reparative phase of an ulcerative proctitis or colitis.

Clinical Features

Colitis cystica profunda has been described in patients of all ages but seems more common in young males. The usual presentation is rectal bleeding and pain sometimes associated with diarrhea and occasionally with rectal prolapse. Digital or sigmoidoscopic examination reveals a rubbery or hard polypoid mass which is often thought to be a cancer.

Roentgen Findings

Radiologic examination is not diagnostic. Most lesions are less than 3 cm in diameter, but they may be so small as not to be seen radiographically. Multiple lesions may suggest multiple polyps or, if there is enough scalloping of the colon, ischemic colitis (Fig. 20.6). Larger lesions may present as a single rectal mass looking like a sessile polyp (Fig. 20.7). Although the mucosa is usually intact, this fact is often not appreciated. The irregular contours and distortions of the overlying mucosa may give the impression of gross ulceration suggesting a diagnosis of adenocarcinoma. In fact, these lesions have been diagnosed as adenocarcinomas at sigmoidoscopy.

Differential Diagnosis

The radiologic differential diagnosis includes adenocarcinoma, villous adenoma, adenomatous polyp, lymphoma, ulcerative or ischemic colitis, and involvement of the colon by disorders of adjacent structures such as endometriosis.

Treatment and Prognosis

Since the disease is rare, management and prognosis are unclear. However, since this seems to be a benign and probably not progressive disorder, treatment should be symptomatic in most cases. In the occasional case in which there is significant bleeding or associated rectal prolapse, surgery may be indicated.

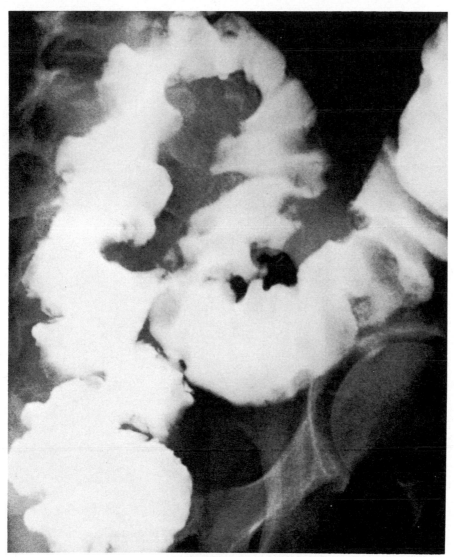

FIG. 20.6. COLITIS CYSTICA PROFUNDA

Multiple submucosal mucus cysts have resulted an irregularity of the bowel wall simulating ischemic colitis.

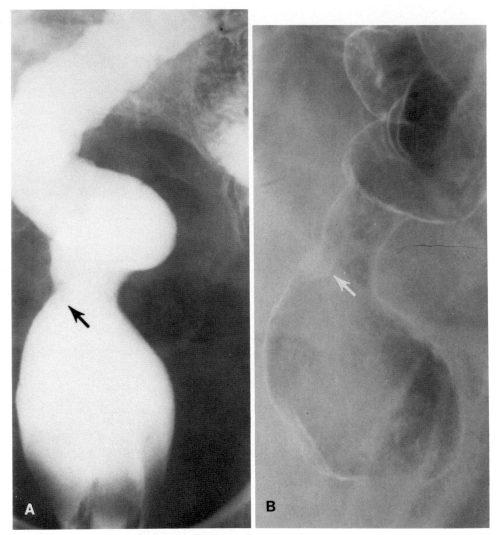

FIG. 20.7. COLITIS CYSTICA PROFUNDA

Barium (**A**) and air-contrast (**B**) exams show a sessile "polyp" which proved to be a submucosal mucus cyst (arrows).

AMYLOIDOSIS

Introduction

Amyloidosis is a multiple system disease which may occur primarily either spontaneously or as a familial disorder, or secondarily in association with chronic inflammatory or immune diseases such as the collagen diseases, lymphoproliferative disorders and chronic infections. The disease is relatively "silent" in the gut but is probably present in 50–70% of patients with both "primary" and "secondary" amyloidosis.

Pathology and Clinical Features

Pathologic examination shows that the amyloid glycoprotein is deposited in the intestinal muscularis and in the lumen of intestinal blood vessels. This results, respectively, in a loss of tissue pliability and alimentary motility; and in ischemia, necrosis, and tissue breakdown. Motility disorders predominate in the esophagus and stomach while in the small intestine malabsorption is more common. In the colon, amyloid disease may present with constipation, diarrhea, ulceration, perforation, or hemorrhage; the clinical picture depends upon whether vascular insufficiency or disordered motility predominates.

Roentgen Findings

While most patients with amyloidosis are likely to have a normal appearing colon when examined by barium enema, the barium-filled colon may show disordered motility, loss of the normal haustral pattern (Fig. 20.8), narrowed and dilated segments (Fig. 20.9), irregularity or nodularity of the mucosa, pseudo-ulcerations or a combination of the above (Fig. 20.10).

Differential Diagnosis

The differential diagnosis must therefore include sclerosing tumors, benign strictue, infarction, adhesions, scleroderma, and ulcerative or Crohn's colitis. In fact, amyloidosis may occur in combination with inflammatory bowel disease. However, the multiple, closely spaced ulcerations, shortening of the colon, and diffuse narrowing of the lumen so characteristic of ulcerative colitis are not found in amyloid disease.

Prognosis

In general, when amyloidosis of the colon is symptomatic, multiple organs are already affected. If colonic amyloidosis is associated with intestinal infarction or hemorrhage, it may be life-threatening, but the usual cause of death is involvement of the kidneys or the heart.

SCLERODERMA

Introduction

Scleroderma, preferably called progressive systemic sclerosis to emphasize the generalized nature of the disorder, is a disease of middle age more common in women than men, in which cutaneous and gastrointestinal symptoms predominate. The skin abnormalities are familiar: subcutaneous edema is followed by induration which is in turn followed by atrophy, fibrosis and tissue breakdown, sometimes with ulceration. The gastrointestinal pathology follows roughly the same progression.

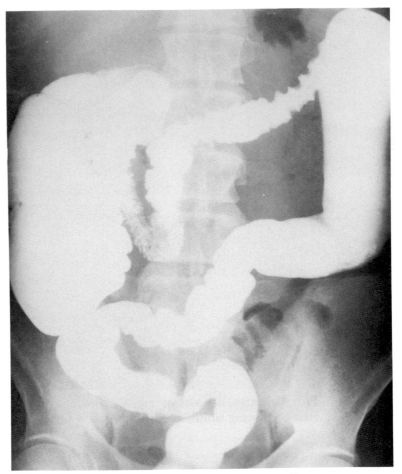

FIG. 20.10. AMYLOIDOSIS OF THE COLON

Note the scalloping and nodularity of the transverse colon. At postmortem examination, this proved to be due to a combination of amyloid plaques and submucosal hemorrhage.

Roentgen Findings

Plain film examination of the abdomen often reveals colonic distention and fecal impaction. It may be quite difficult to prepare the patient adequately for a barium enema. The characteristic finding is an increase in the size of individual haustra so that they form sacculations or pseudo-diverticula, usually on the antimesenteric border of the transverse colon, often asymmetric with the more normal haustra opposite (Fig. 20.11). These pseudo-diverticula are first demonstrated on postevacuation films since the musculature within the saccules is degenerated and atrophic and does not contract (Fig. 20.12). Sometimes one finds short strictured or ulcerated areas, probably secondary to mucosal ischemia and fecal trauma.

Treatment and Prognosis

The treatment of colonic scleroderma is largely directed toward amelioration of the symptoms. Patients with severe colonic scleroderma usually have extensive disease. Life-threatening disease is more likely to be due to pulmonary involvement.

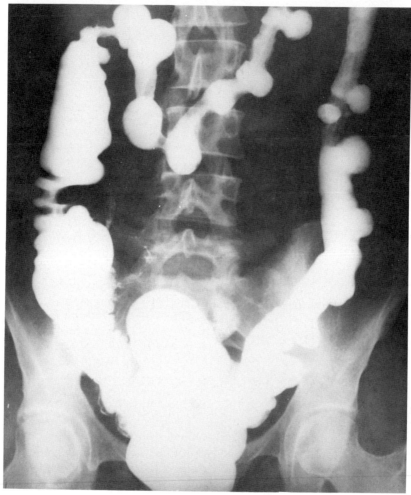

FIG. 20.11. PROGRESSIVE SYSTEMIC SCLEROSIS
Asymmetric, exaggerated haustral pouches form pseudo-diverticula.

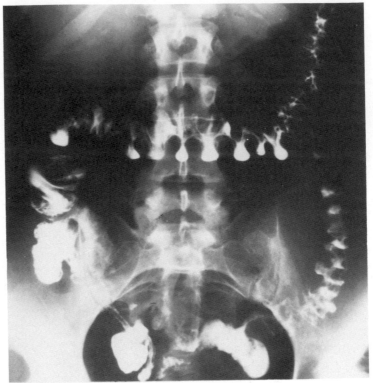

FIG. 20.12. PROGRESSIVE SYSTEMIC SCLEROSIS
A postevacuation film shows the earliest changes of exaggerated haustra along the antimesenteric border of the transverse colon.

CATHARTIC COLON

Introduction

Chronic abuse of "irritant" laxatives such as cascara, podophyllin, phenothalein, and castor oil, over a period of years, can produce severe radiologic abnormalities simulating chronic inflammatory bowel disease. Although "cathartic colon" has been recognized since the 1940's, its precise cause is not known and pathologic descriptions are rare. There is at least one report describing the muscularis as atrophic and the adjacent stroma infiltrated with fat. The myenteric plexuses are present and normal in appearance.

Clinical Features

The clinical history is typically of constipation, but the patient, often of middle age, is not likely to volunteer the information that he or she has been using laxatives in excess. In fact, the patient has usually been using cathartics for longer than 15 years, and a vicious cycle has become established necessitating the continued use of the laxative. Initially, the cathartic results in such good cleansing of the colon that another bowel movement is not possible for several days. The patient mistakenly feels that he is constipated again and repeats the cathartic. Later, the prolonged stimulation of the colon by irritants establishes a neuromuscular incoordination so that the colonic musculature becomes dependent upon external stimulants to produce adequate contractile force. The patient who suffers from this disorder may not complain of constipation, but rather of bloating, gas, or lower abdominal pain. Although some of the irritant cathartics do result in hyperpigmentation of the colonic mucosa, sigmoidoscopy usually reveals little, perhaps some edema of the mucosa.

Roentgen Findings

The radiologic findings may range from a mild loss of haustrations and contractility to a generalized loss of both haustrations and of normal mucosal folds. When collapsed the colon tends to form linear folds rather than the usual pattern. The earliest changes are seen in the right colon, and not infrequently in the terminal ileum (Fig. 20.13). If there has been a coincident abuse of enemas, the descending colon may also be smooth and ahaustral. In severe cases, there is a striking total absence of the normal haustral pattern throughout the colon.

Transient areas of narrowing resembling strictures may be noted at fluoroscopy and may suggest chronic ulcerative colitis or regional enteritis on overhead films. However, at fluoroscopy these areas are seen to be normally distensible and rather than being stiff, the colon distends to a diameter wider than normal without any discomfort to the patient.

Differential Diagnosis

The radiologic differential diagnosis includes ulcerative colitis, Crohn's colitis, and if the disease is limited to the right colon, amebic colitis. The absence of symptoms or signs of colitis, along with the history, are diagnostic.

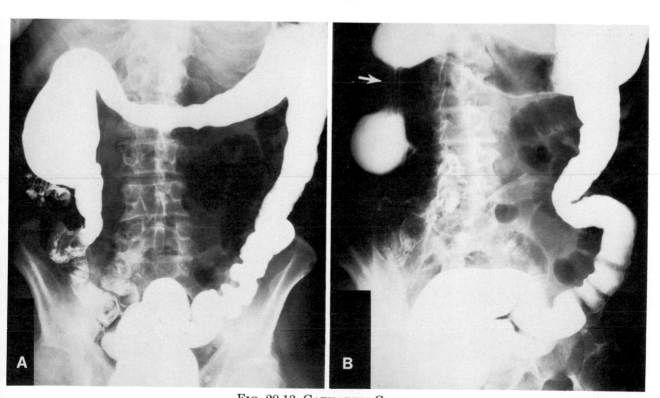

FIG. 20.13. CATHARTIC COLON

(A) The right colon has become smooth and ahaustral. When it collapses (B) it forms linear folds (arrow).

Treatment and Prognosis

Several cases have been reported in which the radiologic abnormalities were reversed, at least in part, by discontinuing the irritant cathartics. This does not seem to be possible in most cases. However, an attempt should be made to switch the patient to a nonirritating bulk laxative.

MEGACOLON

Introduction

The congenital form of megacolon (Hirschsprung's disease) has been described in Chapter 4. Massive distention of the colon may also occur as an acquired lesion on either a functional or an organic basis.

Functional Megacolon

In most cases, functional megacolon is psychogenic in origin. Under normal

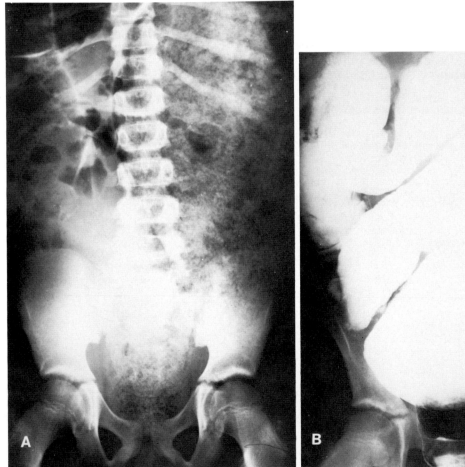
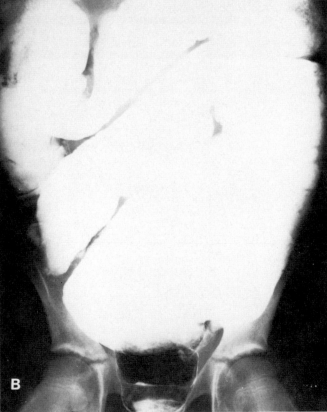

FIG. 20.14. FUNCTIONAL MEGACOLON

This child moved his bowels infrequently and was said by his parents to be constipated. A preliminary film of the abdomen (**A**) shows the colon to be packed with stool. On barium enema, the rectum distends well (**B**), and the colon empties completely (**C**).

circumstances the urge to defecate is perceived when the rectum and rectosigmoid are distended by a semisolid bolus of feces. Activation of this urge also depends on the tone of the surrounding muscle and, as we are all familiar, the urge can be consciously inhibited and will eventually pass. If the stimulus is continually ignored, the rectum and sigmoid will passively distend and it will require additional distention to re-initiate the urge to defecate. Most patients in whom functional megacolon is seen are emotionally unstable or feeble and are often confined to institutions where the combination of the patient's failure to respond to the urge to defecate, or his inability to get himself to a bathroom, combined with the inability of the staff to aid him, results in the first steps which lead to functional megacolon.

The diagnosis is not ordinarily a radiologic one. However, since the patient may have become accustomed to his unusual bowel habits and may be relatively asymptomatic or may be unable to communicate his symptoms, it is not unusual for the diagnosis to be first suggested by a radiologist examining a film of the abdomen or even a film of the chest (Fig. 20.14).

Occasionally, especially in children, the diagnosis is unclear. It may even require rapid sequence fluororadiography to determine whether or not normal rectal peristalsis is present. However, it can be said, in children at least, that if there is significant megacolon without dilatation of the rectum, the lesion is likely to be organic (Fig. 20.15).

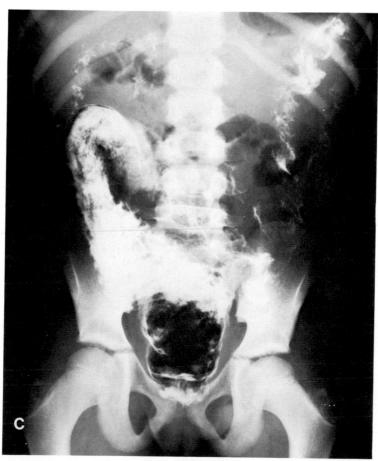

FIG. 20.14. (C)

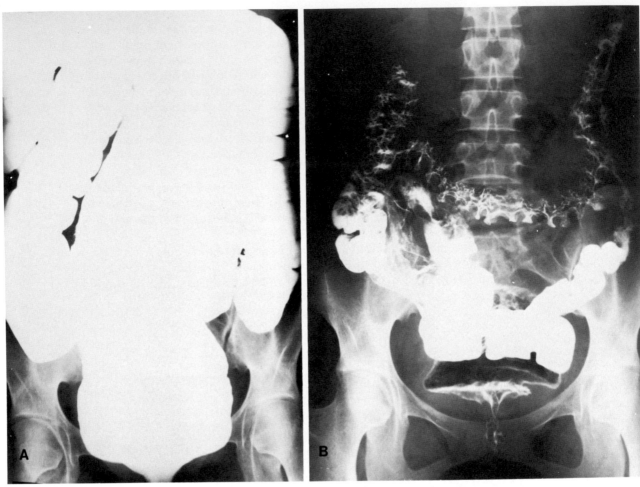

FIG. 20.15. FUNCTIONAL MEGACOLON
Most of the increase in colonic volume in this patient is in the sigmoid and the
rectum is fully distended (**A**). The colon empties well (**B**).

Most patients with functional megacolon tolerate the disorder well, needing little
more than occasional disimpaction. Nevertheless, they do occasionally have complications such as ulceration of the colonic wall by stercoliths and they may even
require surgical emptying of the colon.

Organic Megacolon

Chagas' disease is the best known cause of organic megacolon, but is rarely
encountered outside of South America (Fig. 20.16). The disorder is caused by the
parasite *Trypanasoma cruzi* which enters the body when a Reduviid bug infected
with *T. cruzi* bites the victim and contaminates the wound with its feces. The
parasite multiplies, infests the host, and spreads throughout the body where it
causes a myocardopathy, and results in megaesophagus and megacolon. The parasite
elaborates a toxin which destroys the colon ganglion cells producing segments of
decreased peristalsis with resulting proximal dilatation of the colon. The appearance

may be very similar to Hirschsprung's disease. However, it does not invariably involve the rectum as does Hirschsprung's.

Myxedema is one cause of megacolon which is so insidious in onset that it is often not diagnosed. The colon in myxedema loses much of its muscle tone and may be incapable of adequate peristaltic activity. In addition, the bowel wall may be thickened and stiffened by layers of myxedematous material in the submucosa.

Another cause of organic megacolon is neurologic disease (Fig. 20.17). Patients suffering from paraplegia, poliomyelitis, or tabes dorsalis are at risk to develop megacolon, but happily most of them nowadays receive sufficient medical care to avoid this complication. Occasionally, strictures or tumors of the rectum may cause megacolon but they are much more likely to cause an acute obstruction.

Probably the most common cause of adult organic megacolon in this country is the result of a combination of old age, drugs such as the anticholinergics and phenothiazines, excessive dependence on laxatives and sedentary habits. Elderly patients with Parkinson's disease are an example of this type of organic megacolon.

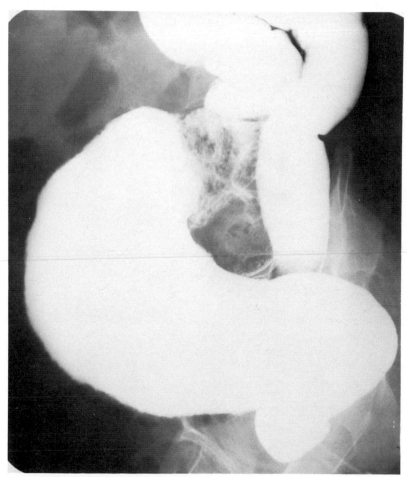

FIG. 20.16. ORGANIC MEGACOLON: CHAGAS' DISEASE
Massive dilatation of the left colon down to the anus.

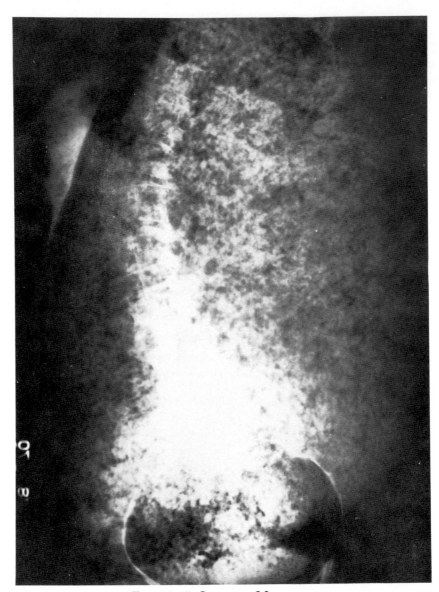

FIG. 20.17. ORGANIC MEGACOLON
An enormous fecal impaction which had to be removed surgically. The patient
was paraplegic.

THE EFFECT OF ADJACENT PATHOLOGY ON THE COLON

The colon, particularly the transverse colon, is in intimate relationship to the pancreas, kidneys and adrenals, stomach, duodenum, spleen and gallbladder. Diseases of these organs may therefore present with colonic symptoms and may displace or deform the colon on barium enema examination.

To deduce the extracolonic source of these deformities, one must be familiar with the relationships of the colon to the adjacent viscera and to the fascial planes of the retroperitoneum and mesentery (Figs. 20.18–20.20).

The mesentery of the transverse colon, the transverse mesocolon, has at its base a "bare area" where it arises from the peritoneum of the posterior wall of the abdominal cavity. As illustrated, the mesocolon arises in a roughly diagonal line extending from the lower pole of the right kidney, across the second portion of the duodenum, along the body and the tail of the pancreas to the upper portion of the left kidney where it terminates in the fascial attachments of the phrenicolic and lienocolic ligaments. Pancreatic lesions spread through the root of the transverse mesocolon to the undersurface of the transverse colon where they characteristically lift and distort the posterior-inferior wall of the distal transverse colon (Figs. 20.21 and 20.22).

The stomach is connected to the anterior-superior surface of the distal transverse colon by the gastrocolic ligament which forms another route for spread of tumor to the colon. It has been shown that the tenia of the colon tend to limit the spread of the disease in the colonic serosa and that disease spreading via the gastrocolic ligaments characteristically effaces the haustra of the superior border of the transverse colon (Fig. 20.23) and may exaggerate the sacculations of the haustra of the inferior border. It should be realized, however, that if the involvement of the colon is extensive, the deformity will be such that it is not possible to deduce whether the route of spread was through the transverse mesocolon or through the gastrocolic ligament (Fig. 20.24).

The kidneys, which lie posterior to the ascending and descending colon, are surrounded by several fascial layers. However, these layers blend together and become weakened inferiorly so that it is not unusual for renal infections to spread caudally along the colon in the flanks (Fig. 20.25). It should be remembered, however, that since the mesocolon is continuous, far-spreading lesions such as pancreatic phlegmons may present in the flanks just as would a renal lesion (Fig. 20.26).

The gallbladder usually lies nestled on the superior surface of the proximal transverse colon. There is no anatomic fascial plane joining the gallbladder to the colon, but the two may become adherent and peritoneography shows that there is often a potential intraperitoneal space between the two which may serve as a route of spread of infection or tumor (Fig. 20.27).

Very large masses such as large tumors or pseudocysts may cause displacement of the colon so striking as to make the point of origin of the mass unclear. Hepatomegaly and splenomegaly are usually obvious. However, it is to be noted that masses arising from the right kidney tend to displace the ascending colon anteriorly and may depress the proximal transverse colon since much of the right kidney lies superior to the transverse mesocolon (Fig. 20.28). On the other hand, left renal masses tend to elevate the splenic flexure and displace the descending colon laterally since most of the left kidney lies inferior and medial to the transverse mesocolon (Fig. 20.29). One interesting variation in the relationship of the descending colon to the left kidney is that when the left kidney is absent, the descending colon tends to lie medial to its normal position (Fig. 20.30).

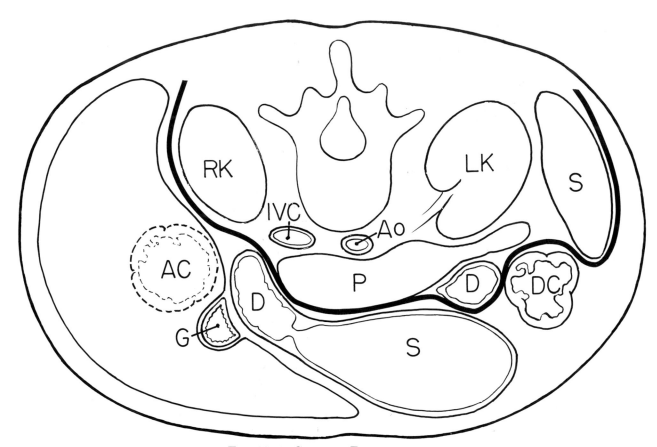

FIG. 20.18. COLONIC RELATIONSHIPS
A transverse section at about T12. The ascending (AC) and descending (DC) colon are marked. This section would be just above the transverse colon.

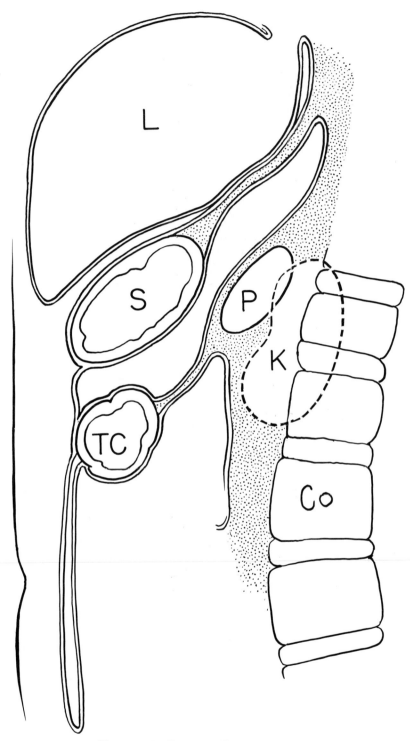

FIG. 20.19. COLONIC RELATIONSHIPS
A sagittal section through the abdomen showing the retroperitoneal structures
and the relationship of the transverse colon to the stomach and pancreas.

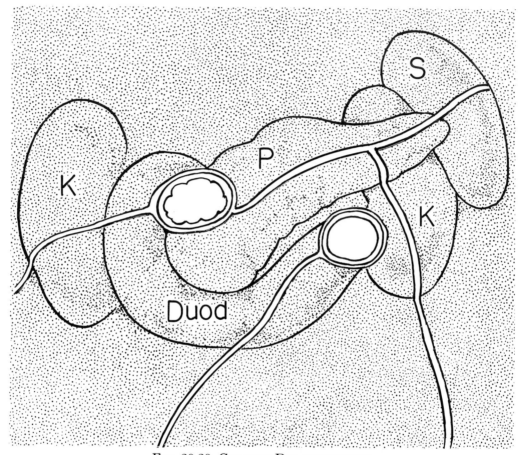

FIG. 20.20. COLONIC RELATIONSHIPS

The "mesentery" of the transverse colon, the transverse mesocolon arises in a roughly diagonal line extending from the lower pole of the right kidney, across the second portion of the duodenum, along the body and tail of the pancreas, to the upper pole of the left kidney where it terminates in the phrenicolic and lienocolic ligaments.

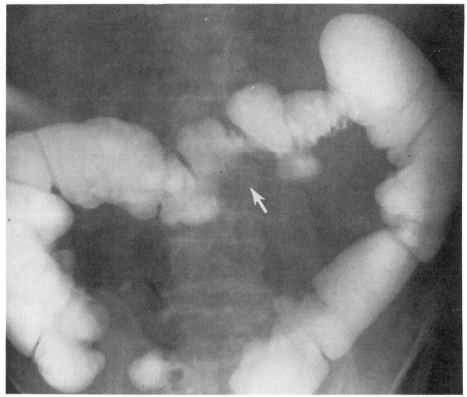

FIG. 20.21. COLONIC RELATIONSHIPS: PANCREAS

Carcinoma of the pancreas invading the transverse colon (arrow). Note the irregularity of the distal transverse colon, also due to invasion. (Courtesy of Dr. Herbert Gramm, New England Deaconess Hospital, Boston, Mass.)

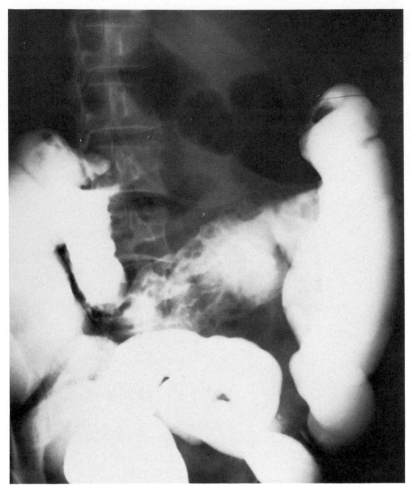

FIG. 20.22. COLONIC RELATIONSHIPS: PANCREAS

Pancreatitis. A large phlegmon has spread through the tissue planes of the transverse mesocolon to the transverse colon.

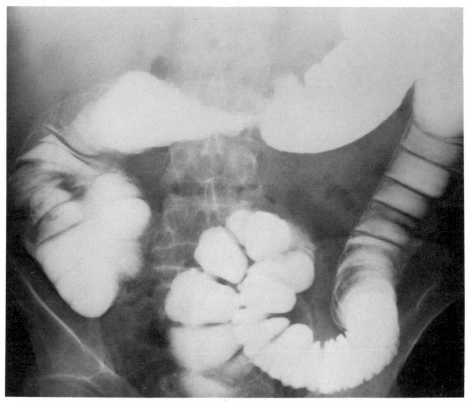

FIG. 20.23. COLONIC RELATIONSHIP: STOMACH

Carcinoma of the stomach. The tumor has spread through the gastrocolic ligament primarily deforming the superior surface of the transverse colon.

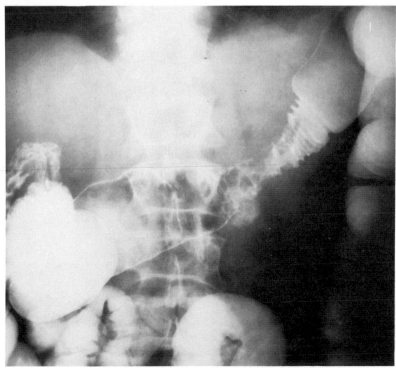

FIG. 20.24. COLONIC RELATIONSHIPS: STOMACH

Carcinoma of the stomach. The nodular encasement of the transverse colon could be due to tumor spread from either the stomach or the pancreas.

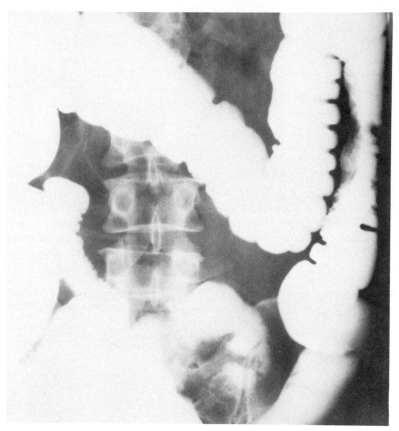

FIG. 20.25. COLONIC RELATIONSHIPS: LEFT KIDNEY

Perinephric abscess. The proximal descending colon is deformed medially by the abscess.

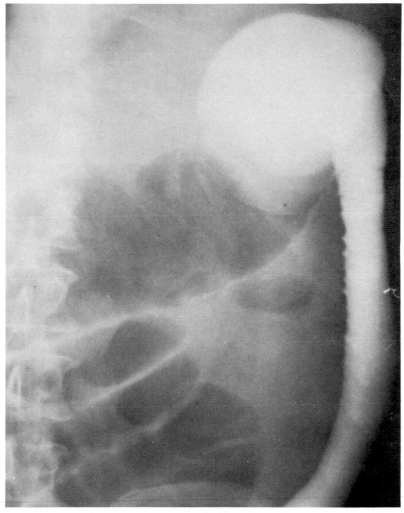

FIG. 20.26. COLONIC RELATIONSHIPS: TRANSVERSE MESOCOLON AND FLANK
Pancreatitis. A pancreatic phlegmon has extended from the transverse mesocolon
into the flank, scalloping and compressing the descending colon.

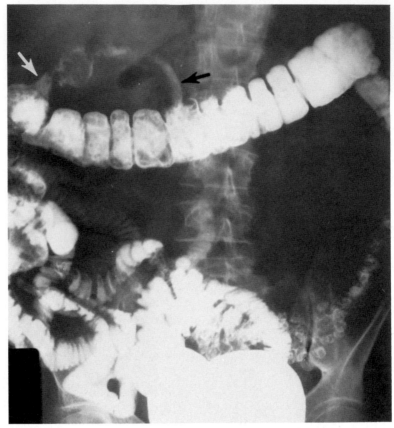

FIG. 20.27. COLONIC RELATIONSHIPS: GALLBLADDER

Cholecystocolic fistula. There is a fistula from the gallbladder to the hepatic flexure (white arrow). The curvilinear barium collection running medially is in the cystic and common ducts (black arrow).

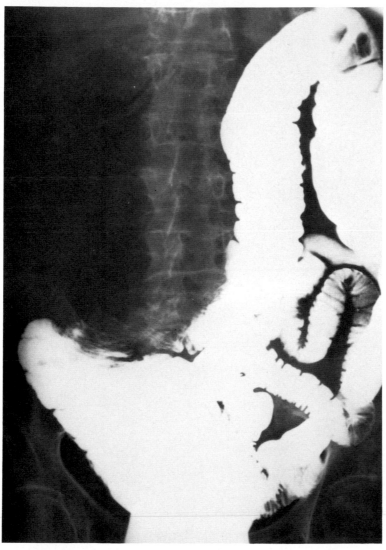

FIG. 20.28. COLONIC RELATIONSHIPS: RIGHT KIDNEY
A large right renal abscess depresses the proximal transverse colon.

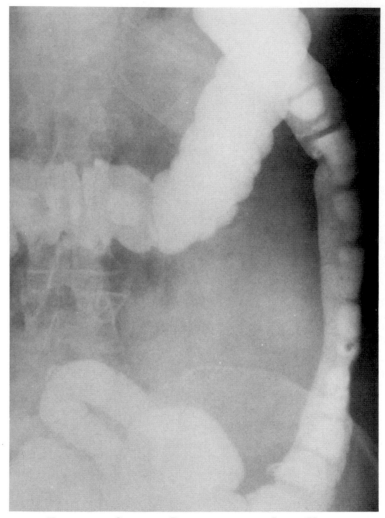

FIG. 20.29. COLONIC RELATIONSHIPS: LEFT KIDNEY
A large renal cell carcinoma lies inferior to the transverse colon and displaces the descending colon laterally.

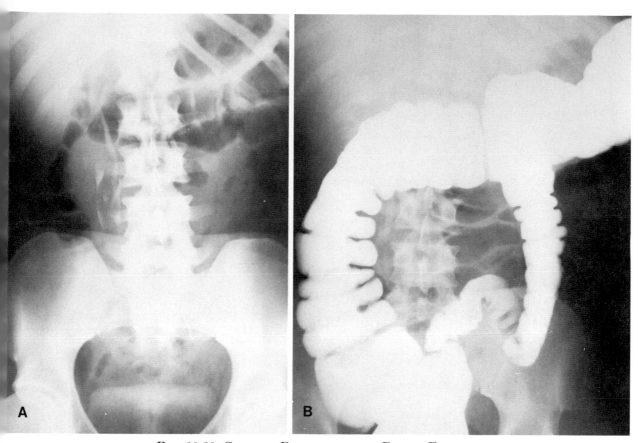

FIG. 20.30. COLONIC RELATIONSHIPS: RENAL ECTOPIA

Crossed renal ectopia is often associated with a more medial location of the descending colon than normal. (**A**) Intravenous pyelogram showing both kidneys on the right side. (**B**) Barium enema showing a medially located descending colon.

The pattern of distortion of the colon by tumor or infection which has spread along the pathways described above is not characteristic. One may see anything from a local flattening or disruption of the normal haustral pattern to spasm, scalloping, puckering, nodularity, fistulas, to gross strictures or encasement of the colon. Except in extensive spread of infection or tumor, however, the mucosal pattern of the colon is usually preserved. This allows differentiation from intrinsic colonic lesions. Sometimes, the extrinsic nature of the deformity will be more obvious on a postevacuation film than on the filled films from a barium enema. This is particularly true of lesions of the rectosigmoid (Fig. 20.31).

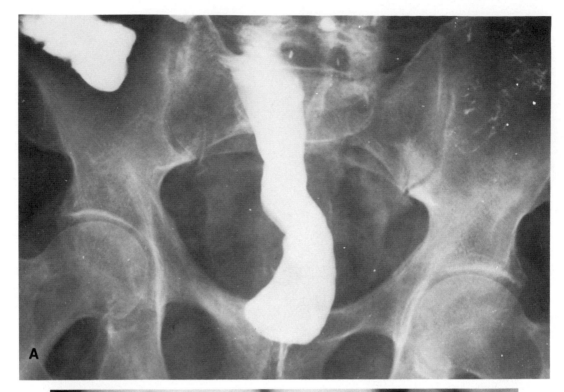

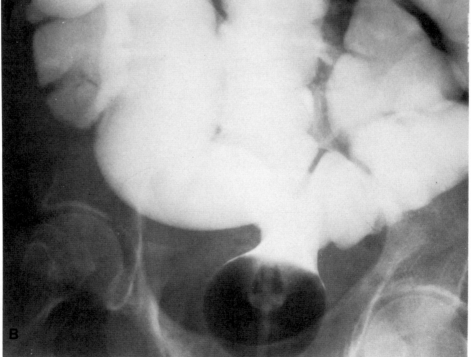

FIG. 20.31. COLONIC RELATIONSHIPS: PELVIS

Frozen pelvis: carcinoma of the prostate. The rectum and rectosigmoid do not collapse on the postevacuation film (**A**). The rigid deformity is less obvious on the barium-filled film (**B**).

BIBLIOGRAPHY

Pneumatosis Coli

Bloch, C.: The natural history of pneumatosis coli. Radiology, *123:* 311, 1977.

Colquhoun, J.: Intramural gas in hollow viscera. Clin. Radiol., *16:* 71, 1965.

Ecker, J., William, R., and Clay, K.: Pneumatosis cystoides intestinalis—Bullous emphysema of the intestine. Am. J. Gastroenterol., *56:* 125, 1971.

Gruenberg, J. C., et al.: Treatment of pneumatosis cystoides intestinalis with oxygen. Arch. Surg., *112:* 62, 1977.

Keyting, W., McCarver R., Kovarik, J., et al.: Pneumatosis intestinalis: A new concept. Radiology, *76:* 733, 1961.

Koss, L. P.: Abdominal gas cysts (pneumatosis cystoides intestinorum homins). Arch. Pathol., *53:* 523, 1952.

Colitis Cystica Profunda

Friedman, E., et al.: Colitis cystica profunda: Colonoscopic and pathological findings. Gastrointest. Endosc., *22:* 40, 1975.

Garner, J. L.: Colitis cystica profunda. Radiology, *89:* 85, 1967.

Grant, K. B., and Roller E. J.: Colitis cystica profunda. Radiology, *89:* 110, 1967.

Wayte, D. M., and Helwig, J. B.: Colitis cystica profunda. Am. J. Clin. Pathol., *48:* 159, 1967.

Amyloidosis

Brandt, K., Cathcart, E. S., and Cohen, A. S.: Clinical analysis of the course and prognosis of 42 patients with amyloidosis. Am. J. Med., *44:* 955, 1968.

Chernekoff, R. M., et al.: Gastrointestinal manifestations of primary amyloidosis. Can. Med. Assoc. J., *106:* 567, 1972.

Cohen, A. S.: Amyloidosis. N. Engl. J. Med., *277:* 522, 628, 1967.

Kyle, R. A., and Bayrd, E. D.: Amyloidosis: A review of 236 cases. Medicine (Baltimore), *54:* 271, 1975.

Legge, D., Carlson, H., and Wollaeger, D.: Roentgenologic appearance of systemic amyloidosis involving the gastrointestinal tract. Am. J. Roentgenol., *110:* 406, 1970.

Wang, C. C., and Robbins, L. L.: Amyloid disease: Its roentgen manifestations. Radiology, *66:* 489, 1956.

Systemic Sclerosis

Hale, C. H., and Schatzki, R.: Roentgenologic appearance of the gastrointestinal tract in scleroderma. Am. J. Roentgenol., *51:* 407, 1944.

Heinz, E. R., Steinberg, A. J., and Sackner, M. A.: Roentgenographic and pathological aspects of intestinal scleroderma. Ann. Intern. Med., *59:* 822, 1963.

Meszaros, W. T.: Systemic sclerosis (scleroderma). Am. J. Roentgenol., *82:* 1000, 1959.

Siegel, R. C.: Scleroderma. Med. Clin. North Am., *61:* 283, 1977.

Cathartic Colon

Heilbrun, N., and Bernstein, C.: Roentgen abnormalities of the large and small intestine associated with prolonged cathartic ingestion. Radiology, *65:* 549, 1955.

Rutter, K., et al.: Diseases of the alimentary system. Constipation and laxative abuse. Br. Med. J., *2:* 997, 1976.

Sleisenger, M. H., and Fordtran, J. S.: *Gastrointestinal Disease*, p. 1817 W. B. Saunders, Philadelphia, 1978.

Megacolon

Atias, A., et al.: Megaesophagus, megacolon and Chagas disease in Chile. Gastroenterology, *44:* 432, 1963.

Lane, R. H., et al.: Idiopathic megacolon: A review of 42 cases. Br. J. Surg., *64:* 305, 1977.

Effect of Adjacent Disease on the Colon

Ghahremani, G. G., and Meyers, M. A.: The cholecystocolic relationships. Am. J. Roentgenol., *125:* 21, 1975.

Meyers, M. A., et al.: Haustral anatomy and pathology: A new look. Radiology, *108:* 497, 1973.

Whalen, J. P., and Riemenschneider, P. A.: An analysis of the normal anatomic relationships of the colon applied to roentgenographic observations. Am. J. Roentgenol., *99:* 55, 1967.

Index

Page numbers in *italics* refer to illustrations.